ADVANCES IN CLINICAL REHABILITATION
Volume 1

Advances in
CLINICAL
REHABILITATION

Volume 1

Myron G. Eisenberg, Ph.D.
Editor-in-Chief

Roy C. Grzesiak, Ph.D.
Associate Editor

SPRINGER PUBLISHING COMPANY
NEW YORK

Springer Publishing Company, Inc.

536 Broadway
New York, NY 10012

87 88 89 90 91 / 5 4 3 2 1

ISBN 0-8261-5060-8
ISSN 0892-8878

Printed in the United States of America

Contents

Contributors

SERIES EDITORS

Myron G. Eisenberg, Ph.D., is Chief of the Psychology Service at the Veterans Administration Medical Center in Hampton, Virginia, and has joint appointments at the Associate Professor level in the Eastern Virginia Medical School's Departments of Physical Medicine and Rehabilitation, and Psychiatry and Behavioral Sciences, Norfolk, Virginia. He obtained his Ph.D. from Northwestern University and received postdoctoral training at the University of Toronto's Clarke Institute. Dr. Eisenberg has published extensively in the area of rehabilitation, holds editorial board positions on several journals, and is a member of several national task forces charged with investigating various quality of life issues of importance to persons with chronic disabling conditions. In addition, he serves as a grant reviewer for the Paralyzed Veterans of America's Research and Technology Foundation. Dr. Eisenberg has received recognition at the local, regional, and national levels acknowledging contributions he has made to the rehabilitation of physically impaired persons. A Past President and Fellow of the American Psychological Association's Division of Rehabilitation Psychology, he is actively involved in heightening the public's awareness of the importance of rehabilitation through the promotion of research. In addition, he is interested in the development of standards that will establish a more effective and consistent basis for evaluating the performance of individual rehabilitation service providers.

Roy C. Grzesiak, Ph.D., is Director of Psychology and Co-Director of the Pain Management Program at the Kessler Institute for Rehabilitation, Inc., in West Orange, New Jersey. He is also Clinical Assistant Professor of Rehabilitation Medicine and Psychiatry at the University of Medicine and Dentistry of New Jersey, New Jersey Medical School, Newark. Dr. Grzesiak received his Ph.D. from Texas Tech University, did his internship at the Rusk Institute for Rehabilitation Medicine, New York University Medical Center, and has a certificate of specialization in psychotherapy and psychoanalysis from the New York University Postdoctoral Program. He is author or co-author of more than 50 papers, articles, and book chapters, the majority addressing psychological aspects of pain problems. In 1985-1986, he was President of the Division of Rehabilitation Psychology of the American Psychological Association. He is on the editorial board o *Rehabilitation Psychology* and is a panel reviewer in behavioral science for the *Archives of Physical Medicine and Rehabilitation.* Dr. Grzesiak is a Fellow of the American Psychological Association. His clinical and research interests include the psychological management of pain, rehabilitation, and health psychology; and the integrative dimensions of cognitive–behavior therapy interpersonal psychotherapy, and post-Freudian psychoanalysis.

SECTION EDITORS

Michael Allen Alexander, M.D., is Medical Director of the D.T. Watson Rehabilitation Hospital, Director of the Children's Handicapped Unit at Children's Hospital of Pittsburgh, and a Clinical Associate Professor of Pediatrics at the University of Pittsburgh. He is a Diplomate of the American Boards of Pediatrics and Physical Medicine and Rehabilitation. Dr. Alexander's major interests have been in the rehabilitation of children, particularly in issues relevant to the comprehensive management from early diagnosis on through evaluations into adulthood. He has authored a number of research publications and book chapters on issues related to pediatric rehabilitation.

Frederica Bowden, Ed.S., is a consultant in the Washington, D.C. area in rehabilitation and special education. She has written and edited a number of publications in that field, as well as in earth science and social studies, and has taught at high school and university levels in a number of different disciplines. A graduate of the University of Arizona (M.Ed., 1982; Ed.S., 1983), she is a doctoral candidate in special education at the University of Arizona. Her bachelor's degree (B.Sc., 1971, McGill University) was in geology and physical geography and she worked in the Canadian arctic as an exploration geologist. A member of rehabilitation and special education professional associations, she is particularly interested in providing those in different disciplines the tools to bridge information gaps.

Robert Allen Keith, Ph.D., is Professor of Psychology at Claremont Graduate School and Director of the Center for Research and Planning at Casa Colina Hospital for Rehabilitation Medicine, both in California. He is a Diplomate in Clinical Psychology of the American Board of Professional Psychology. His research and writings have focused on the organizational analysis of the rehabilitation hospital, program evaluation, functional assessment, and patient data systems. He is a member of the joint task force of the American Academy of Physical Medicine and Rehabilitation and the Amercan Congress of Rehabilitation Medicine on a Uniform National Data System for Rehabilitation Hospitals.

Susan J. Middaugh, Ph.D., is an Associate Professor and Director of the Chronic Pain Rehabilitation Program and Biofeedback Laboratory in the Department of Physical Medicine and Rehabilitation at the Medical University of South Carolina in Charleston. She is a graduate of the University of Kansas, with a B.S. in Physical Therapy, and the University of Tennessee at Knoxville, with a doctorate in Experimental Psychology in 1972. Her primary interest is clinical research in biofeedback with an emphasis on neuromuscular re-education, chronic musculoskeletal pain, and incontinence.

AUTHORS

Edward W. Aberger, Ph.D., is Clinical Coordinator of the Miriam Hospital Chronic Pain Treatment Program in Providence, Rhode Island. He is also an Assistant Clinical Professor of Psychiatry in the Department of Psychiatry and Human Behavior at Brown University. Dr. Aberger received his doctorate in clinical psychology from the University of Kansas. His primary clinical and research interests pertain to the assessment and treatment of chronic pain, with particular emphasis on the role of operant factors.

Augustus Adams, Ph.D., is a Staff Psychologist and Coordinator of Disability Management Services for the Miriam Hospital Chronic Pain Treatment Program in Providence, Rhode Island. He is also a Clinical Instructor of Psychiatry (Psychology) in the Department of Psychiatry and Human Behavior at Brown University. In addition to his clinical work with chronic pain patients, Dr. Adams is involved in ongoing research on etiological factors and treatment outcomes in chronic low back pain. He received his doctorate in psychology at Southern Illinois University.

David K. Ahern, Ph.D., is Program Coordinator of the Miriam Hospital Chronic Pain Treatment Program in Providence, Rhode Island. He is also an Assistant Professor of Psychiatry in the Department of Psychiatry and Human Behavior at Brown University. Dr. Ahern received his Ph.D. from Nova University and completed his clinical internship training at the Brown University Internship Consortium. He has published numerous articles in the area of chronic pain. His other interests include psychophysiology and computer applications.

David H. Ahrenholz, M.D., is an Instructor in the Department of Surgery at the University of Minnesota and Assistant Director of the

Regional Burn Center at St. Paul-Ramsey Burn Center in St. Paul, Minne-sota. He received his M.D. from the University of Iowa Medical School and completed residency training at the University of Minnesota, including 3 years as a National Institutes of Health Research Fellow. Dr. Ahrenholz's research interests include infectious complications after trauma, pathophysi-ology of peritonitis, and pain management. He has authored multiple publi-cations, including several book chapters.

Michael J. Follick, Ph.D., is an Associate Professor in the Department of Psychiatry and Human Behavior, Brown University Program in Medicine. He is also Director of the Division of Behavioral Medicine and of the Chronic Pain Treatment Program at the Miriam Hospital in Providence, Rhode Island. He received his doctorate in Clinical Psychology from the University of Iowa and completed his internship at the University of Minnesota in 1977. He is a Fellow of the Society of Behavioral Medicine and a Past President of that organization. One of his primary areas of clinical and research interest has been the behavioral management of chronic pain, and he has published numerous papers and scientific articles on that topic.

Denise J. Frankoff, M.A., C.C.C., is the former Director of Communi-cation Disorders at D. T. Watson Rehabilitation Hospital, Sewickley, Penn-sylvania. She is currently at the Courage Center, Golden Valley, Minne-sota, as the Coordinator of the Communication Resource Center. The program provides multidisciplinary augmentative communication system evaluations and technical assistance with augmentative systems. Ms. Fran-koff received her master's degree from Northwestern University.

Carl V. Granger, M.D., is Professor of Rehabilitation Medicine, State University of New York at Buffalo and has been on the faculties of Yale University School of Medicine, Tufts University School of Medicine, where he was Professor and Chairman of Physical and Rehabilitation Medicine, and Brown University. Dr. Granger is an active member of the American Congress of Rehabilitation Medicine, Past President of the American Association of Electromyography and Electrodiagnosis, Past President of the American Academy of Physical Medicine and Reha-bilitation, Past President of the International Federation of Physical Medicine and Rehabilitation, and a member of the Medical Advisory Board of the National Multiple Sclerosis Society and of the American Medical Association. He has authored over 60 publications, one of which was awarded the Elizabeth and Sidney Licht Award for Excellence in Scientific Writing.

Byron B. Hamilton, M.S., Ph.D., is a member of the National Task Force to Develop a Uniform Data System for Medical Rehabilitation and principal investigator of the National Institute of Handicapped Research-supported project. He was previously Director of Research at the Rehabiliation Institute of Chicago and is currently Clinical Associate Professor of Rehabilitation Medicine, State University of New York at Buffalo. His doctoral degree is from the State University of New York, Syracuse.

William Given Kee, Ph.D., is a Clinical Psychologist on the faculty of the Medical University of South Carolina. He is the Clinical Director of the Chronic Pain Rehabilitation Program at the University. A graduate of Emory University and the University of Ohio, Dr. Kee's publication and research interests have been in rehabilitation psychology, biofeedback, behavioral medicine, and cognitive therapy.

Jeanne Pelensky, M.D., received her medical degree from Jefferson Medical College and completed an Internal Medicine residency at Bryn Mawr Hospital and a Physical Medicine and Rehabilitation residency at Thomas Jefferson University Hospital. She currently is Assistant Professor of Rehabilitation Medicine, Temple University School of Medicine and Chairman, Department of Rehabilitation Medicine, Fox Chase Cancer Center, Philadelphia. Her specialty interests include cancer rehabilitation and neurophysiology.

Jerrold S. Petrofsky, Ph.D., is a Professor of Biomedical Engineering at Wright State University in Dayton, Ohio and Director of the University's National Center for Rehabilitation Engineering. He has received numerous awards for his work, including those from the Institute for Electrical and Electronics Engineers, the ADD (Abilities Demonstrated by the Disabled) 1982 Research Project of the Year award, and the Spinal Cord Society's 1982 Scientist of the Year award. Dr. Petrofsky has published nearly 200 scholarly papers and holds numerous patents. In addition to his research into programmed electrical stimulation of paralyzed muscles, his current interests include investigation of fatigue factors resulting from exercise, cardiorespiratory responses to exertion, and the influence of space flight on exercise performance.

Elizabeth Rivers, O.T.R., R.N., is a Burn Rehabilitation Specialist at the St. Paul-Ramsey Regional Burn Center, St. Paul, Minnesota, and a part-time clinical instructor on the faculty of the University of Minnesota and the College of St. Catherine, St. Paul, Minnesota. Ms. Rivers has authored several papers and participated in numerous symposia. In addition, she invented the transparent face mask for facial scar control, originated the use of an overhead walker for early upper extremity rehabilitation, and developed the prosthetic foam/elastomer/elastic wrap postoperative dressings as a means of immobilizing body areas. In recognition of her accomplishments in rehabilitation, Ms. Rivers was named recipient of the 1986

Curtis P. Artz Distinguished Service Award from the American Burn As
sociation and the 1985 Communication Award from the Minnesota Occu
pational Therapy Association.

Frances S. Sherwin, M.A., is Academic Coordinator for the Han
Center of Western New York. Previously she was Technical Editor an
Writer for the Department of Social and Preventive Medicine, School o
Medicine, State University of New York at Buffalo and Assistant to th
Dean, School of Health Related Professions. Ms. Sherwin has publishe
extensively and has served as Technical Writer and Editor of the Nationa
Longitudinal Study of Nurse Practitioners, from which numerous bool
chapters and articles emanated.

Lynn D. Solem, M.D., is Director of the Burn Center at St. Paul
Ramsey Burn Center in St. Paul, Minnesota, and Assistant Professor in th
Department of Surgery at the University of Minnesota. She attended medica
school at the University of Minnesota and completed residency trainin
at the University of Minnesota's affiliated hospitals and at the St. Paul
Ramsey Medical Center. Dr. Solem is a member of the American Burr
Association's Committee on the Organization and Delivery of Burn Care
Her major interest areas are burns, including electrical injuries, and rehabili-
tation of the burn patient.

Wen-hsien Wu, M.D., is Professor and Chairman of the Department o
Anesthesiology and Director of the Pain Management Center at UMDNJ-
New Jersey Medical School in Newark, New Jersey. He received his M.D
from the National Taiwan University and his M.D. in Pharmacology-
Physiology from Creighton University. He completed his internship and
anesthesiology residency and research fellowship at University of Pennsyl-
vania, following which he joined the Anesthesiology faculty at Temple
University Medical School, where he developed the Critical Consultation
Respiratory Care Service. Dr. Wu also has held various academic and
clinical positions at West Virginia University, New York University Medical School, and the Veterans Administration Medical Center in Manhattan
(New York).

Rodger L. Wood, Ph.D., is Consultant Neuropsychologist and Head of
the Department of Clinical Psychology at St. Andrew's Hospital, Northampton (Great Britain). He is also a Consultant in Brain Injury Rehabilitation to Casa Colina Hospital for Rehabilitation Medicine, Pomona, California. Dr. Wood has been an invited speaker at a number of international
conferences in Europe, America, and Australia and has published several
chapters and journal papers on brain injury rehabilitation. He received his
Ph.D. from the University of Leicester. In addition to his clinical work,
Dr. Wood is a Senior Research Fellow at the Institute of Health Care
Studies attached to the University of Wales, Swansea.

Acknowledgments

Appreciation is extended to Ann Randall, who typed and retyped many parts of the manuscript and assisted us in meeting the formidable challenge of complying with publication deadlines.

The Editors

Introduction to the Series

This is the first volume in a new series designed to provide practical and current information about rehabilitation interventions from a multidisciplinary perspective. This present book covers four topical content areas: aspects of health and disease that influence rehabilitation, approaches to rehabilitation, rehabilitation in various diseases, and specific rehabilitation therapies. Its focus is on practice, not theory, and it emphasizes clinical applications that can be instituted in work settings with immediate positive impact.

Future volumes of *Advances in Clinical Rehabilitation* will appear at 18-month intervals, and each will review the status and recent progress in several main areas of rehabilitation. It is not our intention to provide in a single volume an accurate representation of activity in each of the many subfields of rehabilitation—space would not permit this. Rather, we try to follow a master plan, according to which some topics will appear in each volume, some in every other volume, and some less frequently. In this way, a few successive volumes, taken together, will present an accurate portrayal of the most recent findings by experts in a particular area of rehabilitation. A cumulative index of chapter titles will show the frequency of coverage of each of these topical areas. Major areas covered by the *Advances* series will be identified in consultation with an Advisory Board comprised of persons considered to be experts in their respective fields.

Like its predecessor, *Annual Review of Rehabilitation*, this series will have as its primary goal the dissemination of information on developments in theory, practice, and technology. However, unlike the *Annual Review*, *Advances* will concentrate on innovations in the practice of rehabilitation across a broad spectrum. While much of the information to be considered in the series will not be designed to "make experts" out of readers in all areas of rehabilitation, the series will heighten the practitioner's awareness of state-of-the-art techniques as they are used by colleagues in disciplines different from their own.

The decision was made by the Series Editors and Advisory Board members to divide *Advances in Clinical Rehabilitation* into sections and appoint a Section Editor to oversee the development of each topical unit. This person is given the authority (and responsibility) to develop a presentation that accurately represents current thinking about the area under consideration. The Section Editor is best able to identify emerging trends and developments and direct the individual contributor to address these relevant and timely issues.

The content of *Advances in Clinical Rehabilitation* will be multidisciplinary in composition. No matter how dedicated the individual practitioner, he or she cannot be expected to deal competently with the whole array of problems that the patient requiring rehabilitation often presents. The much heralded "health care team" has to be something more than a figure of speech if the results of rehabilitation treatment are to be health effective, let alone cost-effective.

While much of the methodology and many of the procedures used in rehabilitation have been known for years, what continues to be lacking are the resources and professional interests necessary to translate these practices into general application. For example, as late as 1980 only half of U.S. medical schools had departments of physical medicine and rehabilitation headed by a physiatrist. Indeed, "it is still possible for an American medical student to complete four years of medical education with little or no exposure to that field" (Somers, 1981). There is also a shortage of therapists and other personnel trained in rehabilitation techniques. Thus, while the importance of introducing rehabilitation techniques into treatment is acknowledged by most physicians and other health care professionals, this has not occurred in any systematic and widespread manner.

The principal reasons underlying the relative lack of attention paid to the importance of introducing a rehabilitation focus to treatment may be related to the nature of the treatment itself; the length of time involved; the need for nonphysician personnel, with a resulting diminution of a physician's role; the importance of motivation and other patient factors as opposed to technological factors; and the frequently disappointing outcome. In short, the treatment, after the first acute phase is over, does not fit neatly into our dominant technology- and specialist-oriented model of health care.

Three decades ago a great majority of the medical profession viewed rehabilitation as an extracurricular activity, an adjunct to proper medicine. Since then there has been a growing realization that the capacity to function in daily work and play and fulfill family responsibilities is a matter of crucial importance. This changing attitude is the result of several diverse factors, including the rapid expansion of rehabilitation facilities in the 1960s and a concomitant expansion of the concept of rehabilitation to include not only the restoration of lost physical function but also assistance to persons with mentally and emotionally handicapping conditions and those who were socially disadvantaged (Brieland, 1971). In addition, a heightened social consensus among consumers of rehabilitation services, the development of self-help groups, and the discovery of new life-sustaining and life-extending techniques tended not only to lengthen the life span and increase the visibility of persons with disabling conditions but also served to heighten this target population's need for assistance in mastering the new technologies available to them. In turn, these developments appear to have led to an increased recognition of the need for rehabilitation services.

It is not difficult to understand the reasons for the changing attitude toward persons with disabling and physically incapacitating conditions if one considers a number of social, political, and medical developments that have occurred over the past 20 years. First, there are more disabled individuals surviving the initial traumatic incident or medical crisis. The 1980 census indicated that one out of every eleven Americans, over 9% of the total population, has some kind of disability. Advances in medical procedures continue to save lives. It is no longer a rare occurrence when a disabled person is seen on the street. In fact, the disabled are coalescing into an identifiable group. They are finding each other and beginning to identify themselves as having much in common regardless of the precise nature of their disability.

Another factor underlying the increased visibility of the disabled is related to the type of person who now may find him or herself disabled. Consider the old stereotype of the disabled person—a frail, perhaps elderly, individual unable to be very active, slowly deteriorating as he or she moves toward death. Now, with the discovery of antibiotics and the development of new technologies, younger persons are surviving the trauma that will leave them disabled. The kinds of lives that these younger, mentally alert, and active individuals want to lead and the opportunities they seek are vastly different from those previously sought by the frail, elderly, or sickly disabled person.

Most recently, an awareness of the need for rehabilitation programs appears to have assumed economic dimensions. Current problems plaguing the entire health care economy are related to runaway benefit coverage provided for long-term care and failure of the health care industry to control the price of these custodial services. Health care administrators have indicated considerable interest in supporting any effort that can reduce the need for long-term care. In addition, the utilization of the concept of Diagnostic Related Groups (DRGs) is further contributing to the viability and attractiveness of adopting a rehabilitation perspective. This costing system, designed to cover 467 principal diagnoses, has been adopted as a means of controlling the upward spiral of health care costs.

The DRG costing system has and will continue to profoundly impact the practice of medicine, especially in relation to its ability to forcefully demonstrate the cost-effectiveness of services rendered. The literature clearly indicates that the next several years will see changes that will virtually revolutionize thinking concerning medical care, reimbursement, and allocation of resources. It is in this changing environment that rehabilitation procedures, techniques, and processes have become cost-effective interventions. The reason underlying this observation is related to the number of weighted work units (WWUs) that the DRG formula assigns to "rehabilitation" interventions. The number of WWUs assigned to services that are rehabilitative in nature far exceeds that given to nonrehabilitative functions. Put simply, WWUs translate directly into revenue. For example, the dollar amount provided for treatment of the diagnosis "alcohol abuse" is $2,300 per admission (WWUs = 74), while $4,500 is allocated for the DRG diagnosis of "rehabilitation, alcoholism" (WWUs = 150). Similar funding levels are assigned to virtually all treatments labeled as rehabilitation (*DRG Handbook*, 1985). Thus, the potential ability of practitioners who employ rehabilitation procedures to generate revenue is significant and will inevitably lead to their increased use in hospital settings. In fact, the job market for rehabilitation professionals appears to be expanding. For example, the number of advertisements for "rehabilitation," "health care," or "medical" psychologists in such publications as *Archives of Physical Medicine and Rehabilitation* and the APA's *Monitor* is steadily increasing. Further evidence of this trend is found in the increased number of advertisements for physical therapists, occupational therapists, speech and hearing therapists, and, perhaps most noteworthy, physiatrists.

While theory and practice go hand-in-hand, the Editors of *Advances in Clinical Rehabilitation* saw a dearth of readily available materials that cogently presented current and practical rehabilitation interventions that could be integrated into daily practice. This practical side of the field often appears to suffer at the expense of more theoretical or conceptual considerations. *Advances in Clinical Rehabilitation* is designed to help redress this deficit by providing the practicing rehabilitation professional with current information about where the field is and where it appears to be going. By so doing, the selection of materials presented in the text hopefully will help us come one step closer to the goal of developing an informed cadre of rehabilitation practitioners.

Preface

This first volume of *Advances in Clinical Rehabilitation* is divided into four sections, each of which has its own Section Editor who reviews its content in the Section Introduction. Section I, "Advances in Assessment," was selected for inclusion in the text because of its centrality to the entire rehabilitation process. Any strategy for altering the health status of patients requires a technology for first assessing that health status and then detecting increments of progress. Rehabilitation practitioners require accurate and appropriate assessment tools. Once rehabilitation services have been marshalled on behalf of the individual, program accountability also depends on regular assessment of the program recipient. Integral to this process is an ability to make accurate measurements of factors selected as important.

Section II, "Advances in Rehabilitation Technology," was selected because of the impact technological advances have had on rehabilitation interventions. Its importance to the field can be assessed in part by the emphasis placed on this topic area by the Section Editors. This section is comprised of three lengthy chapters. The clinical literature is replete with examples of applications of sophisticated electronic devices that are designed to assist in the rehabilitation process and in optimizing the patient's continued independence and functioning in the community. The virtual explosion of such devices appears in part to be related to the general extension of scientific knowledge and applications for consumer use and to the "computerization" of our society. Within the medical arena, this development has been facilitated by biomedical engineers. Their goal is to foster and extend the man–machine interface. Indeed, some of the most exciting and dramatic advances in rehabilitation are occurring in the technological area.

Discussion of selected disease entities and rehabilitation techniques utilized to ameliorate their deleterious and/or noxious side effects is the focus of Section III. Chosen for discussion in this volume are rehabilitation techniques specific to the treatment of burns and cancer. It is anticipated that other conditions will be considered in future volumes of this series.

The text's final section, "Advances in Rehabilitation Research," was included in order to highlight useful information that would assist practitioners in their attempts to validate and extend the current knowledge base in rehabilitation theory and practice. At least one major theme recurs throughout many of the text's chapters, that being the lack of empirically derived studies that justify and effectively demonstrate the use of many treatment strategies currently in use. Included in Section IV is information that can facilitate the initiation of investigations that can help advance rehabilitation practice. Problems in obtaining funding are considered in this chapter, as is information the researcher will find useful in developing sound, comprehensive, and competitive research proposals.

Subject matter considered in this volume is not intended to provide a comprehensive overview or evaluative summary of all aspects of the rehabilitation process occurring across the spectrum of incapacitating and debilitating conditions. Rather, its content is designed to provide detailed information about selected rehabilitation principles, practices, and procedures. If readers begin to consider incorporating some of these concepts into their daily work, the purpose of the text will be fully met. However, its contribution to the rehabilitation literature also will be confirmed if this material encourages readers to critically evaluate what it is they are doing and question, rejustify, and reconfirm the appropriateness of activities practiced and treatments dispensed.

Myron G. Eisenberg
Roy C. Grzesiak
Editors

REFERENCES

Brieland, D. (1971). Rehabilitation psychologists: Roles and functions. In W. S. Neff (Ed.), *Rehabilitation psychology.* Washington, DC: American Psychological Association.

DRG handbook. (1985). Salt Lake City, UT: 3M of the Code 3 Health Information System.

Somers, A. R. (1981). *The geriatric imperative.* New York: Appleton-Century-Crofts.

Contents of Volume 2

(Tentative)

SECTION I
Advances in Clinical Assessment

Robert Allen Keith
Section Editor

Introduction

Robert Allen Keith

Although assessment plays a prominent role in most health services, it has a particularly crucial place in clinical rehabilitation. Rehabilitation deals with both the structural impairments from disease or injury and the cognitive and behavioral consequences of such impairment. Consequently, assessment and treatment must have a perspective that includes most aspects of a patient's life. The appraisal of functional status has a long history in remedial treatment, although measures have concentrated on the simpler tasks associated with the activities of daily living. Such scales are not the only assessment activity in rehabilitation, however, as the chapters here on low back pain and brain injury will demonstrate.

This section on assessment begins with a chapter on functional status measurement, a traditional theme, but the authors emphasize that many others have a stake in assessment measures in addition to practicing clinicians. Administrators, epidemiologists, clinical researchers, health planners, and government agencies are also interested in the characteristics of the rehabilitation caseload.

One obvious gap in the rehabilitation field has been the lack of a common metric. Although there is widespread agreement in the research literature on the primacy of self-care and mobility in the measurement of function, there has been no consensus about which instrument to use. The Functional Independence Measure (FIM) was designed deliberately to fill this gap. A product of the Task Force on a Uniform National Data System, the FIM and an accompanying data set of patient and treatment information are intended to provide industry-wide statistics on rehabilitation populations.

Many scales in use in rehabilitation lack sufficient attention to their development, so that information on reliability, validity, and other such properties are missing. The originators of the FIM, with a three-year grant from the National Institute of Handicapped Research, have planned out a series of stages in which clinicians from a widespread group of facilities have provided judgments and information regarding the content and application of the scale. The grant, under the direction of Carl V. Granger and Byron B. Hamilton of the State University of New York at Buffalo, will ensure that there are sufficient trials in the hands of professionals to establish the feasibility of the adoption of the FIM in facilities across the country. Dr. Granger is well acquainted with clinical applications of functional assessment and is well known for work with the Barthel Index and for his Long-Range Evaluation System.

One of the most perplexing and often one of the most frustrating conditions in rehabilitation is that of chronic low back pain. The assessment perspective presented here by researchers at the Miriam Hospital Chronic Pain Research Unit in Providence, Rhode Island, is one in which the pain experience is part of a syndrome of interrelated problems that combine to interfere with the patient's ability to function. The authors begin with a delineation of the chronic low back pain syndrome. They then turn to the strategies that can be employed for assessment, what issues they address, and what research evidence there is regarding their validity. Finally, they look at how assessment findings can be integrated and the implications for treatment.

The third selection deals with neuropsychological assessment in brain injury, a topic with which many clinicians in rehabilitation still have limited experience. The neuropsychologist is one of the newest additions to the treatment team and brings an orientation and a set of skills that can be of considerable value to other professionals. The arrival of this specialty on the clinical scene coincides with a rising interest in the rehabilitation of the brain-injured. Rodger Wood, Director of the Kemsley Unit, St. Andrews Hospital, in Northampton, England, integrates both behavioral and neuropsychological principles in his work.

It has always been a formidable task for the clinical psychologist to generalize from test performance to other situations, particularly those involving the competencies of everyday living. Dr. Wood draws a distinction between the type of neuropsychological assessment directed toward differential diagnosis and the better understanding of brain–behavior functioning and that which addresses remedial application. The former stems from both experimental and psychometric orientations in which quantification is paramount. While Dr. Wood does not reject quantitative measurement, he is more interested in behavior change as a major goal of rehabilitation. In this perspective, assessment becomes a way of discovering the best ways of improving learning and for controlling dysfunctional behaviors that affect both learning and social relations.

In this chapter the author pays considerable attention to the major areas of behavior that are most commonly affected by brain injury. A successful plan of rehabilitation must be based on an understanding of such deficits, not only by the neuropsychologist but by all members of the treatment team. An additional requisite for success is that the principles involved must be applied regardless of the discipline of the clinician. Thus, the shaping of ambulation and speech behavior become the responsibility of all clinicians, not just the physical therapist and the speech therapist.

It is no accident that the theoretical orientation of both Rodger Wood and the Miriam Hospital group is behavioral in nature. One strength of this perspective is the attention to detail. Records of the patient's behavior and an inventory of environmental influences are an essential part of the assessment process. While careful clinicians have long understood the importance of such records, these authors present systematic frameworks for the gathering of such information.

1

The Functional Independence
Measure: A New Tool
for Rehabilitation

Robert Allen Keith
Carl V. Granger
Byron B. Hamilton
Frances S. Sherwin

The systematic assessment of patient performance has a long tradition in rehabilitation. This is not surprising since improvement of functional ability is a major goal of rehabilitation treatment. Functional status measures, a consistent set of tasks to measure patient proficiency, are a part of that tradition. Although clinicians have been the major users of such measures, others with a stake in the rehabilitation are increasingly interested in them. The emphasis on evaluation and accountability has focused attention on the outcomes of service. More discrete measures than those contained in the usual medical record are needed. Furthermore, judgments regarding the results of treatment require aggregation of data on patient performance into forms conducive to statistical analysis. This shift from individual to pooled information requires uniform and reliable measures. With the advent of cost containment and the need for more efficient and effective programs, managers and administrators are looking to patient improvement as an indicator of organizational productivity. Functional status measures are also used to identify patient characteristics and treatment outcomes in multiple sites for health care planning. In the past, such information has not been available. The advent of prospective payment has heightened the pressures to obtain data that can be used to differentiate among various services and to establish the efficacy of delivery systems.

A serious deterrent to the compilation of comparative statistics has been the lack of an assessment measure that persons who work in the field of rehabilitation could agree upon. Literally dozens of scales have been constructed for use in rehabilitation, but only a few merit serious consideration as a durable tool for clinical, evaluation, and research purposes.

If functional assessment measures are looked at in the larger context in which rehabilitation takes place, their multiple uses become clearer. For performance measures to be available to this larger community, however, an instrument that is used extensively is needed. The Functional Independence Measure (FIM) was designed to fulfill that need. Both the FIM and a data set of patient and treatment information are part of the Uniform National Data System for Medical Rehabilitation. The system, under development from a grant from the National Institute of Handicapped Research, has been subjected to trials by many different kinds of clinicians in facilities throughout the country.

BENEFITS OF FUNCTIONAL STATUS MEASURES

Clinical Management

Understandably, busy clinicians are reluctant to add the rating of patient performance to already heavy schedules. Assessment scales have sufficiently significant advantages, however, to justify the time involved. The clinical team is responsible for determining the patient's initial status, designing a treatment plan, carrying it out, and monitoring progress. A functional assessment scale provides a common framework and terminology for team members to conceptualize and communicate about the effects of impairment. The patient's initial status, in addition to being the focus for a treatment plan, is also a baseline against which to gauge future gains. Rating scales provide objective and explicit documentation of functional performance throughout the treatment regimen. Such indexes aid in determining readiness for discharge; the patient's proficiency can be viewed in relation to the environment in which he or she is to be living. Research has also shown that functional performance is a useful predictor of outcomes, for example, the patient's ability to manage outside the treatment setting (Gresham & Labi, 1984).

Although rehabilitation has taken on the task of dealing with virtually all aspects of a patient's life, the skills involved in self-care and mobility are assumed to be basic for higher levels of functioning. Functional status scales have therefore concentrated on the measurement of self-care and mobility. Most scales do not claim to be comprehensive measures of all of the possible facets of a patient's existence. Several authors have lamented that even though there is agreement about the primacy of self-care and mobility, there has been no agreement on a common set of measures that could be used throughout rehabilitation (Keith, 1984; Labi & Gresham, 1984).

Even though functional status ratings have many other uses, as will be discussed below, it is the clinical team and individual clinicians who are the primary source and users of the information generated. Unless these individuals are committed to the competent use of ratings, the utility of the measures for other purposes will be compromised.

Administrative Management

Although the research literature does not emphasize the administrative use of functional scales, they can be a valuable source of management information. When functional scales are used for this purpose, aggregated data are grouped according to programs or other units of administrative interest. By monitoring patient characteristics the administrator knows where to adjust the use of personnel and equipment according to severity of disability in the caseload. The advent of Diagnostic Related Groups (DRGs) in acute care hospitals and the potential for the discharge of more severely impaired populations into rehabilitation makes monitoring of severity particularly critical. With uniform functional scales the populations to be served can be described to referral sources and to potential markets. The effectiveness of programs can be compared with the institution's previous history, with other facilities, or with published results, and adjustments in programs can be made accordingly.

External Accountability

Diverse groups have an interest in the process and outcome of rehabilitation treatment. The Commission on the Accreditation of Rehabilitation Facilities (CARF) has included program evaluation in its accreditation standards as a way of ensuring that rehabilitation agencies will operate under an accountability mandate. The CARF evaluation model compares program outcomes with goals projected by facility staff. Functional assessment measures play an obvious role in such evaluations.

The value of a common metric that could be used across facilities and regions would be helpful in other ways as well as in the management of single programs. It would provide a shared framework with which to regard patient progress. A data base of admission and discharge scores would help to identify the nature of rehabilitation caseloads, information that is now missing. The impact of rehabilitation programs across a wide set of populations and regions could be determined. The way in which functional assessment measures can be used in program evaluation has been dealt with in more detail elsewhere (Keith, 1984).

Clinical and Epidemiological Research

Research on disability, of whatever variety, is concerned with establishing the occurrence and prevalence of disability, its natural history, and its amenability to change through natural circumstance or intervention. A more extended discussion of the use of functional measures within this context can be seen in Labi and Gresham (1984). Traditional measures of health status used in epidemiology, such as mortality and morbidity, are of limited use with chronic conditions, since they do not deal with the functional consequences of those conditions. Functional status measures can provide a means of determining the impact of disease on a study population, such as the citizens of Framingham (Gresham et al., 1975; Gresham et al., 1979). The prevalence of impairment in the general population has also been determined with the use of functional tests (Jeffreys, Millard, Hyman, & Warren, 1969).

In the clinical setting functional assessment scales are an obvious means of studying the relationship of treatment strategy to patient progress, particularly in relation to the stages of recovery or skill acquisition that patients go through. These indicators are also a proxy measure for functioning outside of the treatment setting and for establishing the extent of independence in such environments. Eventually, functional status measures need to be placed within the larger framework of health status measures that can be applicable to populations outside of rehabilitation (Jette, 1980, 1984). In this way we can more closely relate the goals of rehabilitation to the usual environments in which people function.

A UNIFORM NATIONAL DATA SYSTEM

Medical rehabilitation is the product of traditions in both medicine and rehabilitation. That heritage has resulted in an uncertain identity not only in the mind of the general public but also in the perceptions of some health care professionals. Until recently the number of rehabilitation facilities in existence was not known with certainty. Surveys by the American Hospital Association (Mullner, Killingsworth, Matthews, & Byre, 1980; Mullner, Nuzum, & Matthews, 1983) have helped to establish the number of units in service, although the determination was by self-identification. The Health Care Financing Administration (HCFA) has established criteria for hospitals exempt from DRGs. These criteria enable us to monitor the number of rehabilitation hospitals and units, at least those that expect Medicare reimbursement under exempt status.

There are precedents for several facilities cooperating in the collection of patient information and in the use of a common functional assessment measure. The PULSES and the Barthel Index were used in a study of 10 comprehensive centers, an inquiry that established the feasibility of using standardized measures across settings (Granger, Albrecht, & Hamilton, 1979). The Long Range Evaluation Summary, which incorporates both of these scales as well as other patient information, is used in multiple facilities (Granger & McNamara, 1982; Granger, Sherwood, & Greer, 1977). The Revised Level of Rehabilitation Scale (LORS-II), designed by Carey and Posavac (1982) for program evaluation, is currently in use by a number of hospitals. Likewise, the Patient Evaluation Conference System, a method of using patient profiles with an array of patient information, is the system of choice in many midwestern facilities (Harvey & Jellinek, 1983).

The nature of the population served, for example, the characteristics of patients admitted, are key statistics in any description of the rehabilitation industry. There have been few patient samples, however, that have been large enough or representative enough to show what the population looked like. Probably the largest sample outside of government archives has been the report on 3 years of cases at 40 hospitals in the Hospital Utilization Project (HUP) (Keith & Breckenridge, 1985). With a sample of 52,400 cases, the HUP study does shed some light on the proportion of various diagnoses seen, lengths of stay, and a number of other measures of patient caseload, but the number of facilities is too small to identify with confidence regional differences in case mix.

One of the most urgent reasons to collect reliable patient statistics is to provide information that could be used in developing models for prospective payment. Several efforts have been under way to gain such information: the National Association of Rehabilitation Facilities study, the survey by the rehabilitation section of the American Hospital Association, and the HCFA-funded grant to the Medical College of Wisconsin and the Rand Corporation. One or several of these projects may form the basis of HCFA policies regarding prospective payment under Medicare for rehabilitation hospitals, but none will provide a continuous source of data from which to monitor trends in rehabilitation. Therefore, there must be a way to follow patient characteristics on an ongoing basis, since populations and services change.

Task Force Formation

During a discussion at a forum on functional status at the 1983 annual meeting of the American Congress of Rehabilitation Medicine, it became obvious to those present that the time had come to make a significant effort to start a national patient data system. A group of those present formed a committee to explore the possibilities. In March 1984 the Boards of Governors of the American Congress of Rehabilitation Medicine and the American Academy of Physical Medicine and Rehabilitation authorized the formation of a joint task force. A group of professionals with skills in clinical management, research, evaluation, and patient information was formed with Steven Forer as co-chairman from the Congress and Carl V. Granger as co-chairman from the Academy.

At a series of meetings in Las Vegas, Chicago, Orlando, Boston, and Kansas City over a span of nearly 2 years the Task Force laid out the data elements, devised a scheme for grouping impairments, and designed a simple functional assessment scale. A 3-year grant from the National Institute of Handicapped Research in the fall of 1984 provided support for development and implementation. The grantee institution is the State University of New York at Buffalo with the project location at the Buffalo General Hospital, a major affiliated teaching hospital. Carl V. Granger, M.D., is project director and Byron B. Hamilton, M. D., Ph.D., is principal investigator.

The intent of the Task Force has been to design a patient data set and an assessment instrument that could be used universally among all rehabilitation units. This meant devising data elements that could be easily collected and about which there were clear definitions. An impairment grouping was made that mirrored the 10 patient conditions that HCFA has used in the definition of rehabilitation facilities. The dissemination and use of a uniform set of statistics on patient characteristics, lengths of stay, total charges, and functional status would form the basis for common agreement on the basic elements of information for the industry. It would provide ongoing identification of the population served by rehabilitation, the cost of service, and the outcome. The resulting data base would also be a rich source of information that could be used for research purposes.

The Functional Independence Measure

A crucial specification for an assessment scale is that it has to be simple enough to be adopted throughout rehabilitation but have enough discriminatory power to be useful as an outcome measure. The Task Force reviewed 36 published instruments as well as a number that had not appeared in the literature. Instead of adapting one already in use, the decision was made to construct a new scale, which would allow the simple format that was desired and would also ensure flexibility in the choice of tasks to include.

The first version of the FIM had 16 items in the general areas of self-care, sphincter control, mobility, locomotion, and communication. The rating scheme, shown in Table 1.1, begins with the premise that the first decision involves whether or not the assistance of another person is required. Consequently, Independent (no helper) and Dependent (helper needed) are the gross classifications. Within each level are finer gradations of assistance.

TABLE 1.1. Levels of Function for the Functional Independence Measure

INDEPENDENT: Another person is not required for the activity (NO HELPER).
 4. Complete Independence: Activity typically performed safely without modification, assistive devices, or aids and within reasonable time.
 3. Modified Independence: Activity requires any one of the following: an assistive device, more than reasonable time, safety considerations.
DEPENDENT: Another person is required for either supervision or physical assistance in order for the activity to be performed, or it is not performed (REQUIRES HELPER).
 2. Modified Dependence: When the subject expends more effort than the helper, this constitutes either supervision, minimal assistance, or moderate assistance
  a. Supervision: no more help than cuing or coaxing, without physical contact.
  b. Minimal assistance: no more help than touching.
  c. Moderate assistance: more help than touching, but the subject expends more effort than the helper.
 1. Complete Dependence: When the helper expends more effort than the subject, this constitutes maximal assistance.

Modified Dependence, the level at which therapists commonly would like finer distinctions, has three categories, which can be used to reflect smaller differences in status. Each level of the scale has descriptions of several tasks appropriate to that grade of proficiency.

Between piloting and trying out the scale, two additional items were included: Social Adjustment/Cooperation and Cognition/Problem Solving. The measurement of cognitive functioning, in any sort of simple form, has always eluded rehabilitation specialists, so a subcommittee was formed to work on this area further. The group, headed by Wayne Gordon of the Task Force, also included Harvey Jacobs, James Mikula, and Thomas Kay representing the American Head Injury Foundation. They continued the four-point scale format with five items: Memory, Cognition/Problem Solving, Visual Perception, Emotional Behavior, and Social Behavior. Two of their items could replace those added in the trial phase, so the ultimate version of the FIM would have 23 items. The original 18 items of the trial phase are shown in Table 1.2. The added measures will require testing and trial before a final decision for inclusion can be made.

Trial and Implementation Stages

Pilot Phase

During the 14 weeks of the Pilot Phase professionals from 11 facilities (primarily those of task force members) tested both the patient information set and the FIM. The purpose of this phase was to obtain the reactions of

TABLE 1.2. Functional Independence Measure Items

SELF-CARE

EATING: All aspects of eating and drinking, including opening containers, pouring liquids, cutting meat, buttering bread.

GROOMING: Oral care, hair care, washing hands and face, shaving, applying make-up.

BATHING: Bathing the entire body from the neck down (tub, shower, or bed bath) and skin inspection.

DRESSING, UPPER BODY: Dressing above the waist, donning and removing prosthesis or orthosis, when applicable.

DRESSING, LOWER BODY: Dressing from the waist down, donning or removing prosthesis or orthosis, when applicable.

PERINEAL CARE: Maintaining perineal hygiene, adjusting clothing after toileting.

SPHINCTER CONTROL

BLADDER MANAGEMENT: Complete intentional control of urinary bladder, management of equipment necessary for emptying.

BOWEL MANAGEMENT: Complete intentional control of bowel movement, use of laxatives, suppositories, and manual evacuation.

MOBILITY

TRANSFERS, BED, CHAIR, WHEELCHAIR: Management of all aspects of transferring to and from bed, chair, or wheelchair; or coming to a standing position, if walking is the typical mode of locomotion.

TRANSFERS, TOILET: Getting on and off toilet.

TRANSFERS, TUB OR SHOWER: Getting into and out of a tub or shower stall.

LOCOMOTION

WALKING: Walking 50 meters (about 150 feet) on a level surface once in a standing position. (Not applicable if the subject uses a wheelchair)

WHEELCHAIR: Propelling a wheelchair 50 meters (about 150 feet) and maneuvering through doorways and over thresholds, managing brakes, adjusting leg rests. (Not applicable if the subject walks)

STAIRS: Going up and down 12 to 14 stairs (one flight).

COMMUNICATION

COMPREHENSION: Clear comprehension of visual and auditory communication.

EXPRESSION: Clear expression of language.

SOCIAL AND COGNITIVE SKILLS*

COOPERATION: Skills related to working cooperatively with others.

PROBLEM SOLVING: Skills related to using previously learned information to solve problems of daily living.

---

*Additional items are under development.

staff to the ease of data gathering and the clarity, appropriateness, and completeness of items. Eight different health care disciplines involving 114 clinicians evaluated 110 patients at discharge. Questions were asked not only about the face validity of the material but also about the length of work experience of each clinician, the time to collect information, and suggestions regarding corrections or additions.

Clinicians averaged a little less than 6 years of experience. An average of 3.5 clinicians partially assessed each patient. Only 12% found any FIM items difficult to understand, but 31% felt that items should be added. An average of 6.7 minutes was needed to record demographic data. The data gathering effort per patient averaged 45.2 minutes. The comments from clinicians were reviewed by both project staff and Task Force members; where appropriate, changes were made.

Trial Phase

The Trial Phase began in July 1985 and is to run for at least 6 months. Currently, over 50 facilities are gathering information on 10 patients each for admission, discharge, and follow-up periods. At every assessment two clinicians are to rate each patient on all items of the FIM to establish interrater agreement. In this phase only physicians, physical therapists, occupational therapists, and nurses are being used. A major aim is to determine the reliability of the FIM and the feasibility of implementing both the Uniform Data Set and the FIM.

Implementation Phase

During this phase, to begin in mid-1986, software for provider use is to be developed and a means of central data processing identified. The number of system users will be expanded, the quality of data monitored, and additional work instituted on reliability, validity, and scale descrimination. The Task Force will review both the data set and the FIM to determine if any further modifications should be made before full implementation. The final stage in the development process is to decide what sort of organization should provide data processing services, either by contract with an existing agency or with the formation of a new entity devoted exclusively to the operation of the Uniform National Data System. In any event, a governing board will be set up to control the operation and output of the system.

Scale Development

A common criticism of instruments used in medical rehabilitation has been that too little attention has been paid to the measurement properties of such scales, particularly standardization, discriminatory power, reliability, and validity. Careful consideration was given in the development of the FIM to

he instructions and conditions of use. Both the Pilot and Trial Phases
provided for responses from clinicians concerning ease of use and utility.
From such comments it was possible to reduce some sources of ambiguity
and to ensure standardized administration. The widespread use of the FIM
will yield, for the first time, an accumulation of functional performances
from a variety of facilities and impairment groups that can be used for
normative and comparative purposes.

Discriminatory Power

The discriminatory power or precision of a measure is the extent to which it
is able to detect change in performance in one individual or differences in
performance among populations. Precision is first of all a function of the
scaling properties of a measure. Subcategories of independence and dependence that require judgments that can be made with reasonable certainty
should increase the power of the instrument. It is possible, of course, to
construct a measure of greater discrimination by increasing the length, but a
balance has to be struck between the need for precision and stability and ease
of administration.

Precision can be enhanced by maximizing the internal consistency of
items, that is, the extent to which they measure the same thing. When a
sufficiently large population has been tested, item analysis and intercorrela-
tions will reveal redundant or nondiscriminatory items. Then factor analysis can be employed to identify the clusters of abilities that are tapped.

Reliability

Even though reliability is one of the basic properties of a performance
measure, it is commonly not reported in accounts of new scales (Keith,
1984). The principal means of assessing reliability of the FIM will be by
interrater agreement. Since a variety of professionals will be using the scale,
principally nurses, physical and occupational therapists, and physicians, this
strategy for establishing reliability is most appropriate.

The Trial Phase, which has a target of over 500 patients to be assessed by
two professionals at admission, discharge, and follow-up, will yield a sufficient number of observations to establish the reliability of the FIM in the
hands of practicing clinicians. The interclass correlation coefficient (or
K coefficient) that corrects for chance agreement will be used as the reliability index (Fleiss, 1981).

Validity

Determining the validity of a functional status measure is a long-term
pursuit that will extend past the life of the Task Force and the NIHR grant.
The content of the scale, that is, the abilities it measures, is one form of

validity. From the scrutiny of many experienced clinicians as well as researchers, it is possible to determine the appropriateness of the tasks that are assessed. Since many of the facilities participating in the development phases routinely use other functional assessment instruments, it will be possible to compare the FIM with other measures. Analysis of scores collected during various stages of treatment would help to determine how sensitive the scale is to change. If the FIM is a valid measure, it should reflect improvements seen by other methods during the course of hospitalization. The number of facilities that are collecting data should make it possible to do validity studies on a scale hitherto unknown in rehabilitation.

PATIENT INFORMATION IN THE CURRENT HEALTH CARE CLIMATE

Health care in the United States is going through a period of restructuring of both services and methods of payment. The federal government, the largest single purchaser of services, has imposed a complicated series of regulations aimed at curbing the flow of money into services through Medicare and Medicaid. The DRG system and its attendant prospective payment arrangements are having a profound impact on the health care industry. Commercial insurance companies are also seeking ways to cut the costs of their coverage or to revise coverage.

In such volatile times organizations at all levels, from single facilities to large government agencies such as HCFA, are finding that they lack the necessary information to make informed decisions. The HCFA has the task of recommending policies to Congress regarding those hospitals still exempt from DRGs, including rehabilitation hospitals. Such recommendations should be based on factors that will predict resource consumption with reasonable accuracy. Otherwise rehabilitation facilities will be at considerable financial risk. So far they do not have the basis on which to make recommendations.

Both the Coopers and Lybrand study for National Association of Rehabilitation Facilities and the Medical College of Wisconsin-Rand study for HCFA went through thousands of records in rehabilitation hospitals. A unanimous finding from these two projects was that information from records was generally of poor quality. The lack of uniformity of data was a particular problem. It was impossible to compare or combine functional status measures because facilities did not use the same scales. The Wisconsin-Rand project finally inferred levels of functioning from records using a three-level scale. Even with such crude measures, however, it was found that functional status was one of the best predictors of length of stay or total charges. It is possible then that such measures could contribute to a formula for prospective pricing.

As part of its financing strategies, HCFA will also be examining evidence concerning the differential effectiveness of various systems. One issue of interest is the cost effectiveness of rehabilitation hospitals in relation to skilled nursing facilities and whether some disabled individuals might be treated at a lower and less costly level of care. Again, functional status measures could play a role in this policy determination.

It might appear that the basis upon which the government decides how much to pay for services is far afield from issues in the measurement of functional status. However, such is not the case. The measures taken by the clinical team, of vital use in treatment decisions, are now the foundation of a set of patient descriptors that are necessary for decisions at multiple levels. The individual clinician must be aware of how indispensable this information is for the future of medical rehabilitation and assume responsibility for its accuracy.

REFERENCES

Carey, R. G., & Posavac, E. J. (1982). Rehabilitation program evaluation using a revised Level of Rehabilitation Scale (LORS-II). *Archives of Physical Medicine and Rehabilitation, 63,* 367–370.

Fleiss, J. L. (1981). *Statistical methods for rates and proportions* (2nd ed.). New York: Wiley.

Granger, C. V., Albrecht, G. L., & Hamilton, B. B. (1979). Outcome of comprehensive medical rehabilitation: Measurement by PULSES and the Barthel Index. *Archives of Physical Medicine and Rehabilitation, 60,* 145–154.

Granger, C. V., & McNamara, M. Stroke Outcome Study. Paper presented at the 59th Annual Session, American Congress of Rehabilitation Medicine. Houston, November, 1982.

Granger, C. V., Sherwood, C. C., & Greer, D. S. (1977). Functional status measures in a comprehensive stroke care program. *Archives of Physical Medicine and Rehabilitation, 58,* 555–561.

Gresham, G. E., Fitspatrick, T. E., Wolf, P. A., McNamara, P. M., Kannel, W. B., & Dawber, T. R. (1975). Residual disability in survivors of stroke—The Framingham Study. *New England Journal of Medicine, 293,* 954–956.

Gresham, G. E., & Labi, M. L. C. (1984). Functional assessment instruments currently available for documenting outcomes in rehabilitation medicine. In C. V. Granger & G. E. Gresham (Eds.), *Functional assessment in rehabilitation medicine* (pp. 65–85). Baltimore, MD: Williams & Wilkins.

Gresham, G. E., Phillips, T. F., Wolf, P. A., McNamara, P. M., Kannel, W. B., & Dawber, T. R. (1979). Epidemiological profile of long-term stroke disability: The Framingham Study. *Archives of Physical Medicine and Rehabilitation, 60,* 487–492.

Harvey, R. F., & Jellinek, H. M. (1983). Patient profiles: Utilization in functional performance assessment. *Archives of Physical Medicine and Rehabilitation, 64,* 268–271.

Jeffreys, M., Millard, J. B., Hyman, M., & Warren, M. D. (1969). A set of tests for measuring motor impairment in prevalence studies. *Journal of Chronic Diseases, 22,* 303–319.

Jette, A. M. (1980). Health status indicators: Their utility in chronic disease evaluation research. *Journal of Chronic Diseases, 33*, 567–579.

Jette, A. M. (1984). Concepts of health and methodological issues in functional assessment. In C. V. Granger & G. E. Gresham (Eds.), *Functional assessment in rehabilitation medicine* (pp. 46–64). Baltimore, MD: Williams & Wilkins.

Keith, R. A. (1984). Functional assessment measures in medical rehabilitation: Current status. *Archives of Physical Medicine and Rehabilitation, 65*, 74–78.

Keith, R. A., & Breckenridge, K. (1985). Characteristics of patients from the Hospital Utilization Project data system: 1980–1982. *Archives of Physical Medicine and Rehabilitation, 66*, 768–772.

Labi, M. L. C., & Gresham, G. E. (1984). Some research applications of functional assessment instruments used in rehabilitation medicine. In C. V. Granger & G. E. Gresham (Eds.), *Functional assessment in rehabilitation medicine* (pp. 86–98). Baltimore, MD: Williams & Wilkins.

Mullner, R., Killingsworth, C., Matthews, D., & Byre, C. S. (1980). Inpatient medical rehabilitation: 1979 survey of hospitals and units. *Archives of Physical Medicine and Rehabilitation, 61*, 341–345.

Mullner, R., Nuzum, F. J., & Matthews, D. (1983). Inpatient medical rehabilitation: Results of the 1981 survey of hospitals and units. *Archives of Physical Medicine and Rehabilitation, 64*, 354–358.

2

Clinical Assessment of Chronic Low Back Pain

Edward W. Aberger
Augustus Adams[1]
David K. Ahern
Michael J. Follick

Chronic low back pain (CLBP) is defined as nonmalignant pain that has persisted for 6 months or longer despite repeated treatment attempts, is usually experienced daily, and is accompanied by disruption of one or more aspects of the individual's daily functioning. Chronic low back pain is a major health care problem with exceedingly high costs in terms of individual suffering and its drain on the fiscal and health care resources of society as a whole. For years the dominant conceptual approach to chronic pain was the medically oriented "specificity" model. As viewed by this model, pain is a sole function of, and directly proportional to, tissue damage. In those cases where a patient presents with pain but has little or no discernable tissue pathology, the pain is conceptualized as functional or "psychogenic." Guided by the specificity model, assessment of CLBP has been strictly dichotomous, consisting exclusively of medical diagnostic procedures designed to detect the physical pathology "causing" the pain, and, if unsuccessful, shifting totally to a psychological perspective.

Many pain experts have directly challenged the traditional specificity theory of chronic pain (e.g., Fordyce, 1976a,b, 1983; Melzack, 1974). Impetus for this challenge has come from a number of sources, including research implicating psychological factors in the experience of pain that has a clear organic basis (cf. Beecher, 1959). Moreover, the organic–psychogenic dichotomy has been found to be conceptually deficient due both to

---

[1]Order of first and second names on the authorship byline was determined by a coin toss, and does not reflect differential contribution to the chapter.

the use of the "psychogenic" label as a diagnosis by exclusion (Follick, Aberger, Ahern, & McCartney, 1984) and by research findings demonstrating a lack of relationship between pain-related impairment and the degree of organic findings (Heaton et al., 1982). Hence, rather than a simple linear relationship between the amount of tissue pathology and the experience of pain, experts in the field have proposed a "biopsychosocial" view of chronic pain, in which the presentation of persistent pain complaints and their sequelae represents a final common pathway reflecting a complex interaction of physical, psychological, behavioral, social, and cultural factors. The biopsychosocial nature of chronic pain is exemplified in the concept of the "chronic pain syndrome" (Black, 1975; Follick et al., 1984; Reuler, Girard, & Nardone, 1980). Linking the chronic pain experience to the concept of a syndrome is based upon the recognition that patients with chronic pain, regardless of whether demonstrable physical pathology is present, frequently evidence a multiplicity of interrelated problems that accompany and contribute to the pain experience. That is, the patient's pain problem includes, in addition to pain per se, the impact that pain has on his or her routine functioning, interpersonal relationships, and emotional status.

Just as the traditional model of pain dictated a specific approach to the assessment of chronic pain, the conceptualization of the chronic pain syndrome similarly has implications for assessment. Within this model assessment of chronic pain, like the chronic pain syndrome itself, is multidimensional in nature and involves not simply an investigation of medical/ physical factors but also of the various ways in which pain has impacted on the individual's life.

The approach to assessment described in the present chapter is a direct product of the biopsychosocial model of chronic pain and the conceptualization of the chronic pain syndrome. Assessment methodologies will be presented as they pertain to evaluation of specific elements of the syndrome, and recommendations will be made concerning a specific assessment protocol. In addition, research relevant to the reliability and validity of the recommended measures will be briefly reviewed.

CHRONIC LOW BACK PAIN SYNDROME

There are a diversity of clinical and research findings documenting psychosocial complications associated with chronic pain in general and CLBP in particular. These findings have been integrated in the concept of the chronic low back pain syndrome (Black, 1975; Follick et al., 1984; Reuler et al., 1980). As discussed by Follick et al. (1984), elements comprising the syndrome may include persistent complaints of pain and other pain behaviors, difficulties with health care utilization, overreliance on pain medication, vocational and financial difficulties, functional impairment and disability, marital and family disruption, and disruption of psychological functioning accompanied by emotional distress.

Persistent Complaints of Pain and Pain Behaviors

Patients with chronic pain typically display a variety of overt "pain behaviors." These can include pain-communicating behaviors (e.g., verbal complaints, grimacing, limping), as well as pain-avoidance and pain-relief behaviors (e.g., lying down, taking medication, use of artificial supports). Fordyce (1976a,b) posits that pain behaviors, while initially a direct response to underlying tissue damage, can over time come under the influence of environmental factors through the process of learning. Pain behavior can thus be maintained, independent of pathophysiology, by positive reinforcement (e.g., attention, sympathy), negative reinforcement (e.g., escape from unpleasant responsibilities), and the extinction or punishment of activity or "well behavior." Support for Fordyce's model is provided by research linking changes in pain behavior and activity levels to specific environmental manipulations (Cairns & Pasino, 1977; Fordyce, 1976a,b) and by identification of specific pain behaviors that reliably discriminate pain patients from "normal" and depressed individuals (Follick, Ahern, & Aberger, 1985; Keefe & Block, 1982).

Difficulties with Health Care Utilization

It is not unusual for CLBP patients to be overutilizers of the health care system, seeking and undergoing a multiplicity of diagnostic and medical/surgical procedures despite repeated treatment failures (Follick, Zitter, & Ahern, 1983; Sternbach, 1974). Research has documented that these patients utilize a disproportionately large percentage of health care resources (Johnson, 1979). Conversely, a smaller, although significant, number of patients with CLBP disengage from the medical system after early treatment failures and, thus, inappropriately underutilize health care resources (Fordyce & Steger, 1979).

Medication Overreliance

The frequent occurrence of excessive or inappropriate use of pain-relief medications in CLBP patients has been widely documented (Black, 1975; Ready & Hare, 1979; Roberts, 1981; Taylor, Zlutnick, Corley, & Flora, 1980; Turner, Calsyn, Fordyce, & Ready, 1982). It has been estimated that 50 to 65% of these patients exhibit analgesic abuse, habituation, or addiction (Maruta, Swanson, & Finlayson, 1979).

Vocational and Financial Difficulties

Disruption of vocational functioning is a nearly universal sequela of chroni pain. Unemployment among chronic pain patients is higher than 80% (Malec, Cayner, Harvey, & Timming, 1981; Painter, Seres, & Newman 1980). In addition, of those CLBP patients who continue working, many are restricted to part-time employment or must take less physically demand ing and lower paid positions. Hence, vocational impairment can result in significant financial difficulties and dependence upon external sources o income support, including employer-funded workers' compensation, gov ernment-sponsored disability compensation, and welfare programs.

Functional Impairment and Disability

Patients with CLBP frequently evidence marked impairment in functiona capabilities characterized by an inability to engage in routine daily activitie considered normal for their age and sex (Fordyce, 1983; Sternbach, 1974 Turner & Chapman, 1982). Often pervasive, these impairments include limitations in social, recreational, and work activities; and restrictions in general mobility, range of motion, muscle strength, and ambulation (Follick et al., 1983; Follick, Smith, & Ahern, 1985). Importantly, Bonica (1981) has observed that it is typically not organic pathology per se but rather pain sensations that interfere with the patient's ability to maintain a normal life-style.

Marital and Family Disruption

Chronic low back pain can have a devastating impact on the structure and functioning of the family system (Ahern, Adams, & Follick, 1985; Flor & Turk, 1984; Maruta & Osborne, 1978; Sternbach, 1974). For the spouse and other family members, CLBP poses significant demands, and is asso-ciated with marital discord (Ahern et al., 1985; Mohamed, Weisz, & War-ing, 1978), sexual difficulties (Maruta & Osborne, 1978), a disproportion-ately high divorce rate (Shealy, 1976), and a higher than normal incidence of emotional difficulties in the spouse (Ahern et al., 1985).

Psychological Disruption and Emotional Distress

A large proportion of CLBP patients display significant levels of emotional distress, characterized primarily by depression and anxiety (Armentrout, Moore, Parker, Hewett, & Feltz, 1982; Bradley, Prokop, Margolis, & Gentry, 1978; Prokop, Bradley, Margolis, & Gentry, 1980; Sternbach, 1974). These patients face an uncertain prognosis and the possibility that they may never recover. At the same time they have often abandoned or dramatically reduced the work, social, and recreational activities that were previously central to their lives and served as major sources of reinforcement. Extensive research on the emotional status of these patients using the Minnesota Multiphasic Personality Inventory (MMPI) has found that their distress is frequently accompanied by somatic overconcern ("hypochondriasis") and a tendency to express stress and conflict through physical symptoms ("hysteria"; Armentrout et al., 1982; Bradley et al., 1978; Fordyce, 1976a; Sternbach, 1974). A smaller subgroup of CLBP patients has been identified as evidencing more severe psychopathology, characterized by disordered thinking, agitation, poor impulse control, interpersonal hostility, and social alienation (Armentrout et al., 1982; Sternbach, 1974).

It is important to note that the specific delineation of syndrome elements is to some extent arbitrary, as these elements likely interact in a reciprocal process. Similarly, assessment instruments geared toward a specific syndrome element are likely to provide information relevant to other aspects of the syndrome. Additionally worth noting is that the assessment approach presented in this chapter, while focusing on the assessment of CLBP, is also applicable to the evaluation of nonmalignant chronic pain affecting other body parts. The critical issue for a given patient is not so much the location of pain as the extent to which that pain is causing life-style disruption and is part of a larger chronic pain syndrome.

PURPOSES OF ASSESSMENT

A major purpose of the clinical assessment of CLBP is to examine the extent to which psychosocial factors are involved in the patient's pain problem. This purpose is not synonymous with, and is in fact quite distinct from, determining whether the pain is organic or psychogenic. The present approach to CLBP assessment questions the utility of the organic–psychogenic dichotomy. This dichotomy implies that identification of organic factors automatically precludes the involvement of psychosocial factors in the presentation of the pain problem. In addition, it is impossible to establish a purely psychogenic etiology to pain, and a "functional" diagnosis is merely a diagnosis by exclusion that does not benefit the patient. Rather than attempting to differentially diagnose whether the pain is organic or functional, it is more useful to focus attention on whether the patient displays signs of the CLBP syndrome, and, specifically, the extent to which syndrome elements represent difficulties influencing the overall presentation of pain complaints. This general approach is biopsychosocial in nature, emphasizing the multiplicity of factors involved in chronic pain states, and has relevance regardless of the original etiology of the pain.

A second, related and equally important purpose of psychosocial assessment of CLBP is to provide data necessary for planning a treatment program. The assessment protocol is designed to establish the presence and extent of specific difficulties associated with the persistence of low back pain. This process permits the development of a problem list around which treatment can be planned and aids the clinician in understanding determinants of specific problems that must be addressed in effective treatment.

CLINICAL ASSESSMENT PROTOCOL

The clinician involved in providing psychosocial assessments of CLBP patients must ensure that these patients have had thorough medical evaluation. Medical evaluation is ideally conducted before the psychosocial assessment so that the clinician is aware of organic factors identified as having a clear impact on the pain problem and can proceed with some assurance that potentially serious medical disorders have been ruled out.

The assessment approach presented herein involves various methodologies designed to supplement each other in providing a comprehensive review of the elements of the CLBP syndrome. Methodologies employed include a structured interview, a self-monitoring instrument, self-report questionnaires, and structured behavioral observation. Each of these techniques provides some information not obtainable from the others. In addition, where assessment instruments overlap in information obtained, there is the opportunity to evaluate the consistency of the data.

Interview

A semistructured problem-oriented interview with the patient and spouse is essential in the assessment of the CLBP syndrome. This interview is the central aspect of assessment, providing detailed information on each of the syndrome elements and their interrelationships and forming a basis for the design of appropriate treatment. Moreover, data from the interview provide a foundation for the interpretation and integration of information derived from supplementary assessment methods.

As with any psychotherapeutic intervention, a critical aspect of the interview of the patient with chronic pain is to establish rapport and a therapeutic relationship. A large proportion of CLBP patients presenting for assessment are likely to have a history of minimal physical findings and/or failed medical treatments and may exhibit concern that the evaluation is directed at establishing a "psychological" etiology to the pain. The clinician should remain aware of this potential concern on the part of the patient, particularly at the outset of the interview. Reassurance can be provided by beginning the interview with an explanation that the purpose is to learn about the pain and how it has affected the patient's functional abilities, life-style, and relationships. This approach will help create a nonjudgmental and nonthreatening environment and will serve to improve the quality of information obtained.

Characteristics of the Patient's Pain and Pain Behavior

A useful means of beginning to assess the pain problem is to commence with a discussion of the area likely of most concern to the patient—the pain complaint. Relevant dimensions to evaluate include location, temporal parameters, fluctuations in intensity, and subjective descriptions of the pain (e.g., sharp-shooting, dull ache). Discussion of the patient's pain complaints also provides a natural starting point for detailed investigation of the patient's pain behaviors in general. This process is of special import in pretreatment assessment, as specific pain behaviors must be targeted and their determinants understood in order to provide a basis for intervention. In conjunction with direct observation of the patient, questions such as "What activities and strategies do you generally use to reduce your pain?" and "What activities and conditions do you find tend to worsen your pain?" are useful in ascertaining the overt manifestations of the pain. As discussed by Fordyce (1976a), assessment of these various dimensions provides information regarding the extent to which operant factors may be important in the patient's pain problem. Fordyce (1983) discusses a number of variations in pain complaints and other pain behaviors that suggest operant involvement, including (1) a diurnal pattern whereby pain interferes with performance of daily responsibilities but does not inhibit sleep, (2) pain is described as constant and unvarying without periods of reduced intensity, (3) pain is described as invariably increased by activity of any sort, (4) a differential tendency for aversive activities or unpleasant responsibilities to increase pain, (5) relief of pain from rest, attention, and medication is immediate and invariable, (6) activity is immediately ceased in response to pain, and (7) pain and associated behaviors are highly visible and/or audible and have a major impact on the behavior of individuals in the patient's environment.

Health Care Utilization

A thorough evaluation of the patient's medical history relevant to the pain problem is essential to establishing whether health care overutilization (or underutilization) is a problem. A review of available records, as well as direct history taking from the patient, provides essential data on the coordination of care among health professionals, diagnostic results and treatment efficacy, possible iatrogenic complications, and potential future medical interventions. This portion of the interview also permits ample opportunity to clarify the patient's general attitudes, beliefs, and expectations regarding the role of the health care system in addressing the pain problem.

One way in which health care utilization can be problematic is if there is a lack of coordination in delivery of services among care providers. This is more likely to be a problem when there are multiple physicians providing care and no single physician is identified as the coordinator of these efforts. Additional indicators of difficulties in this regard include (1) the provision across professionals of overlapping interventions (e.g., two concurrent physical therapy or medication regimens), (2) the provision across professionals of contradictory interventions (concurrent orders for bedrest and exercise), and (3) repetition of medical and surgical procedures, not in response to new neurological/physical findings or specific hypotheses but rather as a stereotyped response to persisting pain complaints.

A second potential health care utilization problem can be the development and accumulation over time of iatrogenic complications. These can be manifested in terms of increased pain, new health problems, and/or decreased functional capabilities subsequent to a given treatment. Prominent examples of iatrogenic complications are surgical scar tissue leading to new or increased pain complaints, gastrointestinal and cognitive difficulties secondary to chronic narcotic use, impaired sexual functioning following surgery, and muscle atrophy and decreased flexibility from prescribed inactivity or use of artificial support devices, such as a back brace. Also important is an assessment of the patient's awareness of iatrogenic complications.

Perhaps most significant as a negative outcome of prolonged, unsuccessful involvement in the health care system is that patients may develop general attitudes, beliefs, and expectations that will complicate future treatment and management efforts. A prominent manifestation of this problem is the patient's rigid adherence to the view that treatment efforts should provide total and permanent pain relief, and a concurrent neglect of the potential necessity for learning to cope with some degree of pain. Inherent in this view is the tendency to externalize onto the health care system responsibility for the pain problem, its treatment, and its impact on the patient's life. This can be manifested in a variety of ways: (1) an affect-laden presentation of pain complaints as unbearable and overwhelming, (2) a passive and helpless stance with regard to coping with pain and its associated life-style disruption, (3) an angry and combative response to health care providers for "failing" to relieve the pain, (4) a pattern of moving on to new physicians, or "doctor-shopping," when total pain relief is not obtained, and (5) continued use of pain-relief treatments despite waning efficacy, instructions to cease use, and accumulating iatrogenic effects.

Medication Overreliance

Assessment of this component of the syndrome requires collecting detailed information on the history and parameters of the patient's medication use. Data to obtain on each medication include average daily use, maximum daily use, impact on pain level, impact on activity level, effect on emotional status, and, in particular, patterns of use. A good starting point for evaluating usage patterns is to ascertain from the patient those factors he or she employs in deciding when to take medication and how much medication to take. Among the decision factors frequently employed by patients are time of day and current or anticipated pain intensity level. Also helpful in determining usage patterns is to look for environmental factors that may be associated with medication use, such as presence or absence of significant others, encouragement or discouragement of use by significant others, and changes in the behavior of significant others in response to medication use.

While the major focus of this assessment is medications known primarily for their analgesic properties, it is also important to identify all medications being taken by the patient, including antidepressants, anxiolytics, sedative-hypnotics, and medications for other health problems. Particularly important in this regard is to identify which medications the patient reports are useful in reducing the pain. Similarly, alcohol and nonprescription drug use by the patient, including whether such usage is associated with pain reduction, should be evaluated.

There are a number of indicators that medication use is complicating the pain problem. These include (1) a trend toward increased frequency and quantity of medication use without corresponding, sustained improvements in pain level, thereby suggesting the development of habituation, (2) obtaining prescriptions for pain medication from multiple physicians and combining use of these medications, (3) withdrawal symptoms associated with reduction of, or prolonged abstinence from, use of pain medication, (4) a pattern of emergency physician visits in which medication is dispensed, (5) a prior history of, or current difficulties with, alcohol and substance abuse, (6) primary effect of medication use is not analgesia but rather improved emotional status (e.g., reduced anxiety), (7) medication use results in a reduced activity level, and (8) discordance between patient's report of medication use and data from other sources (e.g., spouse report, self-monitoring instruments, medical records).

An additional concern in assessment is that use of medication, like other pain behaviors, is often maintained and promoted by environmental contingencies. This is particularly likely to be true when pain medication is not taken on a time-contingent basis, but rather is dispensed based upon the occurrence of pain behavior—when the patient complains about pain or requests pain relief. This sets up a state of affairs in which pain behavior is strongly reinforced by the analgesic and sedative-hypnotic effects of medication. This interrelationship between medication use and pain behavior is illustrated by clinical observations of a marked decline in pain complaints and pain intensity once medication withdrawal and control are established (Black, 1975; Fordyce & Steger, 1979; Sternbach, 1974; Taylor et al.,

1980). Another problematic conditioning process sometimes involved in medication use is avoidance learning. This occurs when the patient begins to use medication based upon cues, usually a time of day or specific activity, believed to precede the onset or exacerbation of pain. As with any avoidance learning process, this pattern of behavior is particularly resistant to change and very susceptible to generalization (Fordyce, 1976, 1983).

Vocational and Financial Difficulties

Assessment of this domain first involves ascertaining the nature, extent, and history of any work limitations the patient may have. For the patient who has continued working, but with restrictions, it should be determined whether these restrictions are sanctioned by the employer, or if the patient is trying to "keep up" with no formal changes in the job description. In addition, the duration of the restrictions, whether they involve time and/or duty restrictions, what duties have been abandoned or altered, and the effect this has had on others in the work environment need to be addressed. For the patient who has stopped working, issues of concern are the duration of unemployment, the consequences associated with any attempted return(s) to work, and the patient's perceptions of the conditions necessary to successfully resume work.

Vocational issues have the potential for complicating the chronic pain problem, particularly when pain-related vocational impairment has some reinforcement value to the patient. Identification of any reinforcers of vocational impairment is critical insofar as these may interfere with treatment attempts aimed at returning the patient to full work functioning. A direct determination of benefits associated with impaired vocational functioning may be difficult because of patients' fears of being unfairly perceived as "malingering." However, indirect assessment of the reinforcement value of not working can be made by inquiry into the financial consequences of changes in work status, as well as the patient's preinjury work adjustment/satisfaction and current relationships with employer and co-workers.

Factors suggesting that the patient's reduced vocational functioning may be accruing reinforcement include (1) equal or increased net income subsequent to the pain problem because of disability-related income supplements (workers' compensation, disability insurance), (2) the potential for future financial gain associated with the pain problem (e.g., a patient involved in litigation or seeking a lump-sum compensation settlement), (3) a history of adverse work experiences such as frequent job changes and extended periods of unemployment, (4) discordance between the patient's employment level and his or her perceived qualifications, (5) discordant relationships with co-workers and employer either preceding or subsequent to the pain problem, (6) punishment of the patient's working by significant others (e.g., the patient's husband wants her to be a full-time homemaker rather than work), (7) workers' compensation provides an alternative preferable to potential impending forced changes in earning potential (required retirement, layoffs), and (8) limited educational background and job skills such that retraining or replacement in less physically demanding work is unlikely or would result in markedly reduced earnings.

Traditionally, major importance has been attached to the potential role of financial factors (i.e., receipt of workers' compensation, involvement in litigation) in maintaining excessive disability levels in chronic pain patients (Fordyce, 1976a,b; Sternbach, 1974; White, 1969). Recent research (Dworkin, Handlin, Richlin, Brand, & Vannucci, 1985; Melzack, Katz, & Jeans, 1985) has suggested that such factors may not be as overridingly influential as generally believed. Nonetheless, clinical experience and observation indicate that financial issues are of major significance for certain patients and thus merit careful assessment in all cases.

Functional Impairment and Disability

Assessment of this domain is in actuality an extension of the assessment of pain behavior, as functional impairment and disability represent the generalized manifestation of the effects of specific motoric pain behaviors. For example, assessment of pain behavior might identify that the patient is lying down for extended periods of time; assessment of functional impairment would then focus on specifying those activities limited or precluded by the patient's lying down.

The general goal in assessing functional impairment and disability is to be able to describe the patient's current typical day and how it differs from his or her prepain lifestyle. A more specific goal is to obtain information concerning the topography and determinants of disability that will be relevant in designing treatment. One way to begin this process is to ask the patient in an open-ended fashion to identify those activities that have been affected by the pain. The patient's responses in this regard can give an indication of the relative importance of specific forms of disability; those areas stressed are probably of special significance. However, the patient will likely neglect other areas of impairment that may be critical in the overall pain problem, and the clinician should exercise care to ensure that a standardized review of major areas is provided. Among important areas to review in detail are household/maintenance chores, recreational pursuits, and social activities. (Activities in which the spouse participates are also important to assess and are certainly often a component of functional impairment, but for heuristic purposes this area will be discussed in the section on marital functioning.)

Within each area of functioning, emphasis is placed on identifying specific activities that have changed in frequency and/or quality since the onset of the pain problem. For instance, evaluation of the area of household/maintenance chores would look at such diverse activities as vacuuming, dusting grocery shopping, auto maintenance, shoveling snow, etc. For each activity identified as part of the patient's functional impairment, the following questions should be addressed: Is the patient totally or partially unable to complete the activity? Is the limitation self-initiated or a response to explici medical instructions? Are there particular circumstances under which the limitation is more or less likely to be manifested? What is the desirability (reinforcement value) of the activity—how frequently was it performed prior to the pain problem? What are the responses of others in the patient' environment to the limitation? Has the patient made any recent attempts to overcome the limitation? Obtaining answers to these questions across area: of restriction provides an accumulation of data permitting generalization: concerning the temporal and situational consistency of the patient's overal functional impairment.

As with pain behaviors and other elements of the chronic pain syndrome, functional impairment and disability can be influenced by social, environmental, and learning factors (Follick et al., 1985; Fordyce, 1976). Clearly, where operant influences have been identified for specific pain behaviors, the same is likely to hold true for the patient's functioning and disability in general. Additional indicators that conditioning factors are playing a contributory role include (1) a differential tendency toward restriction in unpleasant versus pleasant activities, (2) a differential tendency toward restriction in activities that were low-frequency versus high-frequency prior to the pain problem, (3) high cross-situational variability in one or more of the patient's limitations, (4) a pattern of periodic overextension involving sudden, brief bursts of activity immediately followed by prolonged, marked inactivity, (5) a pattern suggesting avoidance learning, whereby the patient rigidly accepts an activity restriction as unchanging, never attempting to test out the presumed linkage between a given activity and increased pain, (6) a pattern suggesting generalization of avoidance learning, in which the patient's prior experience of increased pain associated with an activity leads to abandonment of a larger set of similar activities, (7) a social–familial milieu that differentially reinforces the patient's limitations through direct provision of attention and nurturance, assumption of the patient's former responsibilities, or punishment of the patient's attempts at overcoming the limitations, and (8) an increase in pleasant or positive activities as replacements or substitutes for restricted activities. Where conditioning factors are identified, it is necessary to include provisions for systematically altering them if treatment is to be successful.

Marital and Family Disruption

There are four major areas to evaluate in the assessment of the impact of the pain problem on marital and family functioning: documenting the extent of marital/family disruption, establishing the current level of marital/familial discord, examining the extent of marital/familial reinforcement of pain behavior and disability, and evaluating whether pain behavior and disability are serving as a means of communication in the marriage. Clinical experience and prior research have suggested that the marital relationship is generally paramount in its potential to exert a direct influence on the pain problem (Ahern et al., 1985; Block, Kremer, & Gaylor, 1980). Hence, current discussion will highlight marital issues with the understanding that attention should be devoted to similar concerns in the family as a whole.

Documenting marital disruption involves a determination of the various ways in which the pain problem has been associated with changes in the couple's interactions and routine functioning. The term disruption does not necessarily imply a negative quality to changes in the couple's relationship, but rather that these changes have been forced by the pain problem. Ways in which disruption may be manifested include the redistribution of responsibilities (e.g., a change in primary breadwinner or person handling household chores or parenting), a change in frequency and/or nature of shared activities (e.g., social and recreational pursuits, sexual relations), and altered communication patterns.

Assessment of marital discord involves ascertaining the valence of pain-related disruptions in the relationship. Clearly, this first requires brief evaluation of the couple's satisfaction prior to the pain problem, followed by a more in-depth investigation of current satisfaction. On a rational-intuitive level, one would anticipate decreased satisfaction but should remain open to possible increased satisfaction associated with pain-related disruption. Direct, open-ended inquiry of both partners regarding their satisfaction with the marriage can provide information on the couple's willingness to openly discuss problems, their agreement about problems, and their adjustment to pain-related changes in the relationship. This inquiry also provides a behavioral sample of the couple's style of communicating and interacting with one another. With couples who provide minimal information in response to open-ended questioning, it may be necessary to point out specific marital changes that have occurred, and query for reactions to these changes. Some authors also recommend that conjoint marital assessment be supplemented with separate meetings with each partner (Fordyce, 1976; Sternbach, 1974).

Spousal reinforcement has been documented to be an important factor influencing pain behavior and functional impairment (Block et al., 1980; Flor, Kerns, & Turk, 1985). This can occur in the form of increased attention and nurturance contingent upon exhibition of pain behavior, allowing the patient to avoid unpleasant duties contingent upon pain behavior, and criticism or punishment of the patient's attempts at increased activity or well behavior. Much of the data relevant to these conditions will hopefully have been obtained during the preceding assessment of pain behavior and disability; however, should questions remain, it can be useful at this point to follow up on earlier data suggesting spousal reinforcement with a more directed inquiry. Moreover, the couple's interactions during the interview itself may provide information regarding spouse responses to pain behavior.

An additional issue of concern is the extent to which pain behavior and disability are serving as a major method of communication within the relationship and have become integral to maintaining the stability of the marriage (Waring, 1977). The pain problem can provide a basis for avoiding confrontation or decision making on critical marital issues (e.g., having children is delayed due to the patient's disability). In a related vein, pain behavior may also be a way for the couple to indirectly express aggression and disagreement, as well as to indirectly exert control in the relationship (e.g., "Not tonight dear, my back hurts"; "Not tonight dear, I don't want to hurt your back"). In some relationships the pain problem may provide one of the few acceptable means of communicating and accepting nurturance (e.g., the spouse who has difficulty saying "I love you," but readily provides massages to the patient; the patient who is embarrassed by his or her partner's verbal expression of affection, but will accept a massage). In highly discordant relationships, pain behavior and disability may serve as a basis for escalation of conflict, becoming a weapon for the patient and a clearly visible justification for spousal complaint.

There are a number of indicators that the pain problem may be functioning to maintain the stability of the marriage. One is accommodation to the patient's disability as reflected by indications of continuing or increased marital satisfaction despite marked pain-related disruption of the relationship. Similarly, denial by the couple of any problems in their relationship except as a direct outcome of pain suggests that pain serves the function of deflecting marital conflict. An additional indicator is when the couple identifies critical relationship-development issues (e.g., having children, buying a home) as inevitably put on hold because of the pain problem. Where assessment indicates that pain is serving a communicative or stabilizing function in the marriage, the clinician will need to make provisions to address these issues in any planned treatment. Attempts at intervention that do not take into account the role of pain in the marriage will likely be unsuccessful and could lead to destabilization of the couple's relationship.

Emotional Distress and Psychological Difficulties

Patients with CLBP are frequently beset by pervasive life-style changes, and the attendant stresses are likely to impact on their emotional and psychological adjustment. This impact can range from mild transient reactions to sustained, diagnosable major psychiatric disorders. Hence, a thorough review of symptoms involved in making these differential diagnoses is required as well as a comparison of current psychological functioning to adjustment preceding the pain problem. Of particular import is for the clinician to glean an understanding of the sources contributing to the patient's distress, and of the role the patient's prior psychological adjustment may be playing in the pain problem. This assessment is accomplished using standard psychological interview techniques, which incorporate a mental status examination and a review of major affective and psychiatric symptoms. The purpose of this section is not to review these standard evaluation procedures (for such a review, see Korchin, 1976), but rather to discuss specific psychological issues relevant to CLBP.

A typical reaction for many CLBP patients is development of emotional distress in the form of depression and anxiety. Factors that may contribute to the development of depressive symptoms include loss of reinforcement through reduced ability to engage in pleasant activities (Lewinsohn, 1974), perceived loss or lack of control in accruing reinforcers (e.g., compensation payments) (Lewinsohn, 1974), increased exposure to aversive stimulation such as constant nociception (Ferster, 1973), and loss of social reinforcement resulting from deteriorating interpersonal relationships (McLean, 1976). Learned helplessness (Seligman, 1975) may also result from the patient's repeated exposure to treatment failures and ongoing inability to obtain sustained pain relief. Further, other features of depression, including self-depreciation, lowered self-esteem, and pessimism, may arise from the CLBP patient's experiences. For instance, increased dependence on others while having less to offer in return can lead the patient to view himself or herself as inadequate and useless. Delineation of the factors contributing to the patient's depression will guide conceptualization and treatment recommendations. Nevertheless, the clinician should remain aware that, even in the presence of these factors, depressive symptomatology can become endogenous and persist independently of original causal factors (Carson & Adams, 1981). Conversely, the clinician should recognize that pain complaints sometimes develop secondary to an endogenous depression, and ensure that this hypothesis is adequately evaluated.

Difficulties with anxiety, including heightened tension and obsessive rumination, are also often integrally related to the chronic pain experience. The CLBP patient may develop fears and anxiety connected with the anticipation of events and activities that could cause further injury or increased pain. The patient can become preoccupied with avoiding pain, and, over time, fears of specific pain-exacerbating activities may generalize so that progressively more activities and events are shunned as potentially painful. In addition, for the patient whose pain is episodic and/or variable, uncertainty about when pain will worsen can lead to generalized anxiety. Other conditions of the CLBP patient's circumstances, including uncertainties about prognosis, finances, and the future, may also contribute to increases in anxiety and tension. Interestingly, Dolce & Raczynski (1985) cite prior research that suggests that anxiety and attendant increases in muscle tension can contribute to the development and maintenance of musculoskeletal pain; therefore, attention must be devoted to this possibility in the evaluation. Detection of the presence or absence of these conditions is important in understanding the source and manifestations of the patient's anxiety and will guide in the conceptualization and development of treatment plans.

In addition to emotional distress, hypochondriasis and hysteria are commonly noted to be among the psychological difficulties of CLBP patients (Sternbach, 1974). While researchers disagree on whether these personality features are precursors or effects of CLBP, there is evidence suggesting that pain is associated with increased manifestation of these attributes (Roberts & Reinhardt, 1980; Sternbach & Timmermans, 1975). The clinician's concern is the extent to which current expression of hysteria and hypochondriasis may be complicating the patient's adjustment to the pain and associated problems. Rather than focusing on the theoretical significance of these constructs, assessment is most productively geared toward identifying their behavioral correlates. The term hysteria, as generally used, refers to a pronounced tendency to utilize the defenses of denial, repression, and somatization as primary means of dealing with stress and conflict. In the CLBP patient this is often behaviorally manifested as rejection of the suggestion that emotional distress, interpersonal conflict, or other life difficulties may be a part of the pain problem. A related difficulty is the behavior often associated with hypochondriasis; specifically, a very strong somatic focus with accompanying rumination about current symptoms and hypersensitivity to minor bodily changes. Hysteroid and hypochondriacal behaviors may be problematic insofar as they are associated with the patient's identification of painful sensations as the sole problem, attendant failure to recognize and deal with life-style disruption related to the pain, and continued passive reliance on medical solutions.

Concluding the Interview

The conclusion of the interview involves evaluation of the extent to which the patient and spouse recognize each syndrome element that was identified by the clinician and express a willingness to deal with these problem areas. This evaluation can often be accomplished by asking the couple to list the goals that they have in seeking treatment. Identification of goals that acknowledge the range of the patient's particular chronic pain syndrome (e.g., increase my activity level, get off medication, improve my sex life, do more with my wife and kids, return to work) suggests the patient and spouse will be amenable to active participation in the multicomponent treatment approach that is warranted. Conversely, identification of pain relief as the exclusive goal suggests that the patient and spouse are not yet ready for such an approach, and that an immediate aim of the clinician should be to assist them in recognizing the need to address the full range of difficulties connected with the pain. Concurrent with this, it is necessary to plan for appropriate referrals or interventions for those problems that the patient and spouse are willing to address (e.g., psychiatric referral for severe depression).

Reliability and Validity of the Interview

There has been relatively little investigation of the reliability and validity of psychological interviews, and the limited available research has yielded conflicting findings (Haynes, 1978; Matarazzo, 1965). Interview-derived data have been variously found to be temporally reliable (Sobell & Sobell, 1975) and unreliable (Summers, 1970). Similarly, while a number of investigators have demonstrated acceptable correspondence between specific items of information obtained via interview and external verification (Ball, 1967; Dirk & Kuldau, 1974), other investigators have documented marked discrepancies between interview-derived data and data from other sources (Honig, Tannenbaum, & Caldwell, 1968; Schnelle, 1974).

The only study to date empirically evaluating a chronic pain assessment interview yielded evidence supporting its reliability and validity (Heaton et al., 1982). These authors developed a structured interview, the Psychosocial Pain Inventory (PSPI), that included 25 items rated on four-point or two-point scales, designed to yield a total score reflecting the magnitude of psychosocial influences on the presentation of the patient's pain problem. The scoring system possessed high interrater reliability, and PSPI scores were found to discriminate patients independently judged as demonstrating symptom exaggeration beyond documented organic pathology from those not evidencing such exaggeration. In addition, patients with high PSPI scores tended to use more adjectives and adjectives of greater severity on the McGill Pain Questionnaire. Finally, PSPI scores were found to have significant positive correlations with elevations on the hypochondriasis scale of the MMPI.

The PSPI has a level of structure and a scoring system not duplicated in other pain assessment interviews. Hence, Heaton et al.'s (1982) findings cannot be generalized to the interview format suggested in this chapter. Nonetheless, their findings do suggest that important data on psychosocial factors common to both the PSPI and the present interview (e.g., social reinforcement, medication use, financial variables, avoidance of responsibilities) can be reliably and validly obtained.

Ultimately, the clinician conducting an interview of a CLBP patient must remain aware of and take into account factors that may compromise the reliability and validity of the interview. These factors include interviewer skill; differences between the interviewer and patient in age, sex, or race; and the social sensitivity of the various topics discussed (Haynes, 1978; Haynes & Wilson, 1979). In addition, the clinician should take care to examine the correspondence between interview data and information obtained from other assessment methods. Accurate assessment of CLBP will be best ensured when interview data are supplemented and integrated with adjunctive, alternative assessment techniques. The remainder of this chapter will present a recommended battery of supplemental assessment methods for use in evaluation of the CLBP syndrome.

ADJUNCTIVE ASSESSMENT PROCEDURES

Self-monitoring

A self-monitoring behavioral activity diary can be an efficient method of obtaining detailed information on CLBP patients' activity levels and patterns in the natural environment and establishing the extent to which these activities are influenced by pain. This information contributes to understanding the nature and extent of pain-related disability and facilitates the design of appropriate treatment interventions. It also provides objective data with which treatment outcome can be evaluated. Such an instrument, the Daily Activity Diary, has been developed by Follick, Ahern, and Laser-Wolston (1984). Specific syndrome elements addressed using this instrument include pain behaviors and complaints (pain intensity, pain-relief activities), medication usage patterns, functional impairment and disability (lying down, sitting, exercise, routine activities, social interactions), and emotional distress (tension and mood ratings).

The Daily Activity Diary is separated into 48 30-minute intervals (e.g., 6:00 to 6:30 A.M., 6:30 to 7:00 A.M.) that account for the 24 hours of each day. For each 30-minute interval the patient is instructed to record (1) the position (lying, sitting, standing/walking, asleep) maintained most during that time, (2) a brief description of his/her major activity, (3) whether the activity was engaged in for pain relief, (4) any pain medications used, and (5) any other pain-relief activities or devices employed (e.g., hot packs, corset). At bedtime the patient rates his or her pain intensity, tension level, and mood state on three Likert-type scales. The patient is instructed to complete a diary on each of 7 consecutive days.

A variety of other behavioral diaries have been developed for use with CLBP patients (Cairns, Thomas, Mooney, & Pace, 1976; Fordyce et al., 1973; Greenhoot & Sternbach, 1974). The Daily Activity Diary developed by Follick et al., however, has the advantage of being the only instrument of its type with demonstrated adequate reliability and validity. Self-reported lying down and standing/walking times derived from the Daily Activity Diary have been found to correlate significantly with spouse observations of patients' lying down and standing/walking times (Follick et al., 1984). Patients' diary reports of "downtime" (i.e., lying and sitting) have also been demonstrated to correlate significantly with estimates obtained from a portable electromechanical downtime monitor (Follick, Ahern, Laser-Wolston, Adams, & Malloy, 1985). Moreover, diary-derived estimates of medication use were virtually identical to, and correlated significantly with, independently performed pill counts (Follick et al., 1984).

Questionnaires

Questionnaires relevant to the assessment of CLBP will be discussed as they pertain to elements of the syndrome. Due to probable reactive effects of the interview, it is recommended that these questionnaires, insofar as possible, be administered preceding the interview.

Pain Complaints

The McGill Pain Questionnaire (Melzack, 1975) is the most widely known and utilized measure of subjective characteristics of pain. This questionnaire consists of 102 adjectives designed to describe the sensory, affective, and evaluative dimensions of pain, as hypothesized in Melzack and Wall's (1965) gate-control theory. Patients select the one item in each of 20 categories that best describes their pain experience. Examination of these responses provides information on pain quality as well as pain intensity. The McGill Pain Questionnaire has been criticized for a variety of reasons including its length and the difficulty some patients have in understanding the adjectives (Chapman et al., 1985). Nonetheless, there is a wide body of research demonstrating the construct (McCreary, Turner, & Dawson, 1981) and discriminant validity (Dubbison & Melzack, 1976) of this measure.

For the clinician who is particularly interested in collecting highly standardized data on pain intensity and quality, use of the McGill Pain Questionnaire is appropriate. Other, simpler methods worth considering for assessment of subjective pain intensity are numerical rating scales and visual analogue scales (see Chapman et al., 1985).

Health Care Utilization

There are no questionnaire measures of health care utilization presented in the literature. Since the extensive nature of many CLBP patients' contacts with health care providers can make comprehensive interview assessment of medical history unwieldy, clinicians involved in routine evaluation of

CLBP patients may wish to devise their own questionnaire to efficiently survey this area. The authors utilize a questionnaire that collects information relevant to the prior 1-year period on the patient's physician contacts, diagnostic procedures, treatment modalities, surgical interventions, hospitalizations, emergency room visits, medication use, and special pain-relief aids and devices. The format of this questionnaire is designed to facilitate the patient's accurate report by providing, where possible, specific alternatives to select (e.g., lists of specific diagnostic and treatment procedures).

Functional Impairment and Disability

A standardized questionnaire measure of disability can ensure a comprehensive survey of the CLBP patient's functional capabilities, provide a basis for normative and between-patient comparisons, and allow evaluation of pretreatment to posttreatment changes. The Sickness Impact Profile (SIP) is an empirically derived, behaviorally based measure of sickness-related disability that is useful in these regards (Bergner, Bobbitt, Carter, & Gilson, 1981). The SIP consists of 136 items describing activities encountered in routine daily living. The CLBP patient is instructed to endorse any item that describes an activity that he or she presently has difficulty performing because of pain. Items are aggregated to yield percent disability scores on three dimensions—physical, psychosocial, and "other"—as well as an overall impairment percentage. The physical dimension reflects the extent to which the patient is experiencing pain-related disruption in ambulation, mobility, body care, and movement. The psychosocial dimension reflects the extent to which the patient is experiencing disruption of social interaction, communication, alertness, and emotional behavior. The "other" dimension represents a clustering of disparate activity areas including sleep and rest, work, home management, and recreation. Finally, the overall percentage disability index represents the average of disability percentages across all three dimensions.

The SIP has undergone extensive reliability and validity testing. It has been demonstrated to possess high test–retest reliability for the dimension and overall scores across subject samples with differing medical problems (Pollard, Bobbitt, Bergner, Martin, & Gilson, 1976). Validity testing indicates that the overall SIP impairment index correlates highly with patient- and physician-derived estimates of health-related dysfunction and scores on well-validated health status measures (Bergner, Bobbitt, Pollard, Martin, & Gilson, 1976). Perhaps most significantly, the SIP has been validated specifically for use with CLBP patients (Follick et al., 1985). The physical dimension has been found to be inversely associated with standing/walking time and positively correlated with lying down time. In addition, the psychosocial dimension was significantly correlated with emotional distress

nd psychological disturbance as measured by the MMPI. Further, the
hree dimension scores and the overall disability index were sensitive to
pretreatment to posttreatment changes.

In light of its extensive validation, demonstrated utility with CLBP
patients, and available norms to permit comparisons across patient groups,
he SIP is recommended as an integral part of the assessment protocol. It
provides an efficient method for identifying specific areas of impairment, as
well as for monitoring progress during and after treatment.

Marital Disruption

When the interview is conducted with the patient and spouse conjointly,
questionnaire assessment of marital disruption provides a useful adjunct to
interview data in obtaining independent assessments of the marriage from
each spouse. The Locke-Wallace Marital Adjustment Scale (Locke & Wallace, 1959) is a brief 15-item measure yielding an overall index of marital
satisfaction. This questionnaire pertains to adjustment in specific areas of
the marriage such as family finances, recreation, demonstrations of affection, sexual relations, and social relationships. This measure has been frequently used in behavioral research and has been widely used clinically. It
has established norms for adjusted and maladjusted couples, acceptable
criterion-related and discriminant validity (Haynes, 1978; Locke & Wallace, 1959), and is sensitive to treatment-related changes (Haynes & Wilson,
1979).

The Areas of Change Questionnaire (Weiss, Hops, & Patterson, 1973) is
a behaviorally specific instrument assessing desired changes in the marriage
and the accuracy of each partner's perceptions of the other's desires. This
questionnaire is divided into two parts containing identical lists of 34
specific behaviors relating to potential sources of marital conflict (e.g.,
housekeeping, giving attention, spending time with children and/or relatives, spending time together). On the first part the respondent indicates for
each behavior whether he or she wants the partner to change and the
direction and extent of the desired change (on a 7-point Likert scale ranging
from "much less" through "no change" to "much more"). On the second
part the respondent indicates his or her perceptions of the extent and
magnitude of changes desired by the partner. The Areas of Change yields
scores for the total number of changes desired by each partner and the
perceptual accuracy of each partner in identifying the other's sources of
dissatisfaction. There is substantial empirical support for the reliability and
the concurrent, discriminant, and criterion-related validity of this questionnaire (Haynes, 1978; Margolin, Talouie, & Weinstein, 1983; Weiss et al.,
1973).

The Locke-Wallace and Areas of Change questionnaires are recommended for use in the assessment of CLBP as they respectively provide an overall index of marital satisfaction and allow a fine-grained analysis of specific areas contributing to dissatisfaction. These measures may facilitate the linking of particular aspects of the patient's impairment to the marital situation. They are thus useful in guiding and evaluating interventions that target changes in the marriage. In addition, the Locke-Wallace Marital Adjustment Scale has been commonly used in research examining chronic pain patients (Block, 1980; Mohamed et al., 1978), and both the Locke-Wallace and Areas of Change have available norms for CLBP patients and spouses (Ahern et al., 1985). While these are by no means the only or absolutely best marital assessment questionnaires, the authors have found them quite useful. Other well-validated instruments the clinician may wish to consider include the Marital Adjustment Inventory (Snyder, 1979), the Dyadic Adjustment Scale (Spanier, 1976) and the Spouse Verbal Problems Checklist (Carter & Thomas, 1973).

Emotional Distress and Psychological Difficulties

Questionnaire assessment of the patient's psychological status ensures thorough screening for psychiatric illness, provides a basis for normative comparisons, and may identify distress in patients who are reticent in their verbal report. The MMPI is clearly the most widely used questionnaire method for evaluating emotional distress and psychological difficulties in CLBP patients. The MMPI is a 566-item, true/false instrument designed to assess a wide range of psychopathology. It consists of three validity scales and 10 clinical scales. The 10 clinical scales are hypochondriasis, depression, hysteria, psychopathic deviance, masculinity/femininity, paranoia, psychesthenia (anxiety), schizophrenia, mania, and social introversion. The patient obtains a norm-referenced score for each scale as well as an overall profile configuration. Multivariate studies indicate the utility of the MMPI in identifying homogeneous and replicable subgroups of CLBP and other pain patients (Bradley et al., 1978; Prokop et al., 1980). These subgroups differ significantly in such problem characteristics as duration of pain, number of hospitalizations, degree of activity restriction, disruption of marital communication, and social relationships (Armentrout et al., 1982; McGill, Lawlis, Selby, Mooney, & McCoy, 1983). Further, the sensitivity of the MMPI to pretreatment to posttreatment changes in CLBP patients has been widely documented (Follick et al., 1985; Roberts & Reinhardt, 1980).

There have been other instruments utilized clinically and in research with CLBP patients, such as the Symptom Checklist-90 (SCL-90) (Pelz & Merskey, 1982) and the Middlesex Hospital Questionnaire (Woodforde & Merskey, 1972). However, none has achieved the MMPI's broad clinical and research recognition for use with CLBP or is as familiar to health care providers with whom the clinician evaluating CLBP patients will likely be communicating.

Structured Behavioral Observation

Direct behavioral observation is a necessary part of comprehensive assessment of CLBP in that it provides the unique advantage of standardized, objective data independent of the patient's self-report or self-observation. Several structured observation methods have been developed for the evaluation of pain behavior. Two of these methods have been validated specifically for the CLBP population and will be discussed here.

Keefe and Block (1982) developed an observation system consisting of five nonverbal pain behaviors (sighing, grimacing, rubbing, bracing, and guarding). Patients are videotaped during sitting, standing, walking, and reclining. The authors found that these behaviors could be reliably rated by trained observers. They also found that the frequency of occurrence of these behaviors correlated significantly with the pain ratings of both the patients and naive observers. In addition, the frequency of these behaviors distinguished pain patients from normal and depressed subjects and decreased significantly following operant treatment. More recently, this observation system has received further validation for use with in vivo observation (i.e., no videotaping) in the naturalistic setting of the physician's examination room (Keefe, Wilkins, & Cook, 1984).

Follick, Ahern, & Aberger (1985) have developed an empirically derived structured taxonomy consisting of seven verbal and motoric pain behaviors (limitation statements, partial movement, guarding, bracing, position shifts, grimacing, and sounds). Patients are videotaped while undergoing a structured sequence of movements involving sitting, standing, walking, bending, exercising, and a brief standardized interview. The authors found the behaviors could be reliably rated by trained observers and discriminated between CLBP patients and normal controls. Importantly, this latter result was cross-validated using a new sample of subjects. This taxonomy also exhibited sensitivity to pretreatment to posttreatment changes (Follick et al., 1985).

Both of these behavioral observation systems are valuable adjuncts in the assessment of CLBP, allowing for systematic and objective identification of the frequency and intensity of specific pain behaviors to be targeted in intervention. These systems are also useful for evaluation of the efficacy of treatment directed at modifying the presentation of pain behavior. The use of one of these two systems is strongly recommended, with the choice of system dependent upon the clinician's needs and resources. The Follick et al. system has the advantage of being empirically derived, based upon the nominations of patients, spouses, and physicians. The Keefe and Block system has the advantage of being applicable for in vivo observation in the physician's office without the need for videotaping.

SUMMARY

A useful guiding framework for the assessment of CLBP is the CLBP syndrome. This framework recognizes the multidimensional and biopsychosocial nature of chronic pain and emphasizes the need for assessment to target not only pain per se but also the impact that pain has on the individual's life. Thorough evaluation of CLBP addresses a variety of potential syndrome elements, including pain complaints and other pain behaviors, difficulties with health care utilization, medication overreliance, vocational and financial difficulties, functional impairment, marital and family disruption, and psychological/emotional difficulties.

A protocol for assessment of the CLBP syndrome has been recommended, involving a structured interview, a self-monitoring instrument, self-report questionnaires, and structured behavioral observation. Use of this protocol will provide data on the contribution of psychosocial factors to the patient's pain complaints and can serve as a basis for development of interventions and evaluation of treatment outcome.

REFERENCES

Ahern, D. K., Adams, A. E., & Follick, M. J. (1985). Emotional distress and marital disturbance in spouses of chronic low back pain patients. *Clinical Journal of Pain, 1*, 69–74.

Armentrout, D. P., Moore, J. E., Parker, J. C., Hewett, J. E., & Feltz, C. (1982). Pain-patient MMPI subgroups: The psychological dimensions of pain. *Journal of Behavioral Medicine, 5*, 201–211.

Ball, J. C. (1967). The reliability and validity of interview data obtained from fifty-nine narcotic addicts. *American Journal of Sociology, 76*, 650–654.

Beecher, H. K. (1959). *Measurement of subjective responses.* New York: Oxford University Press.

Bergner, M., Bobbitt, R. A., Carter, W. B., & Gilson, B. S. (1981). The Sickness Impact Profile: Development and final revision of a health status measure. *Medical Care, 19*, 787–805.

Bergner, M. Bobbitt, R. A., Pollard, W. E., Martin, D. P., & Gilson, B. S. (1976). The Sickness Impact Profile: Validation of a health status measure. *Medical Care, 14*, 57–67.

Black, R. G. (1975). The chronic pain syndrome. *Surgical Clinics of North America, 55*, 999–1011.

Block, A. R., Kremer, E. F., & Gaylor, M. (1980). Behavioral treatment of chronic pain: The spouse as a discriminative cue for pain behavior. *Pain, 9*, 243–252.

Bonica, J. J. (1981). Preface in *New approaches to treatment of chronic pain: A review of multidisciplinary pain clinics and pain centers.* NIDA Research Monograph 36. Rockville, MD.

Bradley, L., Prokop, C., Margolis, R., & Gentry, W. (1978). Multivariate analyses of the MMPI profiles of low back pain patients. *Journal of Behavioral Medicine, 1*, 253–272.

Cairns, D., & Pasino, J. (1972). Comparison of verbal reinforcement and feedback in the operant treatment of disability due to chronic low back pain. *Behavior Therapy, 8*, 621–630.

Cairns, D., Thomas, L., Mooney, V., & Pace, J. B. (1976). A comprehensive treatment approach to chronic low back pain. *Pain, 2*, 301–308.

Carson, T. P., & Adams, H. E. (1981). Affective disorders: Behavioral perspectives. In S. M. Turner, K. S. Calhoun, & H. E. Adams (Eds.), *Handbook of clinical behavior therapy.* New York: J. Wiley.

Carter, R. D., & Thomas, E. J. (1973). Modification of problematic marital communication using corrective feedback and instruction. *Behavior Therapy, 4*, 100–109.

Chapman, C. R., Casey, K. L., Dubner, R., Foley, K. M., Gracely, R. H., & Reading, A. E. (1985). Pain measurement: An overview. *Pain, 22*, 1–31.

Dirk, S. J., & Kuldau, J. M. (1974). Validity of self-report by psychiatry patients of employment earnings and hospitalization. *Journal of Consulting and Clinical Psychology, 42*, 738.

Dolce, J. J., & Raczynski, J. M. (1985). Neuromuscular activity and electromyography in painful backs: Psychological and biomechanical models in assessment and treatment. *Psychological Bulletin, 97*, 502–520.

Dubbison, O., & Melzack, B. (1976). Classification of clinical pain descriptors by multiple group discriminant analysis. *Experimental Neurology, 51*, 480–487.

Dworkin, R. H., Handlin, D. S., Richlin, D. M., Brand, L., & Vannucci, C. (1985). Unraveling the effects of compensation, litigation, and employment on treatment response in chronic pain. *Pain, 23*, 49–59.

Ferster, C. B. (1973). A functional analysis of depression. *American Psychologist, 28*, 857–870.

Flor, H., Kerns, R. J., & Turk, D. C. (1985). The prediction of pain behaviors in chronic pain patients from spouse reinforcement. Paper presented at the 6th Annual Session of the Society of Behavioral Medicine, New Orleans.

Flor, H., & Turk, D. C. (in press). Chronic pain and the family. In D. C. Turk & R. D. Kerns (Eds.), *Health, illness, and families: A life-span perspective.* New York: Wiley-Interscience.

Follick, M. J., Aberger, E. W., Ahern, D. K., & McCartney, J. (1984). The chronic low back pain syndrome: Identification and management. *Rhode Island Medical Journal, 67*, 219–224.

Follick, M. J., Ahern, D. K., & Aberger, E. W. (1985). Development of an audiovisual taxonomy of pain behavior: Reliability and discriminant validity. *Health Psychology, 4*, 555–568.

Follick, M. J., Ahern, D. K., Aberger, E. W., & Adams, A. E. (1985). *Evaluation of an outpatient-based behavioral management program for chronic pain.* Paper presented at the 19th Annual Convention of the Association for Advancement of Behavior Therapy, Houston, Texas.

Follick, M. J., Ahern, D. K., & Laser-Wolston, N. (1984). Validation of a self-report diary for the assessment of pain behavior and disability. *Pain, 19*, 373–382.

Follick, M. J., Ahern, D. K., Laser-Wolston, N., Adams, A. E., & Malloy, A. (1985). Chronic pain: Electromechanic recording device for measuring patients' activity patterns. *Archives of Physical Medicine and Rehabilitation, 66*, 75-79.

Follick, M. J., Smith, T. W., & Ahern, D. K. (1985). The Sickness Impact Profile A global measure of disability in chronic low back pain. *Pain, 21*, 67-76.

Follick, M. J., Zitter, R. E., & Ahern, D. K. (1983). Failures in the operant treatment of chronic pain. In E. B. Foa & P. Emmelkamp (Eds.), *Failures in behavior therapy.* New York: Wiley.

Fordyce, W. E. (1976a). *Behavioral methods for chronic pain and illness.* St. Louis, MO: Mosby.

Fordyce, W. E. (1976b). Behavioral concepts in chronic pain and illness. In P. O Davidson (Ed.), *The behavioral management of anxiety, depression, & pain.* New York: Brunner/Mazel.

Fordyce, W. E. (1983). Behavioral conditioning concepts in chronic pain. In J. J Bonica, U. Lindblom, & A. Iggo (Eds.), *Advances in pain research and therapy, Vol. 5.* New York: Raven Press.

Fordyce, W. E., Fowler, R. S., Lehmann, J. F., Delateur, B. J., Sand, P. L., & Trieschman, R. B. (1973). Operant conditioning in the treatment of chronic pain. *Archives of Physical Medicine and Rehabilitation, 54*, 399-408.

Fordyce, W. E. & Steger, J. C. (1979). Chronic pain. In O. F. Pomerleau & J. P Brady (Eds.), *Behavioral medicine: Theory and practice.* Baltimore, MD: Williams & Wilkins.

Greenhoot, J., & Sternbach, R. A. (1974). Conjoint treatment of chronic pain *Advances in Neurology, 4*, 595-603.

Haynes, S. N. (1978). *Principles of behavioral assessment.* New York: Gardner.

Haynes, S. N., & Wilson, C. C. (1979). *Behavioral assessment.* San Francisco: Josey-Bass.

Heaton, R. K., Getto, C. J., Lehman, R. A. W., Fordyce, W. E., Brauer, E., & Groban, S. E. (1982). A standardized evaluation of psychosocial factors in chronic pain. *Pain, 12*, 165-174.

Honig, A. S., Tannenbaum, J., & Caldwell, B. (1968). Maternal behavior in verbal report and in laboratory observation. Paper presented at the meeting of the American Psychological Association, San Francisco.

Johnson, A. D. (1979). *Compensation aspects of low back claims.* Technical report, State of Washington, Department of Labor & Industries.

Keefe, F. J., & Block, A. R. (1982). Development of an observation method for assessing pain behavior in chronic low back pain patients. *Behavior Therapy, 13*, 363-375.

Keefe, F. J., Wilkins, R. H., & Cook, W. A. (1984). Direct observation of pain behavior in low back pain patients during physical examination. *Pain, 20*, 69-76.

Korchin, S. J. (1976). *Modern clinical psychology.* New York: Basic Books.

Lewinsohn, P. M. (1974). Clinical and theoretical aspects of depression. In K. S. Calhoun, H. E. Adams, & K. M. Mitchell (Eds.), *Innovative treatment methods in psychopathology.* New York: Wiley.

Locke, H. J., & Wallace, K. M. (1959). Short marital-adjustment and prediction tests: Their reliability and validity. *Marriage and Family Living, 21*, 251-255.

Malec, J., Cayner, J. J., Harvey, R. F., & Timming, R. C. (1981). Pain management: Long-term follow-up of an inpatient program. *Archives of Physical Medicine and Rehabilitation, 62*, 369-372.

Margolin, G., Talouie, S., & Weinstein, C. D. (1983). Areas of Change Questionnaire: A practical approach to marital assessment. *Journal of Consulting and Clinical Psychology, 51*, 220–231.

Maruta, T., & Osborn, D. (1978). Sexual activity in chronic pain patients. *Psychosomatics, 19*, 231–237.

Maruta, T., Swanson, D. W., & Finlayson, R. E. (1979). Drug abuse and dependency in patients with chronic pain. *Mayo Clinic Proceedings, 54*, 241–244.

Matarazzo, J. D. (1965). The interview. In B. B. Wolman (Ed.), *Handbook of clinical psychology*, New York: McGraw-Hill.

McCreary, C., Turner, J., & Dawson, E. (1981). Principal dimensions of the pain experience and psychological disturbance in chronic low back pain patients. *Pain, 11*, 85–92.

McGill, J., Lawlis, F., Selby, D., Mooney, V., & McCoy, C. E. (1983). The relationship of Minnesota Multiphasic Personality Inventory (MMPI) clusters to pain behaviors. *Journal of Behavioral Medicine, 6*, 77–92.

McLean, P. (1976). Therapeutic decision-making in the behavioral treatment of depression. In P. O. Davidson (Ed.), *The behavioral management of anxiety, depression, and pain*. New York: Brunner/Mazel.

Melzack, R. (1974). Psychological concepts and methods for the control of pain. In J. J. Bonica (Ed.), *Advances in neurology* (Vol. 4, pp. 275–280). New York: Raven Press.

Melzack, R. (1975). The McGill Pain Questionnaire: Major properties and scoring methods. *Pain, 1*, 277–299.

Melzack, R., Katz, J., & Jeans, M. E. (1985). The role of compensation in chronic pain: Analysis using a new method of scoring the McGill Pain Questionnaire. *Pain, 23*, 101–112.

Melzack, R., & Wall, P. (1965). Pain mechanisms: A new theory. *Science, 50*, 971–979.

Mohamed, S. N., Weisz, G. M., & Waring, E. M. (1978). The relationship of chronic pain to depression, marital adjustment, and family dynamics. *Pain, 5*, 282–292.

Painter, J. R., Seres, J. L., & Newman, R. I. (1980). Assessing benefits of the pain center: Why some patients regress? *Pain, 8*, 101–113.

Pelz, M., & Merskey, H. (1982). A description of the psychological effects of chronic pain lesions. *Pain, 64*, 293–301.

Pollard, W. E., Bobbitt, R. A., Bergner, M., Martin, D. P., & Gilson, B. S. (1976). The Sickness Impact Profile: Reliability of a health status measure. *Medical Care, 14*, 146–155.

Prokop, C., Bradley, L., Margolis, R., & Gentry, W. (1980). Mulitivariate analysis of the MMPI profiles of patients with multiple pain complaints. *Journal of Personality Assessment, 44*, 246–252.

Ready, L. B., & Hare, B. (1979). Drug problems in chronic pain patients. *Anesthesiology Review, 6*, 28–31.

Reuler, J. B., Girard, D. E., & Nardone, D. A. (1980). The chronic pain syndrome: Misconceptions and management. *Annals of Internal Medicine, 93*, 588–596.

Roberts, A. H. (1981). The behavioral treatment of chronic pain. In J. M. Ferguson & C. B. Taylor (Eds.), *The comprehensive handbook of behavioral medicine, 2*. New York: Spectrum.

Roberts, A. H., & Reinhardt, L. (1980). The behavioral management of chronic pain: Long-term follow-up with comparison groups. *Pain, 8*, 151–162.

Sanders, S. H. (1985). Chronic pain: Conceptualization and epidemiology. *Annals of Behavioral Medicine, 7*, 3–5.

Schnelle, J. F. (1974). A brief report on invalidity of parent evaluations of behavior change. *Journal of Applied Behavioral Analysis, 7*, 341–343.

Seligman, M. E. P. (1975). *Helplessness: On depression, development, and death.* San Francisco: Freeman.

Shealy, C. N. (1976). *The pain game.* Millbrae, CA: Celestial Arts.

Snyder, D. K. (1979). *Marital Satisfaction Inventory.* Los Angeles: Western Psychological Services.

Sobell, L. C., & Sobell, M. B. (1975). Outpatient alcoholics give valid self-reports. *Journal of Nervous and Mental Disease, 161*, 32–42.

Spanier, G. B. (1976). Measuring dyadic adjustment: New scales for assessing the quality of marriage and similar dyads. *Journal of Marriage and the Family, 38*, 15–28.

Sternbach, R. A. (1974). *Pain patients: Traits and treatment.* New York: Academic Press.

Sternbach, R. A., & Timmermans, G. (1975). Personality changes associated with reduction of pain. *Pain, 1*, 177–181.

Summers, T. (1970). Validity of alcoholics' self-reported drinking history. *Quarterly Journal of Studies on Alcohol, 31*, 972–974.

Taylor, C. B., Zlutnick, S. I., Corley, M. J., & Flora, J. (1980). The effects of detoxification, relaxation, and brief supportive therapy on chronic pain. *Pain, 8*, 319–329.

Turner, J. A., Calsyn, D. A., Fordyce, W. E., & Ready, L. B. (1982). Drug utilization patterns in chronic pain patients. *Pain, 12*, 357–363.

Turner, J. A., & Chapman, C. R. (1982). Psychological interventions for chronic pain: A critical review. I. Relaxation training and biofeedback. *Pain, 12*, 1–21.

Waring, E. M. (1977). The role of the family in symptom selection and perpetuation in psychosomatic illness. *Psychotherapy and Psychosomatics, 28*, 253–259.

Weiss, R. L., Hops, H., & Patterson, G. R. (1973). A framework for conceptualizing marital conflict, a technology for altering it, some data for evaluating it. In F. W. Clark & L. A. Hamerlynck (Eds.), *Critical issues in research and practice: Proceedings of the 4th Banff International Conference on Behavior Modification.* Champaign, IL: Research Press.

White, A. W. (1969). Low back pain in men receiving Workmen's Compensation: A follow-up study. *Canadian Medical Association Journal, 101*, 61–67.

Woodforde, J., & Merskey, H. (1972). Personality traits of patients with chronic pain. *Journal of Psychosomatic Research, 16*, 167–172.

3
Neuropsychological Assessment in Brain Injury Rehabilitation

Rodger Llewellyn Wood

Over the last 5 years several excellent textbooks have been published that review neuropsychological testing procedures. These have described a wide range of tests, the relationship between test performance and types of brain damage, the influence of behavior on test performance, and the relationship between neuropsychological assessment and certain aspects of behavior (Fiskov & Boll, 1981; Heilman & Valenstein, 1984; Levin, Benton, & Grossman, 1982; Lezak, 1983; Kolb & Wishaw, 1980; Walsh, 1985). In some respects there is little to add to these reviews, except perhaps to point out that these texts necessarily adopt a broad perspective toward neuropsychological assessment, whereas a more specific approach is necessary when such assessments are carried out as a preliminary to the rehabilitation of a brain-damaged patient. A neuropsychological assessment for rehabilitation is essentially based upon the same tests described in the above texts. The procedures for applying these tests in rehabilitation may differ, however, and it may even be necessary to interpret these tests in a different way.

The nature of a patient's neuropsychological disorder can often determine the process of rehabilitation. This may require the neuropsychologist to adopt what Walsh (1985) describes as the "educational role." He suggests that the neuropsychologist often stands in a "central position" in the multidisciplinary team dealing with the brain-impaired patient. Development of the team approach requires a need to assume an "educational role." One could go as far as to say that, in the rehabilitation team, the neuropsychologist is *uniquely* placed to integrate information obtained from a variety of clinical sources and offer an explanation as to why a particular kind of disability exists. In order to do this it is necessary to determine what cognitive, perceptual, or psychomotor deficits underly the functional dis-

ability or disorder of behavior that forms the focus of attention for th
rehabilitation team (Goldstein, 1983).

How such information is obtained and its usefulness in determining th
rehabilitation process remains a matter of debate. Conventionally, we obtai
a measure of the patient's performance on a range of tests, organized eith
as standard batteries or ad hoc clinical measures of neuropsychologic
ability. This index of performance is presumed to help the rehabilitatio
specialist understand how cognitive and/or personality factors may impos
constraints on behavior or the relearning of functional and other skills tha
promote personal independence. Such knowledge is expected to help th
rehabilitation team devise the best approach for the remediation of thos
skills that are fundamental to activities of daily living (ADL).

Restricting neuropsychological assessment in rehabilitation to an analysi
of test data presents several problems. One is that the ability to obtai
information, which is both clinically relevant to the rehabilitation team an
capable of being presented in a sensible and goal-directed way, depend
largely on the attitudes toward assessment adopted by the neuropsycholo
gist. Unfortunately, many neuropsychologists style their assessment in sucl
a way that the data generated by tests are difficult to use by rehabilitatio
therapists. This is because the test results do not answer the questions tha
form the basis of their treatment procedures. One reason for this is tha
rehabilitation is concerned with *behavior*, while neuropsychological assess
ment has been preoccupied with the analysis of *ability* (Diller & Gordo
1981). While the two are inevitably linked—behavior being an end produc
of a number of specific abilities—there are also important distinctions. On
distinction possibly forms the basis for differentiating psychological an
neuropsychological assessment. The former concentrates on personality (i
the shape of behavior or expressed ideas) and environmental determinants o
personality change, while the latter focuses on specific cognitive skills an
how they vary relative to one another and in response to organic variable
that are known to determine cognitive disorders.

Crockett, Clark, and Klonoff (1981) regard this as an artificial division i
the clinical assessment of human characteristics that may have a bearing o
treatment in rehabilitation. They suggest that to describe a patient's behav
ior solely in terms of cognitive deficits is misleading because it denies th
intricate interactions among cognitive factors, personality, and the variet
of coping strategies exhibited by patients who have sustained brain injury
These coping strategies may reflect the patient's premorbid style of behav
ior as well as reflect a response to the brain injury. More importantly, sucl
strategies seem to represent a response to the type of cognitive dysfunctio
that the individual has sustained. In this respect, it is somewhat ironic t
note the number of neuropsychological reports on patients in rehabilitatio
units that comment on the patient's behavior as a preliminary to describin

he nature and extent of cognitive dysfunction in order to state how the
behavior may have interfered with test performance and subsequent results.
t is far less common to see this process turned around in the conclusions of
he report in order to formulate an explanation for certain behavior or
personality disorders or inappropriate coping strategies on the basis of
specific cognitive deficits.

This style of assessment, which focuses on artificial cognitive ability at
he expense of other aspects of behavior, owes something to the historical
development of neuropsychology as a branch of the neurosciences. The
original task of neuropsychology was to analyze brain–behavior relationships in an attempt to map the functional organization of the brain. To do
his it used the tools of experimental psychology to systematically measure
and differentiate specific cognitive skills while observing alterations in the
levels of such skills as a result of circumscribed lesions. Once the relationships between certain types of areas of cerebral pathology and subsequent
forms of cognitive impairment had been established there was a natural
extension of neuropsychological investigation into the clinical field.

Probably one of the first roles for the clinical neuropsychologist was
providing a differential diagnosis to distinguish behavior that was neurologically mediated from behavior that occurred as part of a psychological or
psychotic reaction. The systematic evaluation of cognitive components of
behavior was derived from the experimental method employed in working
on normal human subjects, a procedure that has more in common with
research conducted under the ambit of general experimental and cognitive
psychology than behavioral neurology. This approach to the measurement
of "brain function" became established as a foundation for the developing
science of neuropsychology. However, while *measurement* may be the pre-
dominant feature of any emerging scientific discipline (Lezak, 1983), *application* must be its goal. Consistent with this philosophy, neuropsychologists
are beginning to find ways of applying their skills in a treatment capacity.
So far there are two major areas of application. The first is in the form of
treatment approaches to remediate specific cognitive deficits, which result
from brain trauma, vascular lesions, or neurological disease. Another application involves the neuropsychologist acting as an advisor to other therapy
specialties, the educational role, helping them to understand the effect of
neurological deficits on behavior and suggesting ways to improve the potential of individual patients for rehabilitation and vocational retraining.

Unlike other sciences, however, there appears to be some discontinuity
between the neuropsychological process of measurement and the practical
application of information derived from such measurement. The indications
are that the form of assessment that proves successful in neuropsychological
diagnosis does not appear to generate the same type of useful information
for the purpose of rehabilitation. In view of this apparent imbalance be-

tween the historical or conventional approach to neuropsychological assess ment and the information required by the rehabilitation team to form th basis of a treatment model, it may be necessary for neuropsychologists t consider the range of applications involved in a neuropsychological assess ment, and, if necessary, review the concepts upon which their clinica practices are based. This chapter attempts to examine why the conventiona neuropsychological approach to diagnostic assessment may not provide th best foundation for assessment in rehabilitation.

THE PSYCHOMETRIC APPROACH TO NEUROPSYCHOLOGICAL ASSESSMENT

A neuropsychological assessment is capable of providing a range of infor mation concerning the type and severity of cognitive impairment, the rate o recovery, and the nature of the cognitive sequelae that are likely to interfer with independence. Procedures for obtaining a profile of cognitive abilitie have been available in a variety of forms for a number of years. They includ a range of individual and specialized tests, organized either as "informa composite batteries" (Kolb & Wishaw, 1980) or standardized batteries o tasks, designed to evaluate a range of cognitive skills and identify any abnormal variation in the individual's pattern of ability (e.g., the Halstead–Reitan Battery; see Boll, 1981). Data from such neuropsychological proce dures can be qualitative and descriptive, such as that provided by Luria's Neuropsychological Investigation (Christensen, 1975), or arranged numer ically, according to some quantitative analysis of different skills (Golden, 1981). Both methods require experience and training, but the former de mands that the practitioner has a far greater *clinical* acumen than does the latter.

Because the evolution of clinical psychology has been, on the one hand, dynamic and nonphysical (Boll, 1981), and, on the other hand, experimen tal and psychometric, there has not been much emphasis placed on either the neurophysiological or neuroanatomical systems that underlie many of the clinical problems presented to the neuropsychologist. Many neuropsychol ogists have tended, therefore, to rely on test data that provide some "cook book" interpretation of neuropsychological abnormalities, rather than try ing to find clinical interpretations to explain how a cognitive anomaly might produce some behavior disorder. This can lead to the dubious practice in clinical neuropsychology of finding ways to translate observations of be havior, which may have some neurological basis, into a numerically based profile of abilities, presumably in the hope of short-circuiting the need to understand brain–behavior relationships. One example is the quantitative ersion of Luria's test referred to earlier: the Luria-Nebraska Neuropsychological Battery (see Golden, 1981, for a review). This does not mean that quantitative data have no value in clinical examinations. It does mean, however, that too much reliance can be placed on psychometric methods at the expense of developing an adequate knowledge base for an understanding of brain-behavior relationships.

Problems with the Psychometric Approach

In an important paper describing the problems evaluating psychological deficits after brain injury, Newcombe and Artioloa i Fortuny (1979) state that "conventional psychometric testing has inevitable shortcomings. In particular, intelligence tests (with or without a risky juggling of test scores) are flagrantly inadequate as measures of intellectual handicap following brain injury." The use of I.Q. and other standardized scores as a measure to determine the presence and effect of brain damage has been criticized more recently by Diller and Gordon (1981) in their discussion on rehabilitation and clinical neuropsychology. They state that "test scores, in and of themselves are lacking, since they provide little insight into the mechanisms/processes of impaired performance." The convenience of the serendipitous distinction between verbal and performance subtests of the Wechsler Adult Intelligence Scale (WAIS) (Kolb & Wishaw, 1980) as an indicator of some lateralized abnormality has been exploited by many psychologists without much thought to the type of brain damage most likely to produce such a discrepancy. This practice continues, even though studies have shown cases where lateralized brain pathology is present without producing any verbal-performance discrepancy on the WAIS (Wood, 1980) and, in some cases, producing no intellectual abnormalities at all.

The reliance on I.Q. scores can have a particularly damaging effect on the assessment of recovery from head injury. This is most likely to occur when a head-injured patient is assessed as having an I.Q. in or above the average range, especially if the contemporary assessment corresponds to some pre-morbid estimate of ability. Such information is frequently assumed to imply that the patient has recovered his or her cognitive faculties or, at least, has the capability to cope with the intellectual demands of daily life and some kind of occupation. Often this is far from the case! After traumatic brain injury there can be a major discrepancy between intellectual *ability* and the person's intellectual *capability*. This results from the fact that the brain injury leads to a separation between a person's established intellectual abilities, which are measured using standardized tests, and the individual's capacity for directing his or her behavior or implementing decisions based on that intellectual ability. This phenomenon is most frequently seen in cases of frontal lobe injury where a high I.Q. level may be recorded bu without the patient being able to perform many routine activities of dail living.

The type of information provided by a psychometric approach in neu ropsychology does not always help rehabilitation therapists formulate tech niques to overcome behavior difficulties imposed by neuropsychologica deficits. Some reasons for this are discussed by Diller and Gordon (1981) They point to an important conceptual difference between neuropsychol ogy and rehabilitation, which enlarges on the earlier comment distinguish ing *behavior change*, a goal of rehabilitation, from *analysis of ability*, which ha been the hallmark of neuropsychology.

Diller and Gordon explain this difference by distinguishing betwee impairment and disability. *Impairment* means that some change has occurre in a cognitive or motor system to alter the function of that system. Th alteration in function can be designated as some form of disability. Th essential difference between the two is that an impairment is a judgment or the integrity of a particular functional system. *Disability*, however, is relative concept because it varies according to the prevailing circumstances the nature of the environment, or the interests of the person who display such impairment. There is another important difference. Impairment refer to a change in some *hypothesized cognitive process*, while disability is base on an *observation of behavior change*. To elaborate on an example given by Diller and Gordon: a concert pianist who suffers a brain injury with subsequent loss of fine motor control to a hand will experience far greater disability than would a manual laborer who sustained the same injury bu whose main occupational function is to dig holes on a building site. Both individuals display a similar impairment but they vary considerably in term of the disability caused by that impairment. On the other hand, two differ-ent patients may show apparently identical difficulties at the behavioral level and yet the reason for such difficulty might be quite different in each case. The underlying reasons for failure at a task may demand different ap-proaches to rehabilitation and management (Brooks & Lincoln, 1984).

Rehabilitation, therefore, is concerned with disability, while clinical neu-ropsychology has been concerned with impairment. Unfortunately, while neuropsychology has been very effective in identifying cognitive impair-ment, it has failed to describe how the impairment relates to general aspects of behavior.

The type of cognitive impairment identified in many neuropsychological examinations seems to bear little correspondence to the type of disability displayed by patients recovering from brain injury. An example of this can be obtained by comparing the performance of patients on cognitive tasks with structured activities of daily living.

It is not uncommon to find that patients who are poor on constructional nd visuospatial tasks fail to show any corresponding difficulty when onfronted with real-life tasks that require visuospatial awareness. One airly dramatic example comes from the author's own clinical practice. A 0-year-old woman who suffered a severe, diffuse brain injury as a result of nerpes simplex encephalitis was seen for assessment to review her progress nd determine her potential for rehabilitation. Six months after the onset of he illness a variety of tests indicated that she had no *measurable* memory unction. Her communication was very limited because of expressive and omprehension problems. The dysphasia was so severe that only a veneer of utomatic speech (limited to social comments such as "hello" or "very well, hank you") was retained. A measure of verbal reasoning and other lan- ;uage-related skills was unobtainable (because of her dysphasia) and she lisplayed great difficulty (recording mentally defective scores) on the Block)esign and Object Assembly subtests of the WAIS, with no ability to draw he Rey complex figure.

On the basis of her age and appalling neuropsychological performance, a)oor prognosis was formed and no formal rehabilitation given. Her hus-)and was advised to employ a housekeeper who could assist with many of he domestic chores while acting as a companion to his wife. After a further ' months (without any rehabilitation) she returned for a follow-up exami- 1ation. No difference was noted in her performance on a variety of cogni- ive, language, perceptual, or psychomotor tasks. It was with some surprise, herefore, that we received the news that this lady was driving her car illegally because of epilepsy), playing golf (albeit with a greater handicap), :ooking, and seeing to nearly all the domestic chores, having dismissed the 1ousekeeper some weeks before.

Newcombe (1981) reports another case of discontinuity between test performance and practical ability. Her patient, a surgeon, sustained a missile wound during World War II. Twenty years later he still had a "large metal fragment . . . lodged in the ventricles of his brain." Psychological test results indicated that he still displayed considerable difficulty with construc- tional and visuospatial tasks, exhibited by his poor performance on the Block Design task of the WAIS. Contrary to expectations this did not interfere with his ability to successfully wield a scalpel as a practicing surgeon. From her considerable experience in the field of neuropsychologi- cal investigation, Newcombe made the remark that the ". . . gaps between scores on laboratory measures and functional independence (Christmas et al., 1974) or job efficiency (Newcombe & Ratcliff, 1979) suggest that the prospects for rehabilitation should be assessed at 'the bench' rather than based solely on psychological test performance."

One does not have to rely on anecdotal evidence for such examples. Brooks (1979), during a 3-month follow-up of head-injured patients, found no association between clinical memory test performance and the kind of memory difficulties observed by the friends or family of the patient. At more general level of behavior, Andrews and Stewart (1979) found that th performance of stroke patients tested in the clinic was far better than it wa at home. Sarno, Sarno, and Levita (1971) noted that children receivin speech therapy failed to show changes on formal language tests that coul correlate with changes of functional language. Eagle (1979) stated tha quadriplegic children who record intelligence test performances at the "de fective" level are often capable of effective behavior. Finally, Diller an Gordon (1981) report that rehabilitation workers found poor vocationa predictive value in traditional testing approaches and that the same tests adapted for industrial psychology, failed to offer "practical" methods fo training in vocational rehabilitation.

Another source of evidence to show that an association between impair ment and disability has not developed can be found by scrutinizing the content of recent textbooks on neuropsychology. The reader will find few references to rehabilitation per se and little direct information to help advise the neuropsychologist on how to relate assessment procedures to clinica forms of treatment. Such discontinuity between measurement and rehabili tation therapy is probably responsible for practitioners of cognitive rehabili tation focusing on artificial skills, such as improving an individual's ability on a block design task or learning a list of words, when the rehabilitation therapist is concerned about far more basic and practical skills, such a whether or not the patient can pick up a spoon and eat with it!

A final problem related to the psychometric approach involves the failure of many neuropsychologists to distinguish between different types of neu ropathology when selecting test procedures. Lezak (1983) reports that different types of brain lesions and etiologies can differentially affect higher cognitive function and the patient's potential for rehabilitation. A similar attitude toward assessment for rehabilitation is held by Brooks and Lincoln (1984). They make the comment that "brain damage of different etiologies, different velocities, different sites, and occurring at different ages can have markedly different effects on cognitive functions." When determining the nature of reported disability after traumatic brain injury the relationship between the type of brain damage and the method of recording subsequent cognitive impairment may be a critical factor determining the clinical utility of the data.

A NEUROBEHAVIORAL APPROACH
TO ASSESSMENT

As early as 1955 Hebb was of the opinion that "neuropsychology should be aimed at explaining complex behavior." More recently, Beaumont (1983) pointed out that "neuropsychology rests entirely upon inferences about brain organization derived from the observation of behavior," while Goldstein (1983) proposed that neuropsychology should form a "productive alliance with behavior therapy in regard to the planning, implementation, and evaluation of individual rehabilitation programs." Diller and Gordon apply such thinking to the rehabilitation of brain injury (which they describe as a procedure designed to "impact" skills used in routine aspects of living) and state that "while the clinical neuropsychologist is concerned with the diagnosis and description of cognitive impairments and their relationship to parameters of brain damage, rehabilitation poses the issue of how descriptions impact the person's skills, environment, activity patterns, and status. To achieve maximum benefit in a rehabilitation setting, clinical neuropsychologists must relate their findings to these aspects of functioning." Diagnostic approaches that identify impairment may therefore offer little to the professional who is concerned with remediating disability because not enough thought has been given to how such impairments affect day-to-day behavior.

How neuropsychology undergoes the metamorphosis from diagnostic neuropsychology to a form of neuropsychological assessment that will describe functional behavior and aid rehabilitation has not yet been defined. A structured approach (if not a model) is needed to help this development and offer a framework within which the clinical neuropsychologist can apply his skills. One such approach has been suggested by Powell (1981) and developed for brain injury rehabilitation by Wood and Eames (1981) and Wood (1984a, 1986a). This combines a behavioral with a neuropsychological perspective for the remediation of those abilities that have become impaired as a result of brain damage. The method attempts to improve the learning potential of severely brain-injured patients and also helps to control many of the behaviors that prevent rehabilitation from taking place. According to Wood (1984a), from this perspective the "role of neuropsychology in the rehabilitation process is that of specifying the *behaviors* that may serve as appropriate targets for treatment." Goldstein (1983) regards the difference between the behavioral approach and the standard neuropsychological report as one that places an "emphasis on rehabilitation rather than diagnosis."

By combining behavioral methods and neuropsychology, a process of assessment can take place that integrates cognitive and personality variables with functional appraisal of the patient's level of independence. The essential difference between this procedure and the traditional neuropsychological assessment is that while the latter often places limited importance on (1) the *nature* of the brain injury, (2) the *time* since the injury, (3) the *environmental influences* on behavior, and (4) the patient's *motivation* for recovery, the neurobehavioral approach makes such information central to the process of evaluating recovery and the patient's potential for rehabilitation.

The implication in this procedure is that all assessments that are presumed to offer treatment in brain injury rehabilitation should have a theoretical and scientific footing. This argument has recently been revived by Baddeley (1984) and supported by Brooks and Lincoln (1984), who criticize the "ad hoc" nature of many cognitive tests used to measure the effects of brain injury. They comment, "the clinical assessment of cognitive function, especially after head injury, has proceeded almost entirely independently of current theoretical views about cognition." This can be avoided by adopting a "neurobehavioral" framework that helps combine observations of brain–behavior relationships in such a way that the neuropsychologist not only describes the nature of a functional anomaly but does so in a way that provides a foundation for rehabilitation. As a procedure and neurobehavioral approach, it emphasizes the learning process implicit in behavioral procedures. Powell (1981) claims that behavior therapy modifies the function of "almost every region of the brain," thereby making it a "legitimate aim of behavior therapy to directly attempt the modification of the brain itself," a process fundamental to the goals of rehabilitation.

NEUROBEHAVIORAL ASSESSMENT IN REHABILITATION

Conventional neuropsychological assessment makes interpretations about specific aspects of (cognitive) behavior, couched in terms or events that take place beyond the actual level of observation. This gives rise to the development of a series of "hypothetical constructs," described in a variety of terms (sometimes referred to as "test jargon"), which present a measure of cognitive activity on a dimension that may have no relevance for routine aspects of day-to-day behavior. In rehabilitation, however, neuropsychological assessment must be related to treatment. Walsh (1985) suggests that the measurement of ability must relate to some functional skill (as opposed to aspects of artificial intelligence). He states that "new psychological measures of function will need to be designed. Many currently used tests probably do not approximate closely enough to the processes involved in performance in occupations or professions."

What is needed for rehabilitation is a form of assessment that spells out the *functional relationship* among (1) observed or recorded cognitive activities, (2) the behavior displayed by the individual, and (3) the environmental demands that exist at the time such behavior is observed. A neurobehavioral assessment provides a way of observing behavior that helps identify the relationships between its antecedents, the behavior itself, and, finally, its consequences in terms of adaptive responses to the environment. Such a process can help discriminate organic influences on behavior from environmental ones. Also, systematic observations based on "time samples" or some other behavioral baseline allow the neuropsychological assessment to become an integrated part of a series of systematic observations, providing a framework for interpreting test results in the context of emotional or behavioral factors.

It would appear, therefore, that the primary need in any assessment for rehabilitation is to specify target behaviors that are appropriate for treatment. Wood (1984a, 1986a) has described behavior problems that may entirely prevent rehabilitation taking place, while Lezak (1983) pointed out how certain behavior problems, such as dependency, passivity, obsessionality, and irresponsibility, can act as major obstacles to a patient whose rehabilitation depends on the active relearning of skills and habit patterns. This does not mean that behavioral observations cannot include psychological phenomena such as attention, organizational thinking, or consciousness. It is true that these "behaviors" have been neglected by the behaviorists because of technical problems involved in recording and controlling them (Davey, 1981). More recently, however, rules that govern the function of such "internal operations" have been established (Bolles, 1979; Plum & Posner, 1982), helping us use such concepts to explain deficits of behavior following brain injury (e.g., Eames & Wood, 1985).

Malec (1983) proposed that "behavior disturbance is most often related to cognitive dysfunction." Some aspect of cognitive impairment affects the patient's ability to "make accurate stimulus-response-outcome predictions and to develop or recall behavior rules, to self-monitor and develop accurate self-efficiency predictions, to engage in appropriate self-reinforcement, and to reason and solve problems." By limiting our explanations of behavior to some hypothesized set of cognitive abilities (essentially unobservable processes) we may divert attention away from those environmental variables that influence or even elicit the behavior that rehabilitation is aimed at correcting. The advantage of integrating aspects of cognitive and behavioral assessment is that we account not only for the *observable* aspects of behavior but also those cognitive processes that *underly* such behavior.

The neurobehavioral procedure uses highly specific measures of cognitive ability to evaluate observations made of the patient during functional or ADL-type activities. The patient's performance on these tasks should provide some understanding of the nature of the cognitive deficit underlying behavior and act as a basis for developing treatment techniques and planning rehabilitation. Goldstein, Lezak, and others have indicated that not all behaviors are likely to respond to treatment and, therefore, one has to select for treatment only those aspects of behavior that are likely to show some importance for personal independence. There is another need for selecting behaviors to attend to any given time in the rehabilitation process. Bond and Brooks (1976) describe how different behaviors recover at different rates following brain injury. Consequently, a more economical use of time and effort may be achieved by the selection of specific behaviors for treatment at specific times during the recovery period.

In some respects, this highlights another essential difference between neurobehavioral assessment and the conventional neuropsychological assessment. The latter commonly uses broad-based cognitive tasks (tasks that rely on several cognitive abilities to achieve a good level of performance) to explain specific brain–behavior relationships. The neurobehavioral approach adopts the contrary perspective, observing broad-based behaviors (such as a complex motor sequence that relies on several cognitive attributes), attempting to explain a dysfunction in that sequence by an analysis of the individual and specific cognitive skills that combine to allow its behavioral expression. In this respect the neurobehavioral approach seems to have an ally in Lezak (1983). She states that "most neuropsychological examination techniques in clinical use elicit complex behavior." She advises, however, that in order to find out what defective functions or capacities enter into an impaired performance a "descriptive" procedure is needed, utilizing "hypothesis testing" to identify specific deficits of behavior.

PRIORITIES FOR ASSESSMENT IN REHABILITATION

There are probably six categories of cognition and behavior commonly affected by brain injury and capable of determining outcome in rehabilitation. They are:

1. Disorders of attention and information processing.
2. Problems of learning and memory.
3. Disorders of language and communication.
4. Difficulties in planning, organizing, or directing behavior.
5. Reduction of drive or motivation.
6. Emotional lability and organically mediated behavior.

An investigation of these abilities should comprise a major part of the neuropsychologist's assessment on any patient being considered for rehabilitation. This list does not necessarily exclude an evaluation of perception, praxis, or any other specific cognitive activity. The emphasis, however, must be to describe the nature of some dysfunction in terms of its effect on behavior. Perceptual functions are common in stroke patients, but, whatever the type of brain injury, perceptual functions may also affect memory for visual material or one's ability to use visually based strategies to cope with memory problems (Brooks & Lincoln, 1984). Disorders of attention may include specific abnormalities of visual or auditory perception, while the ability to organize one's behavior may depend upon the integrity of visuo-praxis. These elements of the problem will need to be described in the context of explaining the nature of behavior dysfunction.

Before proceeding with these aspects of an assessment, a comment should be made concerning the way we collect information on functional behavior within a neurobehavioral framework.

An Observational Baseline of Behavior

Any assessment in rehabilitation needs to take account of the multitude of situations and factors that help initiate, direct, and maintain behavior. We need, therefore, to obtain a behavioral baseline, collected by those members of the multidisciplinary team involved in the patient's management. This will help establish a pattern of the patient's behavior and abilities in (1) different situations, (2) during different activities, (3) at different times of the day, and (4) in response to different staff members. The value of such a comprehensive observation is that one can record the variation in levels of activity as well as the attitudes displayed by the patient toward different members of staff or therapy activities.

Adaptive behavior can be observed and measured by utilizing existing and standardized scales, such as the Adaptive Behavior Scale (Fogelman, 1975) or the Progress Assessment Chart (Gunzberg, 1974). The latter has been developed for the assessment of the mentally handicapped patient but has considerable overlap for the types of functional behavior important to independent living following brain injury. The advantage of such scales is that they offer a comprehensive and systematic method of describing behavior. In some respects, however, it is more meaningful to develop "in-house" measures of patient behavior, showing responses to specific situations. These response patterns can be measured according to single-case design procedures (Hersen & Barlow, 1978) or through the use of the kind of "simple and purpose-built tests" recommended by Brooks and Lincoln (1984). They describe a "bipolar adjective" procedure, used by Brooks and McKinlay (1983) to identify and measure personality change after severe head injury. By contrasting adjectives that describe behavior, for example, talkative–quiet, mature–childish, it becomes possible to rate a patient on different parameters of behavior at different points in time throughout recovery.

More detailed appraisals of adaptive and functional behavior can be designed to suit the specific needs of individual rehabilitation programs. The Kemsley Rehabilitation Unit in England has adopted a behavioral approach to brain injury rehabilitation that utilizes a behavior check list comprising 149 specific behaviors, all of which interfere with rehabilitation and independent living. Those behaviors that are identified as being of relevance to an individual's rehabilitation program are independently rated by eight representatives of the rehabilitation team (nurses and therapists) at intervals throughout the treatment program. This allows us to record changes taking place, not necessarily as a direct result of treatment, but as a consequence of a structured environment and a behavior therapy program. Observations based on these behavior rating scales plus single-case design procedures have been collected over 7 years on over 100 patients undergoing a comprehensive rehabilitation program. They show considerable variation in behavior, level of ability, speed of response, cooperation, and social attitude presented by individual patients, depending upon which staff member happens to be engaged in a therapy activity as well as the type of therapy activity involved. This is the first step in helping to differentiate purposeful and motivated behavior that may be at odds with the goals of the rehabilitation team from behavior that may be organically mediated and therefore less predictable in terms of its association with identifiable environmental situations.

A comprehensive baseline also allows the treatment team to discriminate between *ability* and *performance*. This is an important distinction because it may determine how we perceive the limits of a patient's ability and thereby influence the treatment goals set by the rehabilitation team. *Ability* can be defined as the *best level* of behavior observed of a patient performing any particular skill or activity. *Performance*, on the other hand, describes the *usual level* of activity displayed with regard to that skill. A scale can be devised to give such observations some numerical value, for example, between 0 and 10. This may indicate that an individual's ability to wash and dress spontaneously and without help has been observed at a level close to total independence (numerical value = 8). Such ability may contrast radically with the usual level of performance in washing and dressing if, for example, the patient seeks a lot of attention and assistance (corresponding to a numerical value of 4). The discrepancy between ability and performance ratings can form the basis of a training program. It can help us gauge our expectations of a patient's performance while, at the same time, help us measure progress. Lezak (1983) refers to a similar procedure for assessing performance that she refers to as the "best performance" method. She claims that the advantage of this procedure is that it is not bound to any particular test procedure and can include behavior that is independent of formal methods of testing.

This is the point at which assessment joins evaluation of treatment. Once we have been able to decide how often problems occur, we can begin to implement procedures to change and improve behavior while continuing the same observational analysis to evaluate the effectiveness of our clinical interventions.

Disorders of Attention and Information Processing

Often brain damage does not produce any deficits in intellect per se (especially after frontal lobe lesions; see Walsh, 1985). Instead, it affects the speed at which a person can process information or respond to environmental cues (Wood, 1986b). Problems of focusing and maintaining attention are possibly the most pervasive deficits affecting recovery and rehabilitation following brain injury. There is a considerable literature on this subject. Conkey (1938), Ruesch (1944), Dencker and Lofving (1958), Gronwall and Sampson (1974), Chadwick (1976), van Zomeren, Brouwer, and Deelman (1984), and Wood (1984b) describe attentional problems following traumatic brain injury. Some of these studies show that even mild concussional injuries can produce disorders of attention quite disproportionate to the severity of the original injury, in terms of the degree to which they affect behavior and the protracted time they take to resolve. Lezak (1983) provides a more general description of how attention deficits follow various kinds of brain injury and how these interact with test performance and affect aspects of behavior.

Wood (1984a, b, 1986b) indicates how attention problems can interfere with behavior and relearning in rehabilitation. A clear statement of the patient's attentional capabilities is therefore necessary in order that the rehabilitation team might have an idea of:

1. *The length of time therapy sessions should last*, in order not to exceed the patient's span of concentration.
2. *The processing capacity of the patient*. This will determine the amount of information to present to the patient at any given time.
3. *The speed of information processing*, which determines how fast a person can process information or respond to a particular environmental cue.
4. *The "noise level" of the environment*, in order to minimize distractions that will interfere with the patient's ability to focus attention on the rehabilitation task.

Information concerning the constraints imposed on rehabilitation therapy by these attentional anomalies is vital when it comes to planning therapy activity, the environment in which that therapy takes place, the amount of information to be presented, and even the way it is presented.

Problems of Learning and Memory

Disorders of memory are a common legacy of brain injury and can impose constraints on rehabilitation. For the purpose of advising on treatment it is important for the neuropsychologist not just to measure the *severity* of the memory problem but also to determine its *nature*. This is because it is the nature, not the severity, of memory deficit that will determine the approach to remediating the impairment.

Although a wide range of memory tests are available, their value in rehabilitation depends on how they are used. Lezak (1983) recommends that "at a minimum" we should assess *span of immediate retention; learning*, in terms of the extent of recent memory, as well as learning capacity; the *way* new information is retained, and, finally, the *efficiency of retrieval*, for both recent and remote information. This demands an evaluation of the different sensory modalities involved in learning and memory, as well as different processes of memory, such as recall and recognition.

When an assessment of memory is made in preparation for retraining some aspect of retrieval we should not limit our thinking to a measure of "test memory." Brooks and Lincoln (1984) warn that the results of memory tests do not relate closely to some of the difficulties exhibited by patients in daily life. In order to properly assess such problems, they recommend the use of rating scales and behavioral observations. Some techniques are already available in the shape of questionnaires (Bennet-Levy & Powell, 1980; Sunderland, Harris, & Baddeley, 1983). These record the types of errors made by individuals during their daily activities and include the influence of cognitive difficulties.

The value of assessment procedures that are not based on actual test performance is not restricted to the dubious assumption of a relationship between test performance and behavior but on the fact that many patients who complain of memory problems fail to record abnormal scores on clinical tests. This is probably because the forgetfulness they experience is due to attentional difficulties rather than memory per se. Some patients find that they can remember events or faces but not verbally presented information or names. Others find that they can recall events but not locate them in a temporal context. Another important distinction to help discriminate a memory impairment from an attention deficit is to see to what extent information responds to some form of cuing. Some patients appear to totally lose information, so that no amount of cuing or reminding will help its retrieval. Other individuals retain the ability to respond to a prompt or a cue yet are unable to recall information spontaneously at a time when it achieves some functional purpose. An example of this would be a wife asking her brain-injured spouse to remember to put the dinner in the oven at a certain time. On arrival home, the wife might find that he has forgotten to carry out the request, but, when reminded, the husband has full recall of the request being given. The inability to recall such information at a time when it would be effective is made all the more irritating (to the patient) by the fact that, if not prompted, they often recall the information at other times when it serves no functional purpose. This problem of recall has characteristics in common with certain types of dysphasia, when patients can produce a word spontaneously yet not to command. The implication is that it has more to do with a deficit of attention and some form of *information search*, rather than with a hypothesized memory store. Clinical experience suggests that this type of memory problem is most common following traumatic brain injury.

The assessment of memory should also give consideration to the *order* of recall because this too has implications for the nature of the patient's information processing capabilities and the organizational aspects of memory. One example of this can be found in the way patients respond to the "Anna Thompson Story" of the Wechsler Memory Scale. It is not uncommon to find patients who recall a normal amount of information but in a very fragmented way—one that bears little resemblance to that presented by the examiner. Many of these patients show a considerable loss of information after an interval of 40 minutes. This possibly occurs because the original information was not organized in a logical or coherent manner that would prevent fading or interference effects from other, competing information, presented during the interval between original presentation and delayed recall. The same effect can be seen on the Rey New Word Learning Task (see Lezak, 1983), which requires the patient to learn a list of 15 words over five trials. Some brain-injured patients do not show the primacy-recency effect expected from normal persons who attempt this task. Instead, they exhibit an almost random recall, producing words in various orders, without any sign of organizational thinking to provide a foundation for learning. This has obvious implications for rehabilitation because it is bound to affect the ability of a patient to remember instructions in a coherent form. The neuropsychologist should determine the amount of information a patient is capable of remembering at a given time and then advise the rehabilitation therapists to amend their instructions accordingly.

Disorders of Language and Communication

The importance for this area of assessment is that the neuropsychologist does not get bogged down with the "minutiae" of speech disorders found in the more interesting dysphasias (Brooks & Lincoln, 1984). Instead, a method of evaluating a broad area of interpersonal communication, involving quality of speech, content of language, organization of ideas (the ability to maintain a conversational theme), and, finally, the control of verbal expression is needed. This latter comment refers to the fact that many patients are garrulous, indulging in a form of "ritual prolixity" that can have a detrimental effect on the rehabilitation process as described by Wood and Eames (1981) and Wood (1986a).

The neuropsychological assessment of communication is, generally speaking, both comprehensive and meaningful to real-life behavior. Correspondence between test performance and ordinary conversation can still not be taken for granted, however, as was shown in the studies by Sarno, Sarno, and Levita (1971). They found that an increased score on a language test had limited implications for the patient's spontaneous communicative capacity in the real world. To ensure the relevance of test results we need, yet again, to amalgamate the structured assessment of language disorder with a systematic recording of communicative behavior. The former will help identify mechanisms that underly the communication difficulty, while the behavior analysis will show the strategies used by individuals to express themselves in real situations.

Some procedures have already been developed to try to bridge the gap between test scores and communication in real life. Sarno (1969) produced the Functional Communication Profile, while, more recently, Holland (1980) developed The Communication Activities in Daily Living Scale. The former permits ratings of "practical language behavior," while the latter presents the patient with language tasks in familiar and practical contexts. While this is a good idea, it calls for a degree of role-playing, which may inhibit many patients and cause anxiety to interfere with communication ability.

Communication should not be construed simply as verbal expression. Rehabilitation must often be provided for patients who, having lost the ability for speech, are forced to rely on some other means of communication. In such circumstances the neuropsychologist may need to determine the patient's ability to acquire a form of sign language. To do this it may be necessary to exclude the presence of ideomotor or ideational dyspraxia because either could prevent the organized movement permitting the expression of some sign. There also may be perceptual problems preventing the patient from understanding visual signs or gestures made by members of staff in an attempt at communication. Wood (1986a) has shown how such perceptual problems in the context of language disorders can lead to the development of aggressive behavior. The effect of memory on acquiring a sign language will also need to be assessed to ensure the most efficient learning and maintenance of motivation.

In rehabilitation, patients' social acceptability determines the quality of residential care they can receive far more than their functional state. With this in mind we need to consider the appropriateness of speech, its content rather than production. Some patients suffer from too much language output as opposed to not enough or unclear speech. Verbosity, prolixity, and garrulousness are frequent nouns used to describe the communication styles of patients with frontal brain lesions. Added to this is the inflexibility and concreteness of the patient with a frontal lesion (Bond, 1984), which means that not only is speech characterized by verbosity but also by monotonous repetition of stereotyped phrases. In and of themselves these phrases may be innocuous, and, when first heard, quite acceptable. If, however, the same conversational themes crop up each time one encounters the patient then social interaction with that individual can become a punishing event (for the listener), reducing the social acceptability of the patient. These communication styles need to be described in order to try and find ways of remedying the problem. Wood and Eames (1981) and Wood (1986a) describe two patients whose language content rather than production was the focus for rehabilitation.

Planning, Organizing, and Directing Behavior

Normal everyday life is characterized by a flexible adaptation of behavior in response to environmental demands. For most of us this flexibility is automatic; we only become aware of its importance when we are overloaded with responsibility or face a specific task that stretches our intellectual capability. Following brain injury, however, this adaptive attitude often fails. People find difficulty in organizing their thinking to deal with even routine problems of daily living. They cannot identify the priorities of a situation or the sequence of actions that will allow completion of an activity in the most economical time. These deficits can be broken down into problems of identification, integration, and regulation. These are characteristics of the "frontal lobe syndrome" and become manifest as disorders of planning, organizing, and directing behavior. This cluster of problems often appears in contrast to an individual's recorded level of intelligence and frequently underlies aggressive forms of behavior because of the frustration experienced by the individual at not being able to initiate ideas that are fundamental to independent human behavior.

Luria (1966) considered frontal lesions to provoke a disturbance in the programming of diverse activities. The final intended action is affected because of a lack of information provided during the elaboration of the action. As such, frontal damage deregulates the control of essential elements of a person's intentions, causing a disruption of complex forms of activity. The ability to constantly monitor one's actions in respect to some activity is also impaired. A similar conclusion was reached by Nauta (1971). He claimed that a "derangement of behavioral programming" occurred because the stability of goal-directed behavior was impaired. This meant that the individual could not maintain a continuous idea to underlie and influence decision making.

Some neuropsychological procedures, such as the Porteus Maze Test (Porteus, 1959, 1965), are designed to provide information on planning and foresight because the patient is required to choose alternative courses of action and to follow or reject such choices at strategic states during the action sequence. The Tinkertoy Test (Lezak, 1981; see Lezak, 1983, for a review) has also been designed to examine an individual's ability to initiate, plan, and execute complex decisions. She also recommends the Wisconsin Card-Sorting Test (Berg, 1948) because it requires a patient to repeatedly change a line of reasoning to solve a problem and may elicit difficulties of organization, directing, and planning. Clinical experience would suggest, however, that this task is often completed without too much difficulty by patients who are reported or observed to have planning or organizational problems.

Lezak (1983) provides a range of tests that measure self-regulatory behavior and help identify conceptual inflexibility and stimulus-bound behavior. Both of these characteristics can result in perseverative, stereotyped, and nonadaptive behavior, which can have a detrimental effect on the maintenance of personal independence. She admits, however, that there are "few formal tests" to measure planning, organizing, and goal-directed behavior. She suggests that it is the way a patient *approaches* the test that provides insights into these important conceptual abilities. Most formal tests are structured in such a way that the examiner determines how the patient approaches the task. Any alteration in this procedure is not encouraged because it might affect the test scores and test validity. The restricted number of responses available on most structured tests also limits the observation of unrealistic, irrational, or disorganized thinking. It is important, therefore, that some observation is made on how the patient approaches activities of daily living, such as personal care, money management, and preparing a meal. Lezak makes the important comment that it is not enough to simply question a patient on how such activities can be organized. Many patients with frontal lesions can describe what they are supposed to do, given a particular situation, yet are unable to exhibit such behavior in real situations. This is part of their inability to use good judgment and maintain a realistic perspective toward their behavior.

Drive and Motivation

Rehabilitation requires a great deal of effort and cooperation on the part of the patient. Consequently, motivation is a key factor in successful programs (Golden, 1978; Wood & Eames, 1981). Motivation is affected by a number of factors: how well the patient perceives the success of his efforts; the effects of medication such as phenytoin, phenobarbitone, or the phenothiazine group of drugs; the social rewards available; the nature of personality; and the desire to return to work (not a necessary ambition for many individuals).

An important part of any rehabilitation assessment is to find out what motivates the patients, how they are "turned on" to making a sustained effort. This can be achieved by interviewing the patient and his or her relatives to gain a broader perspective of the social influences that may prevail on behavior. Often the relatives expect too much too soon and their subsequent disappointment, when recovery does not match expectations, is transmitted to the patient, sometimes with disastrous results as far as the patients' attitudes are concerned. By identifying these family dynamics and incorporating them into the assessment of the patient, many potential problems of motivation can be avoided.

It is important to remember that the brain injury itself can exert a serious negative affect on motivation. An important component of motivation is arousal. This determines an individual's level of drive, which, in turn, determines the extent to which a person's ideas, needs, and ambitions can be put into action. Drive is more of a neurophysiological system than a neuropsychological system, but it is often left to the neuropsychologist to determine whether a patient can translate interest (a psychological construct) into effort (a physiological construct). Brain-damaged individuals will often express an interest in a particular activity or commodity and yet make no effort to satisfy that particular need, even when the opportunity is created for them to obtain such a goal (see Wood, 1986b). Drive is, therefore, essential to motivation, and motivation is central to rehabilitation. It would, therefore, seem important that a clear statement on a patient's level of motivation or capacity to maintain a certain level of drive and effort is obtained in order that the rehabilitation team may know how to establish their goals of treatment and expectations regarding achievement of those goals.

Drive plays an important part in maintaining effort. This is vital for obtaining a successful outcome in rehabilitation because many therapy activities need to be presented frequently, over a long period of time, in order to achieve successful results. Patients who suffer from short attention span, disorders of arousal, or a dyshedonic personality will need to be identified in order that adjustments can be made to the rehabilitation program that will accommodate these problems. Eames and Wood (1985) and Wood (1986b) describe how problems of drive and motivation, which are imposed by different forms of brain injury, affect behavior, sometimes to the extent that rehabilitation is made exceedingly difficult, if not impossible, to achieve (see Wood, 1986a).

To some extent motivation can be assessed by a patient's response to test situations. It is probable, however, that the factors that underlie motivation to neuropsychological testing are not the same, either in type or degree, as those determining behavior in rehabilitation tasks or to the demands of social independence. This means that observations of behavior must be made in different environmental settings and during different activities if a complete profile of a person's effort potential as well as effortful behavior is to be obtained.

Emotional Lability and Organically Mediated Behavior

As recovery from an insult to the brain progresses, behavior problems may emerge, either as (1) secondary psychological reactions to an increasing awareness of a residual handicap or (2) behavior problems that are a direct result of the brain injury itself, occurring as neurologically mediated disorders of mood (Wood, 1986a).

Behavior disorders of any kind have long been recognized as presenting a major impediment to rehabilitation planning. It is of some importance, therefore, that the nature of the behavior disorder is properly understood because treatment will vary depending on whether the undesirable behavior has been learned or has some kind of organic basis (Wood & Eames, 1981). The neuropsychologist should be able to discriminate between organic or psychogenic behavior disorders, and, if the behavior problem conforms to the latter type, then the neuropsychologist should advise the treatment team regarding behavior management. This may help avoid the often unfortunate intervention with major sedative drugs that sometimes exacerbate rather than relieve the situation. To make the differential diagnosis between a psychological reaction and an organically mediated reaction, careful observation will be necessary to determine whether the behavior has any pattern in terms of its frequency or whether it occurs in association with certain environmental events. Other indicators would be the circumstances under which the behavior occurs: If it occurs abruptly, being poorly directed or having an aimless, disorganized quality, then it is more likely to be organic. If, on the other hand, the behavior is purposeful, possessing a planned or systematic quality that leads to some form of gratification or reward, a psychological basis for the behavior is more likely. Wood (1986b) discusses the different types of behavior disorders that act as serious constraints on many forms of rehabilitation therapy. For a clearer description of the difference between such behaviors, the reader is referred to Lishman (1978), Bond (1984), Wood and Eames (1981), and Wood (1984a, b).

SUMMARY

Behavior is comprised of a number of cognitive functions. These include reasoning, judgment, planning, directing, computation, ordering, abstracting, and generalizing. Most people consider such abilities as the collective process of "thinking." Thinking may be further defined as "adaptive intelligence" (Lezak, 1983). Many forms of brain injury interfere with the process of thinking without interfering with specific intellectual skills. This suggests that thinking relies on an interaction and integration of many cognitive systems that form the substrate of intelligence. This brings the assessment of neurologically disordered behavior directly into the ambit of the clinical neuropsychologist, but, in order to describe behavior in ways that will be meaningful to other health care professionals, the approach to neuropsychological assessment will need to be changed. It will not be sufficient to assess cognitive ability in terms of specific skills or forms of impairment. An effort must be made to describe the product of these specific functions in terms of their combined action and their application in the process of thinking.

REFERENCES

Andrews, K., & Stewart, J. (1979). Stroke recovery: He can but does he? *Rheumatology and Rehabilitation, 18*, 43–48.

Baddeley, A. D. (1984). Memory theory and memory therapy. In B. A. Wilson and N. Moffat (Eds.), *Clinical measurement of memory problems*. London: Croom Helm.

Beaumont, J. G. (1983). *Introduction to neuropsychology*. Oxford, England: Blackwell Scientific.

Bennet-Levy, J., & Powell, G. E. (1980). The subjective memory questionnaire (SMQ): An investigation into the self-reporting of 'real life' memory skills. *British Journal of Social and Clinical Psychology, 19*, 177–183.

Benton, A. (1982). Spatial thinking in neurological patients. In M. Potegal (Ed.), *Spatial abilities: Development and physiological foundations*. New York: Academic Press.

Berg, E. A. (1948). A simple objective technique for measuring flexibility in thinking. *Journal of General Psychology, 38*, 15–22.

Boll, T. J. (1981). The Halstead-Reitan Neuropsychological Battery. In S. B. Filskov and T. J. Boll (Eds.), *Handbook of clinical neuropsychology*. New York: Wiley.

Bolles, R. C. (1979). *Learning theory* (2nd ed.). New York: Holt, Rinehart, and Winston.

Bond, M. (1984). The psychiatry of closed head injury. In D. N. Brooks (Ed.), *Closed head injury: Psychological, social and family consequences*. Oxford, England: Oxford University Press.

Bond, M. R., & Brooks, D. N. (1976). Understanding the process of recovery as a basis for the investigation of the brain injured. *Scandinavian Journal of Rehabilitation, 8*, 127–133.

Brooks, D. N. (1979). Psychological deficits after severe blunt head injury: Their significance and rehabilitation. In D. J. Osborne, M. M. Gruneberg, & J. R. Eiser (Eds.), *Research in psychology and medicine, Vol. 2*. London: Academic Press.

Brooks, D. N., & Lincoln, N. B. (1984). Assessment for rehabilitation. In B. A. Wilson and N. Moffat (Eds.), *Clinical management of memory problems*. London: Croom Helm.

Chadwick, O. (1976). Conference notes of a meeting of the joint British-Dutch head injury workshop. Oxford, England (unpublished observations).

Christensen, A. L. (1975). *Luria's neuropsychological investigation.* New York: Spectrum.

Christmas, E. M., Humphrey, M. E., Richardson, A. E., & Smith, E. M. (1974). The response of brain-damaged patients to a rehabilitation regime. *Rheumatology and Rehabilitation, 13,* 92–97.

Conkey, R. C. (1938). Psychological changes associated with head injuries. *Archives of Psychology, 232,* 1–62.

Crockett, D., Clark, C., & Klonoff, H. (1981). Introduction—An overview of neuropsychology. In S. B. Filskov and T. J. Boll (Eds.), *Handbook of clinical psychology.* New York: Wiley.

Davey, G. (1981). *Animal learning and conditioning.* London: Macmillan.

Dencker, S. J., & Lofving, B. (1958). A psychometric study of identical twins discordant for closed head injury. *Acta Psychiatrica Neurologica Scandinavica, 333,* Suppl. 122.

Diller, L., & Gordon, W. A. (1981). Criterion for cognitive deficits in brain injured adults. *Journal of Consulting and Clinical Psychology, 49,* 822–834.

Eagle, R. S. (1979). *Cognition and "effectance" in severely involved quadriplegic children.* Paper presented at the American Psychological Association 87th Annual Convention, New York.

Eames, P. G., & Wood, R. L1. (1985). Consciousness in the brain damaged adult. In M. Stevens (Ed.), *Clinical aspects of consciousness.* Oxford, England: Oxford University Press.

Fiskov, S. B., & Boll, T. J. (1981). *Handbook of clinical neuropsychology.* New York: Wiley.

Fogelman, C. J. (1975). *The Adaptive Behavior Scale.* American Association of Mental Deficiency.

Golden, C. J. (1981). A standardized version of Luria's neuropsychological tests: A quantitative and qualitative approach to neuropsychological evaluation. In S. B. Filskov and T. J. Boll (Eds.), *Handbook of clinical neurology.* New York: Wiley.

Golden, C. J. (Ed.). (1978). Issues in neuropsychological assessment. In *Diagnosis and rehabilitation in clinical neuropsychology.* Springfield, IL: Charles C. Thomas.

Goldstein, G. (1983). Methodological and theoretical issues in neuropsychological assessment. In R. Edelstein and E. C. Coutive (Eds.), *Behavioral assessment and treatment of the traumatically brain damaged.* New York: Plenum.

Gronwall, D., & Sampson, H. (1974). *Psychological effects of concussion.* Auckland, New Zealand: Auckland University Press.

Gunzberg, H. C. (1974). *Progress Assessment Chart of Social Development.* Birmingham, England: SEFA Publications.

Hebb, D. O. (1955). Drives and the C.N.S. (conceptual nervous system). *Psychological Review, 62,* 243–254.

Heilman, K. M., & Valenstein, E. (1984). *Clinical neuropsychology.* New York: Oxford University Press.

Hersen, M., & Barlow, D. H. (1978). *Single-case experimental designs: Strategy for studying behaviour change.* Elmont, NY: Pergamon.

Holland, A. L. (1980). *Communicative abilities in daily living: A test of functional communication for aphasic adults.* Baltimore, MD: University Park Press.

Kolb, B., & Wishaw, I. Q. (1980). *Fundamentals of neuropsychology.* San Francisco: W. H. Freeman.

Levin, H. S., Benton, A. L., & Grossman, R. G. (1982). *Neurobehavioral consequences of closed head injury.* New York: Oxford University Press.

Lezak, M. D. (1983). *Neuropsychological assessment.* New York: Oxford University Press.

Lishman, W. A. (1978). *Organic psychiatry.* Oxford, England: Blackwell.

Luria, A. R. (1966). *Higher cortical functions in man.* New York: Basic Books.

Malec, J. (1983). Training the brain-injured client in behavioral self-management skills. In R. Edelstein and E. C. Coutive (Eds.), *Behavioral assessment and treatment of the traumatically brain damaged.* New York: Plenum.

Nauta, W. J. H. (1971). The problem of the frontal lobe. *Journal of Psychiatric Research, 8,* 167–187.

Newcombe, F. (1981). The psychological consequences of closed head injury: Assessment and rehabilitation. *International Journal of Rehabilitation Medicine, 3,* 50–66.

Newcombe, F., & Artioli i Fortuny, L. A. (1979). Problems and perspectives in the evaluation of psychological deficits after cerebral lesions. *International Journal of Rehabilitation Medicine, 1,* 182–192.

Newcombe, F., & Ratcliff, G. (1979). Long-term psychological consequences of cerebral lesions. In M. S. Gazzaniga (Ed.), *Handbook of behavioral neurobiology.* New York: Plenum.

Plum, F., & Posner, J. B. (1982). *Diagnosis of stupor and coma.* Philadelphia: Davis.

Porteus, S. D. (1959). *The Maze Test and clinical psychology.* Palo Alto, CA: Pacific Books.

Porteus, S. D. (1965). *Porteus Maze Test: Fifty-years' application.* Palo Alto, CA: Pacific Books.

Powell, G. E. (1981). *Brain function therapy.* London: Gower.

Ruesch, J. (1944). Intellectual impairment in head injuries. *American Journal of Psychiatry, 100,* 480–496.

Sarno, M. T. (1969). *The Functional Communication Profile: Manual of Directions.* New York: New York University Medical Center.

Sarno, J. E., Sarno, M. T., & Levita, E. (1971). Evaluating language improvement after completed stroke. *Archives of Physical Medicine and Rehabilitation, 52,* 73–78.

Sunderland, A., Harris, J. E., & Baddeley, A. D. (1983). Do laboratory tests predict everyday memory? A neuropsychological study. *Journal of Verbal Learning and Verbal Behavior, 22,* 341–357.

Van Zomeren, A. H., Brouwer, W. H., & Deelman, B. G. (1984). Attentional deficits: The riddles of selectivity, speed, and alertness. In D. N. Brooks (Ed.), *Closed head injury: Psychological, social, and family consequences.* Oxford, England: Oxford University Press.

Walsh, K. W. (1985). *Understanding brain damage.* London: Churchill Livingstone.

Wood, R. Ll. (1980). The relationship of brain damage, measured by computerized axial tomography, to quantitative intellectual impairment. In D. J. Osborne (Ed.), *Research in Psychology and Medicine* (Vol. 1). London: Academic Press.

Wood, R. Ll. (1984a). Behaviour disorders following severe brain injury: Their presentation and psychological management. In D. N. Brooks (Ed.), *Closed head injury: Psychological, social, and family consequences.* Oxford, England: Oxford University Press.

Wood, R. Ll. (1984b). The management of attention disorders following brain injury. In B. A. Wilson and N. Moffat (Eds.), *Clinical management of memory problems.* London: Croom Helm.

Wood, R. Ll. (1986a). A neuro-behavioural approach in the rehabilitation of sever
    brain injury. In A. Mazzucchi (Ed.), *Neuropsychological rehabilitation.* Milar
    Italy: I. L. Mulino.
Wood, R. Ll. (1986b). Clinical constraints affecting human conditioning. In
    G. Davey (Ed.), *Human conditioning.* New York: Wiley.
Wood. R. Ll., & Eames, P. G. (1981). Behaviour modification in the rehabilitatior
    of brain injury. In G. Davey (Ed.), *Applications of conditioning theory.* New
    York: Methuen.

SECTION II
Advances in Rehabilitation Technology

Susan Middaugh
and
Michael A. Alexander
Section Editors

Introduction

Susan Middaugh
Michael A. Alexander

Technology is advancing all around us, in our homes, in our schools, in our hospitals, and at our place of work. As a result, we are becoming comfortable with equipment that computes, monitors, and automates. This provides a very receptive climate for this section on advances in rehabilitation technology. Perhaps for this reason, the technology presented in Chapters 4, 5, and 6 seems interesting and enticing rather than daunting. Perhaps also for this reason, the authors of these chapters clearly expect the technology they describe to be widely employed in clinical settings in the near future. This technology is accessible, and the clinical applications can be carried out right now, in large part, by the interested clinician in a rehabilitation setting with equipment that is available at reasonable cost. It is evident in these three chapters that new technological developments are being incorporated into clinical practice with increasing rapidity. This provides a stimulating clinical and research climate as new treatment options, in turn, raise new questions.

Chapter 4, "The Child and Technology," by Denise J. Frankoff and Michael A. Alexander, considers the impact of computer technology on pediatric rehabilitation. By far the most important advances made in pediatric rehabilitation are those related to computer applications to clinical practice. This chapter is designed to provide a rationale for exposing children to technology at an early age; to review the levels of technology available to children; and to describe the procurement, training, and follow-up process associated with computer use.

Chapter 5, "Functional Electrical Stimulation and the Rehabilitation of the Spinal Cord-Injured Patient," by Jerrold S. Petrofsky, combines research in exercise physiology, orthotics, and computers to bring an old idea, functional electrical stimulation, up to date and also launch it effectively into the future. Since the early days of electricity, electrical stimulation has been used for rehabilitation, and the concepts of electrical exercise and electrical bracing of paralyzed muscles have long been applied. However, it has taken a combination of advances in both technology and physiology to produce the treatment procedures presented in Chapter 5. Once a treatment procedure becomes technologically possible, however, it also must be proven both clinically beneficial and economically feasible in order to be widely accepted. Dr. Petrofsky addresses these very practical issues of cost versus benefit, not only in terms of dollars and cents but also in terms of the physical and mental status of the patient. This has required a great deal of interesting research on exercise benefits and exercise tolerance in spinal cord injured individuals. This body of work has led to the development of treatment procedures that are certainly the most "high tech" in this section but which are, at least in part, within the reach of the interested clinician.

Chapter 6, "Advances in Electromyographic Monitoring and Biofeedback in Treatment of Chronic Cervical and Low Back Pain," by Susan J. Middaugh and William G. Kee, demonstrates how EMG monitoring for muscle evaluation can be combined with site-specific EMG biofeedback procedures and therapeutic exercise principles for treatment of patients with chronic cervical and low back pain. The authors emphasize that advances in technology must be accompanied by advances in treatment technique and treatment rationale in order to be clinically appropriate. EMG biofeedback is highly effective in teaching muscle responses, but there is often a problem with determining what muscle responses need to be taught in order to reach a desired clinical goal. Chapter 6 presents EMG evaluation procedures for accurately assessing muscles in the area of pain in the individual patient and illustrates how such evaluation leads to more appropriate biofeedback training of muscles in the context of movement and daily activities. The chapter also points out the inadequacy of the pain/spasm/pain cycle as an explanatory concept and indicates other factors that appear to be more contributory in the development of chronic pain.

Each of the chapters in this section makes a strong statement that developments in technology have to be accompanied by concurrent developments in treatment procedure and treatment rationale. All three chapters illustrate how new technology leads to new treatment options that force rethinking of precisely what it is we want to do. New technology also has a way of sending us back to basics, which are often our guiding psychological or physiological explanatory concepts, in order to develop the scientific data base that is essential for effective application. All three chapters also point out the necessity, in today's climate of cost consciousness and accountability, of establishing the scientific basis and the clinical efficacy of new treatment procedures, particularly those requiring new instrumentation.

4

The Child and Technology

Denise J. Frankoff
Michael A. Alexander

Computers are constantly used to accomplish daily activities with greater effectiveness and efficiency. They have increased the autonomy of handicapped individuals by performing tasks for them that others have had to do in the past. According to Vanderheiden (1982), personal computers can play a "dual role" for disabled individuals. They can allow the disabled individual to perform functions and compete at the same level as the non-disabled individual. Even more importantly, they can also be used to help remediate sensory, physical, and cognitive deficits.

In recent years information on computer technology and the disabled has appeared in the lay and professional literature with increasing frequency. In newspapers one can frequently read about the influence of technology on the educational and vocational pursuits of the disabled. There remains, however, a discrepancy between the extent to which computers are being used and computer proficiency. Two major factors are responsible for this phenomenon. First, the cost of computer technology has been prohibitive to the general public. Second, the public has felt intimidated by the proliferation of jargon by the technical community. In the 1960s and 1970s computer literacy became a buzzword. However, information and training on microcomputer applications were lacking. Early computers had limited memory and required the user to have some familiarity with computer languages (e.g., "Basic" or "Pascal") and to be able to work with disk operating systems to accomplish even the simplest tasks.

Thomas (1984) contends that educators should move beyond computer literacy to "computer proficiency." Thomas claims computer proficiency implies (1) a basic knowledge of the educational functions a computer can and cannot accomplish, (2) appreciation of the applications of the do's and don'ts of microcomputer–human interaction, (3) eradication of the fear of computers, and (4) an ability to use computerized instruction effectively by analyzing the educational objectives and prerequisite cognitive skills of educational activities.

The purpose of this chapter is to provide a rationale for exposing young children to technology at an early age; review the levels of technology available: toys, communication aids, and personal computers; describe the assessment process; and describe the procurement, training, and follow-up process.

THE CHILD AND TECHNOLOGY: WHY BOTHER?

The Office of Technical Assessment (1983) estimated there are 750,000 to 1.5 million severely disabled nonspeaking children and adults in this country. Each of these persons will experience barriers to social, educational, vocational, and recreational achievement and personal fulfillment. Microcomputer applications can help overcome these barriers.

Bloom (1964) postulated that approximately 50% of intellectual growth is accomplished between birth and the age of 4 years. Cognitive development during these early years is facilitated by environmental interaction. Through movement and change children acquire knowledge of their environment. These experiences provide the framework for perceptual and symbolic information processing. Vocalizations of young infants function to initiate and sustain interaction, satisfy needs, exert control, and establish and maintain contact. Research indicates that early single-word utterances refer to action-based relations (Bloom & Lahey, 1978; McCormick & Schiefelbusch, 1984). For example, early single-word utterances such as "open," "all gone," and "hot" often refer to stimuli that are being acted on or have changed in some designated way.

It is from the knowledge gained through interaction that the information functions of language develop (Muma, 1978). These functions of language, listed by Chapman and Miller (1980), include (1) to give information; (2) to get information; (3) to describe; (4) to get the listener to act, believe, and feel; (5) to express intention, belief, and feeling; (6) to indicate readiness for further communication; (7) to solve problems; and (8) to entertain. Motor disabilities can adversely affect all of these language functions.

Technology can enable the young, multiply handicapped child to interact with his environment in a so-called "normal" manner. With computers, young, handicapped children can learn to identify and categorize sensory input, learn a language system, and develop interpersonal skills. Papert (1980), designer of the programming language "Logo," proposes that computer technology can significantly influence the development of intellectual abilities. He emphasizes that with new materials children can learn

ew skills. He states that "knowledge accessible through formal processes
an now be approached concretely" (p. 21). He labels this the "Power
'rinciple."

THE CHILD AND TECHNOLOGY: WHEN TO START

'he concept of a critical period of learning and positive effects of early
atervention have been suggested by numerous investigators (Behrmann,
984; Bloom & Lahey, 1978; Hagen, 1984; Scarr-Salapatek & Williams,
973; Stevens, 1982). Research indicates that early intervention programs
ave positive effects on psychosocial development of children.

Recently Piaget's model of cognitive development has been questioned
·y several researchers (Behrmann, 1984). Piaget's theory proposes that
adividuals pass through specific developmental stages. During these stages
xperiences are systematically processed, leading to control over one's envi-
onment and problem-solving capabilities. Now it is hypothesized that
afants may be capable of innately perceiving, classifying, and representing
timuli at a younger age than previously thought. Recent research with
nfants using microcomputers has yielded significant gains in functional
tatus. Brinker and Lewis (1982) taught infants as young as 3 months of age
witch activation. These infants learned to activate switches that turned on
·attery-powered toys and tape recordings of music. Behrmann and Lahm
1984) are teaching handicapped infants under 30 months of age to activate
 switch. Infants in their study as young as 11 months of age are using
aicrocomputers for communicative and environmental control purposes.
Thus, through technology children can learn how to affect control over
heir environment at a developmental stage where it was not expected.

LEVELS OF TECHNOLOGY

Toys

One of the first ways children learn to control their environment is through
oys. Often the physically and cognitively impaired child cannot spontane-
·usly explore and manipulate objects in meaningful ways. These children
requently experience failure and fear when attempting to play with toys.
Thus these children frequently become passive observers rather than active
earners.

Social, educational, and therapeutic goals can be achieved using adapted
oys. Jeffrey (1981) has listed skills that can be developed through the use of
oys. These include:

1. Visual skills such as acuity, tracking, and stimulation.
2. Auditory skills involving awareness and discrimination.
3. Tactile skills.
4. Communication skills facilitating interaction and vocal development
5. Gross motor skills.
6. Fine motor skills such as eye–hand coordination and pincer grasp.
7. Perceptual skills.
8. Cognitive skills such as concept development.
9. Social and emotional skills including solitary play, parallel play, group play, imitative play, and imaginary play.
10. Life skills such as self-help.

Adapted toys can be the handicapped child's first introduction to technol ogy. Experiences achieved through play with these toys can prepare the child to understand more sophisticated technology such as an electronic communication device and an electric wheelchair.

Burkhart (1980) reported that a child she worked with generally held hi head up for only 20 seconds but consistently held it up for 30 to 40 second when activating a tape recorder. In addition, educators have noted a reduc tion in self-stimulatory behaviors when children successfully explore toys (Blakely, 1985; Burkhart, 1980).

For some children only simple adaptations to commercially available toys are needed. For children who have difficulty grasping and/or holding toys handles, enlarged knobs, and fabric snaps could be used. Faith Carlson, in her book *Prattle and Play* (1982), outlines the materials needed and steps involved in making these adaptations. In addition, Carlson describes "rec- ipes" for several other types of self-made toys for children with motor- control problems. These include trays and boards with wells and divisions symbol blocks, stuffed symbol toys, clothing with symbols affixed to it and play boards.

The severely handicapped child may not achieve success with these simple adaptations. However, these children can learn to control the numer- ous commercially available battery-operated toys with special switches and adaptors. Some switches and adaptors can be made with minimal effort. Burkhart (1980), Shein and Mandel (1982), and Coker (1984) provide step-by-step instructions for making homemade switches and adaptors. For example, Burkhart (1980) describes a pull switch that can be operated by a single pull. Materials include a potato chip can, jump rope, tennis ball, metal jar lid, popsicle stick, wire, pliers, solder, sandpaper, ear-formed plug, and masking tape. Switches and adaptors can be purchased from several compa- nies (the Prentke-Romich Company, Zygo Industries, Inc., and Toys for Special Children, Steven Kanor, Ph.D.). Some commercially available adapted toys are shown in Figures 4.1 and 4.2.

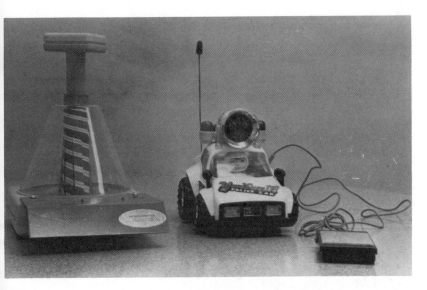

FIGURE 4.1 Adapted toys (photographed with permission from Steven Kanor, Ph.D., 101 Lefurgy Avenue, Hastings-on-Hudson, NY 10706).

Toys can be borrowed from Toy Lending Libraries. Several of these libraries exist within the United States, Canada, and Europe. Many toy libraries have a wide range of commercial toys and a large inventory of switches. For example, the Adriel and Evelyn Harris Toy Library for the Disabled (Canadian Association of Toy Libraries, 1981) serves the New York, New Jersey, and Connecticut areas. It is open to all organizations serving handicapped individuals, as well as their parents. It operates a Mobile Toy Unit using a minibus to travel to individual homes, clinics, schools, hospitals, and other organizations. Thus, given the proper equipment, handicapped children can learn to actively and successfully explore their environment.

COMMUNICATION AIDS

In 1980 the Executive Board of the American Speech-Language-Hearing Association established The Ad Hoc Committee on the Communicative Processes for Non-speaking Persons to address issues related to the diagnosis and treatment of nonspeaking individuals. From this, a position statement was formulated. In this chapter terminology referring to augmentative communication will be used as defined by this position paper.

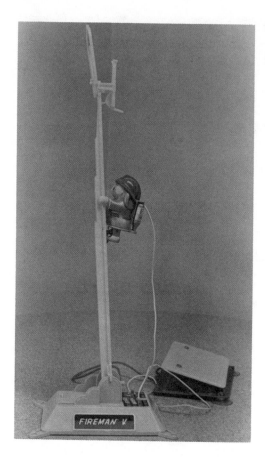

FIGURE 4.2 Adapted toy with plate switch (photographed with permission from Steven Kanor Ph.D.).

The label "nonspeaking" refers to and defines a group of persons for whom speech is temporarily or permanently inadequate to meet all of his or her communication needs and whose inability to speak is not primarily a result of hearing impairment (Ad Hoc Committee, 1980, p. 268). The term *augmentative communication* refers to a system that functions to supplement whatever vocal skills are possessed by the individual.

Several authors have commented on the prerequisites to successful use of an augmentative communication system. (Capozzi & Mineo, 1984; Chapman & Miller, 1980; The Pennsylvania Task Force on Augmentative Communication, 1985). These prerequisites include (1) evidence of cognitive development at Sensory Motor Stage V or beyond, characterized by the recognition of causality and the development of intentional communication; (2) disparity among cognitive abilities, communication abilities, and interactive needs; (3) adequate physical attending skills and auditory and visual tracking and attending skills; and (4) supportive family and/or caretaker(s) actively involved in the training process. Children who do not understand causality and cannot adequately attend to stimuli need a training program focusing on the development of these cognitive/linguistic prerequisites.

TYPES OF AUGMENTATIVE COMMUNICATION SYSTEMS

There are two major types of augmentative communication systems: (1) nonaided communication systems—systems that do not require physical aids such as manual or gestural communication codes, and (2) aided communication systems—techniques involving the use of a physical object or device. An augmentative communication system can provide a nonspeaking individual with a means of interaction. Recent research indicates that the teaching of signs may facilitate language development (Bricker, 1972; Karlan et al., 1982; Poulton & Algozzine, 1980). To effectively use these systems, the individual must have relatively good fine motor control and participants must be within the same visual field and, for any speed, have the use of both arms. Some manual communication systems such as American Sign Language include a set of arbitrary signs that are not understood by the general population. In contrast, Signed English and Ameri-Ind, the latter being an intertribal communication system, involve the use of many symbols that are frequently identifiable by normal adults.

The selection of content is based on a needs assessment, the sequence of language acquisition, and the physical and cognitive capabilities of the individual. These issues will be further discussed in the section on system selection and training.

Aided communication systems utilize symbols or "semantic transfer systems" (Capozzi & Mineo, 1984) through which meaning is communicated. According to Silverman (1980), a symbol is a sensory image that represents something based on association or convention. Silverman states that "the level of abstraction of a picture is a function of the amount of detail present in the object or event depicted, that is included in the picture. The more detail omitted, the higher the level of abstraction" (p. 9). Shane and Blau (1981) suggest three levels of symbolic complexity. Pictographic symbols are concrete pictures directly representing an idea. These may include pictures and photographs. Ideographic symbols are more complex as the symbol does not directly represent its referent. Picsyms© (Carlson, 1985), Blissymbols© (Silverman, 1980), and Minsymbols© (Baker, 1982) are examples of ideographic symbols (see Figures 4.3 and 4.4). The most abstract type of symbol is arbitrary, meaning the relationship between the

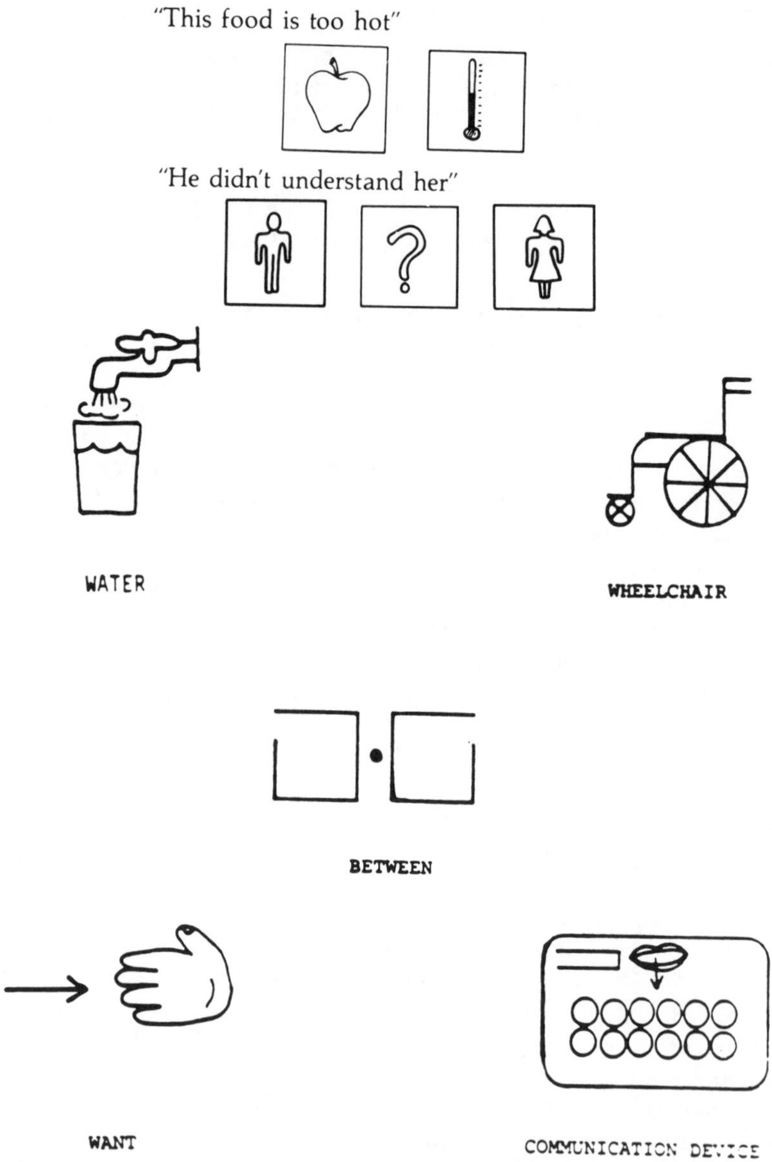

"This food is too hot"

"He didn't understand her"

WATER   WHEELCHAIR

BETWEEN

WANT   COMMUNICATION DEVICE

FIGURE 4.3 *Top*: Minsymbols (photographed with permission from Prentke-Romich Co.) *Bottom*: Picsyms (photographed with permission, *PICSYMS Categorical Dictionary*, written and illustrated by Faith Carlson, copyright 1985, Baggeboda Press, 1128 Rhode Island St., Lawrence, KS 66045).

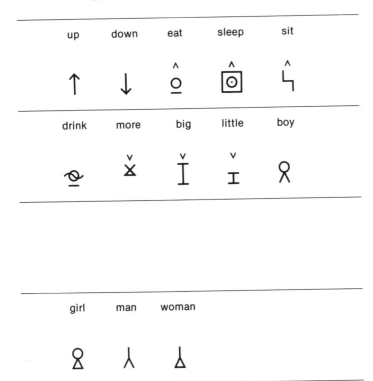

FIGURE 4.4 Typeset Blissymbols (photographed with permission from Blissymbolics Communications Institute).

symbol and referent is not identifiable. These include the written word, Braille, and Morse Code.

The selection of a symbol system is based on the child's needs, cognitive abilities, and linguistic capabilities. Other factors related to symbol selection include size, spacing, boldness to the stimuli, and physical limitations of use. Symbols should be placed such that selecting is made as rapidly as possible, with a minimal degree of involuntary movement and increase in tension.

The type of symbols selected will also affect the quantity of information conveyed and, therefore, the speed. Speed is of the essence when communicating. The normal response time in conversation is less than 3 second (Baker, 1982). As response time increases, anxiety increases (for bot listener and speaker) and interest level (particularly by the listener) deterio rates. Baker (1983) reported that it may take a neurologically impaire person 5 seconds to make a single character selection, thus requiring man minutes to complete a message. Fishman, Timler, and Yoder (1985) re ported that most speakers produce one utterance every time they speak. I contrast, a communication board user as well as the receiver generate severa responses each because of the need for feedback, breakdowns in interaction and breakdown repairs.

Baker (1982) has researched this communication problem extensively. H developed the concept of Minimal Effort Speech or "Minspeak." The Minspeak symbol system is a semantic compaction approach based on the logical coding of concepts and symbols. Images or icons are used to repre sent objects or concepts. Users can design their own icons and icon mean ings. The icons can represent different things depending on how they are used in a sequence. For example, when used together the house and dolla bill icons can be the code for bank. When the icons house and diploma are used together they can refer to school. With Minspeak recognition rathe than recall memory is used. This permits quick and efficient informatio storage and retrieval. When coupled with an electronic memory and speec unit or printer Minspeak allows for rapid and detailed communication.

ACCESSING THE INFORMATION

Information on augmentative communication systems can be accessed in two major ways: (1) direct selection and (2) scanning. According to Shane and Blau (1981), direct selection can be achieved using (1) an extremity; (2) an extremity plus an aid, such as a hand-held pointer; (3) the eyes; (4) a rod; and (5) a light beam. Direct selection is the most rapid means of selection. It is chosen if the user has the motoric capabilities (see Figure 4.5). In contrast, scanning is defined by Vanderheiden and Harris-Vanderheiden (quoted in Vanderheiden & Grilley, 1984) as "any method whereby the selections are offered to the user by a person or display and the user selects the message components by responding to a person or display" (p. 26). This requires an ability to sequence events and a higher cognitive level.

Harris and Vanderheiden (quoted in Vanderheiden & Grilley, 1984) have documented two basic types of scanning: *Linear scanning*—items are pre sented one at a time until entry is selected; and *group item scanning*—an entire group or row is scanned, a group or row is selected and the items are then scanned individually until a selection is made. Grouping the most

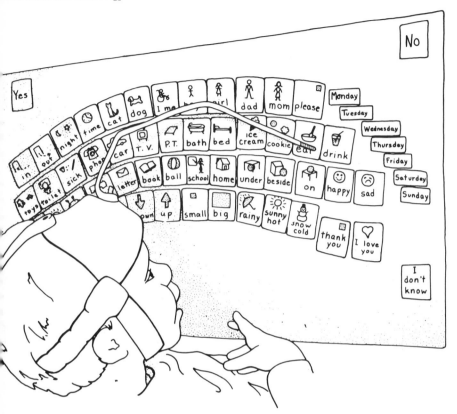

FIGURE 4.5 Direct selection using a head pointer [reprinted with permission from Vanderheiden and Grilley (1984)].

frequently used characters in the top-left quadrant further speeds the process. Scanning is an effective means of access for physically disabled individuals.

Silverman (1980) described a directed scanning method whereby items can be scanned in any direction depending on the shortest distance. This is one of the most rapid scanning approaches. Vanderheiden and Grilley (1984) described another accessing technique called "encoding." This technique is described as "any technique or aid in which the desired choice is indicated by a pattern or code of input signals, where the pattern or code must be memorized or referred to on a chart" (p. 22). A number-, letter-, or color-coding system could be used. The individual would then select the symbol he wanted such as a picture, word, phrase, or letter by indicating the code (see Figure 4.6). Some educators consider encoding to be a cognitive

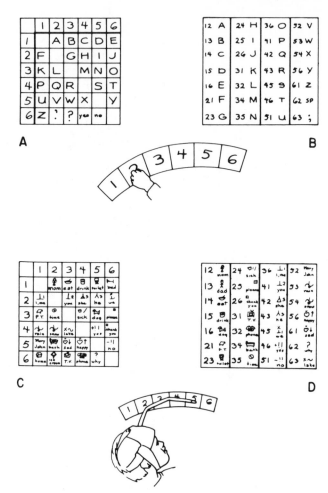

FIGURE 4.6 Encoding strategies [reprinted with permission from Vanderheiden and Grilley (1984)].

strategy as it involves a predetermined code system (Capozzi & Mineo, 1984; Shane & Blau, 1981). Thus it may not be appropriate for a cognitively impaired individual or younger child.

CONTROL INTERFACES

Should the scanning method be chosen, a switch, or interface, is needed. The switch activates the system. When selecting a switch a thorough assessment of the individual's physical abilities is necessary. Switch activation should be rapid and involve minimal effort so as to minimize tone overflow. Capozzi and Mineo (1984) suggested evaluating several switches at more than just one anatomic site. Vanderheiden (1979) proposed assessing range of motion, speed, accuracy of various body parts in various positions, and postures. Ongoing and repeated assessments of the child's physical abilities and task performance are necessary to ensure proper interface selection as the child ages.

There are three major types of control interfaces. *Physical movement switches* are those that require the user to move a part of his or her body. Examples include joysticks, rocking levers, tread switches, and leaf and wobble switches. *Pneumatic switches* use blowing or sucking to activate a relay. *Electromyographic switches* involve the use of surface electrodes to detect the electrical signals from activated muscles. The generated signal is used to close a switch relay. Again, the type of interface selected will depend on the user's physical capabilities. Physical movement switches would be selected if the user was able to move some part of his body such as the head, foot, or hand. Pneumatic switches are frequently used by spinal cord-injured patients where oral motor control is spared. An electromyographic switch is chosen when the person has control over a muscle that does not generate usable movement and where tone overflow is not a problem. Interfaces vary in the type of feedback they provide, such as auditory and visual. This, too, should be considered when selecting switches. In a sensory-impaired person an audible click as the switch closes represents additional feedback.

A wide variety of pointing devices and control interfaces are commercially available (see Figure 4.7). Also, standard interfaces can be modified to accommodate the physically handicapped individual. Information on rental and purchase can be obtained by contacting manufacturers for current catalogs and policies. (See the manufacturers' address list at the conclusion of this chapter for details.)

ELECTRONIC COMMUNICATION DEVICES

Electronic communication aids can be accessed by direct selection or scanning methods. They offer modes of output such as visual, auditory, tactile, or vocal. More than one mode of output may be available with any one system. Electronic communication aids include simple scanning aids, adapted typewriters, portable electronic aids, and advanced communication and control aids (Vanderheiden, 1979). In general, these systems are less portable than are the nonelectronic types. In cost they range from under $200 to in excess of $6,000. Many of these devices are commercially available. It is also possible to modify and customize standard equipment.

A

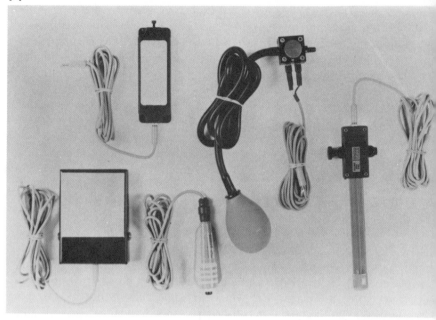

B

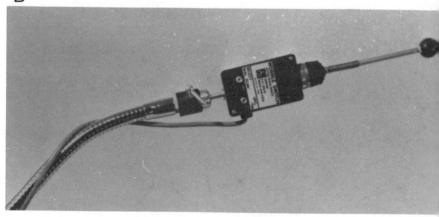

FIGURE 4.7. A: Zygo switches (*l-r*): leaf switch, pneumatic switch with squeeze ball, thumb switch, touch switch, tread switch (photograph courtesy of Zygo Industries, Inc.). B: Wobble switch (photograph courtesy of Prentke-Romich Co.). C: Tongue switch (photograph courtesy of Prentke-Romich Co.). D: Arm slot switch (photograph courtesy of Prentke-Romich Co.). E: Joystick (photograph courtesy of Prentke-Romich Co.).

C

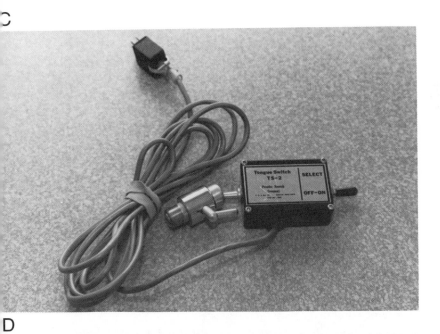

D

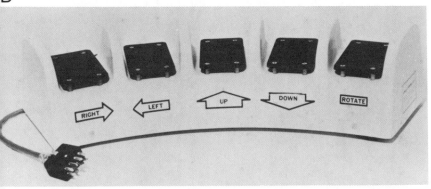

E

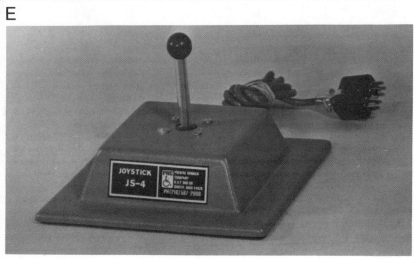

Montgomery (1980) described four modes of output an electronic communication aid may offer. Each has its advantages and disadvantages. These modes include (1) visual, (2) printed, (3) video, and (4) vocal. Another mode is tactile output in the form of raised dots of the Braille system. As stated above, some systems have more than one output mode, offering greater flexibility.

Visual output involves displays that are easily read. Interchangeable overlays may be used, providing access to a wide range of vocabulary. With printed output, a permanent hard copy is available, allowing long-distance correspondence. Symbols are conventional and can include morphological markers and punctuation. Thus, printed output systems can be used in academic settings. Video systems have display flexibility and editing capabilities. They are less portable, requiring hardware, software, and a power source. Vocal output devices provide instantaneous communication using prerecorded or synthesized speech. They are conducive to several forms of interaction, such as telephone conversation and group interactions. A wide range of vocabulary may be accessed.

The Zygo Model 16 (Zygo Industries, Inc.) (see Figure 4.8) is an

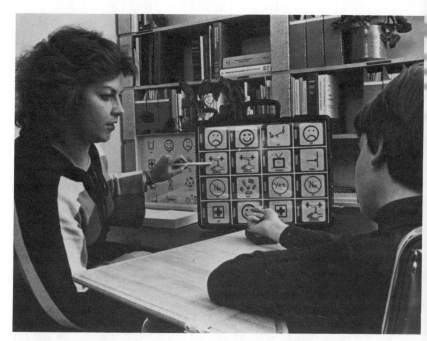

FIGURE 4.8 Zygo Model 16c Communication System (photograph courtesy of Zygo Industries, Inc.).

example of a simple scanning device. The user either directly points to or accesses the information using a switch. When the scanning mode is utilized lights are illuminated in groups or individually. The user activates a switch to make a selection. The Sharp Memowriter (no longer available) and Canon Communicator (Canon U.S.A.) (see Figure 4.9) are examples of keyboard instruments that produce a hard copy.

Typewriters can be adapted by using expanded keyboards and key guards. The P.M.V. system (P.M.V. Systems), Light Writer (Toby Churchill LTD), and the Expanded Keyboard Memowriter (Prentke-Romich Co.) are examples of this type of device.

Numerous electronic portable communication systems and control aids are commercially available. The Express III (Prentke-Romich Co.) is a microprocessor-based communication aid. Printed and vocal output modes are available. The Express III offers programmable vocabulary. It may be operated by direct selection and all scanning methods. Other options for the Express III include a remote display, video display, and a keyboard interface, allowing the user access to standard computers.

The ACS Speech Pac/Epson (Adaptive Communication Systems, Inc.) is another communication and control aid (see Figure 4.10). It is accessed by direct selection via either its keyboard or an ACS Expanded Membrane Board. The ACS Speech Pac/Epson has vocal output, LCD display, and printed output. Information is stored and retrieved by logical letter coding known as the "LoLec" program. The user determines the code based on association. For example, the sentence "I would like a cup of coffee" could

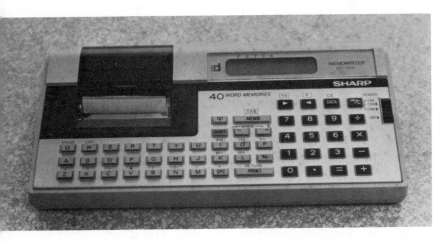

FIGURE 4.9 Sharp Memo Writer (photographed with permission from Zygo Industries, Inc.).

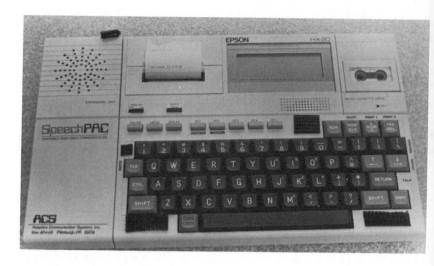

FIGURE 4.10 Epson Speech Pac (photographed with permission from Adaptive Communication Systems).

be assigned the code CC. The Epson interfaces with the Apple computer. The telephone modem permits hook-up to other computers via the telephone. The Control Pac permits control of electrical devices from the keyboard. The ACS Eval Pac is an evaluation, training, and communication device that can be accessed by direct selection or scanning. It too has vocal output. Custom programs can be developed and stored in memory.

The Touch Talker and Light Talker (Prentke-Romich Co.) are portable communication aids with an LCD display and vocal output (see Figure 4.11). They provide auditory and tactile feedback. A programmable vocabulary is available. Information can be programmed according to the Minspeak coding system, which claimed to be the most rapid and flexible coding strategy. The Touch Talker is accessed via direct selection. The Light Talker is accessed via direct selection using the Prentke-Romich Optical Headpointer or via scanning using control interfaces.

Another approach to augmentative communication is the selection of software that can enable a general purpose computer to act as a communication device. The most advanced system of this type is the Words Plus Living Center (Word +, Inc.). It allows communication by selecting from a stored vocabulary and phrase list that can be customized and easily adapted. It is available for the IBM PC and PC, Jr., PC-compatible computers, and the Apple II and IIC computers. It provides vocal as well as printed output. In addition, it permits the following other functions: word processing, drawing, environmental control, calculation, music composition, and

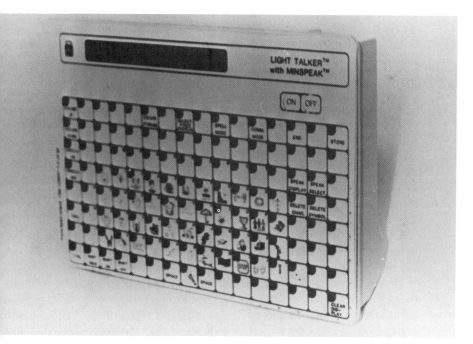

FIGURE 4.11 Light Talker™ (photograph courtesy of Prentke-Romich Co.).

games. Another example of this approach is the Talk II Program (Rusha-koff, 1981) requiring an Apple II computer, Echo Speech Synthesizer, and a printer as an option. The spoken vocabulary can be customized and adapted as needed. This system can accommodate a vocabulary of from 600 to 750 words and phrases, and from 600 to 2,000 sentences. A message can be retrieved with just one key stroke. This approach to augmentative communication may provide greater flexibility and growth. In general, the decision is based on how the system will be used. These issues will be discussed later in this chapter.

OVERVIEW OF MICROCOMPUTER APPLICATIONS

In general, microcomputers can assist the disabled child in performing tasks in the following application areas: (1) academics, (2) recreation and entertainment, (3) telecommunications, (4) environmental control, and (5) environmental manipulation.

Since the mid-1980s computer-assisted instruction (CAI) for the disabled has gained popularity and acceptance among educators. Hagen (1984) attributes this to three major developments: (1) increased access to micro-computer usage, (2) the development of appropriate software, and (3) the development of software review systems. Also, Mahaffey (1985) points out that with new technological advances and the large volume of sales, the cost of technology has now become relatively affordable.

The advantages and disadvantages of CAI have been discussed by Hagen (1984), Schwartz (1984), and Behrmann (1984). In general, computers provide instruction that is active, self-paced, nonjudgmental, motivating, reinforcing, and multisensory. Some computer programs can assist in the development of attending skills, logic, reasoning abilities, fine motor skills, and eye–hand coordination skills. Computer programs can provide immediate feedback and reinforcement. Hagen (1984) contends it is this property that makes CAI superior to traditional paper and pencil drills.

Currently there are four major types of instructional programs (Behrmann, 1984; Hagen, 1984; Larson & Steiner, 1985; Schwartz, 1984): (1) drill and practice, (2) tutorials, (3) games, and (4) simulations.

Drill and practice programs have widespread use in special education today. They are used to facilitate and develop special academic skills such as vocabulary and mathematics. They provide the user with feedback regarding correct and incorrect responses. For example, the software *First Categories* (Laureate Learning System) helps children classify 16 nouns into six categories. It has three levels of complexity and includes a test level. Graphics, speech synthesis, and text are employed.

Schwartz (1984) cautions that some general practice programs can provide "little more than expensive electronic workbooks" (p. 11). Also, Hagen (1984) contends that care should be taken to select software that the learning-disabled child can control. She contends that the best software is the type that can be modified to meet the needs of the individual child through authoring. This concept will be discussed later in this section of the chapter.

Tutorials aim to teach new information through review and testing routines. Instruction is systematically presented based on a hierarchy of skills and adapted based on performance achieved. The format of tutorial programs involves an interaction between the learner and the program. Since the learner is actively involved, the focus of these programs is on learning to apply skills and concepts rather than rote learning. An example of this type of program is the *Comprehension-Main Idea Program* by Unicom. It provides tutorials and practice lessons in reading comprehension related to the main idea of the story for grades 2 through 6.

Games aim to motivate and interest the user. These programs can be exciting to children as they frequently employ animation, sound effects, and graphics. Larson and Steiner (1985) contend that some text or graphic adventure games can be used to develop problem-solving skills and thinking abilities.

Simulations are programs designed to simulate real-life experiences. They aim to facilitate insight and problem-solving skills and can be used to achieve curriculum objectives. Mahaffey (1985) contends that computers can build "insight, intuition, and pragmatic concepts" (p. 7). He claims the clinic, hospital, or educational environment can infrequently model real-life situations efficiently. One such program is *Oregon Trail* (Minnesota Educational Computing Consortium). This program teaches about life in America in the 1800s. The student is asked to make decisions about hunting for food, purchasing supplies, and survival tactics.

Problem-solving skills can also be taught through computer programming. Using the "Logo" language system (Papert, 1980), several educators and researchers have successfully taught programming to learning-disabled children (Hagen, 1984; Huber, 1985; Mahaffey, 1985; Weir, Russell, & Valente, 1982). Educators have discovered that the use of the "Logo" system facilitates self-expression and logic through discovery learning. It can allow a child to conquer abstract problems in a concrete way. Weir et al. (1982) also claim that it assists the educator "in discovering hidden strengths in students" (p. 358).

Microcomputer applications in the field of communication disorders are growing rapidly. The format for commercially available software programs designed for language intervention is similar to the types mentioned above. These include drill and practice, simulation, tutorials, instructional games, and problem-solving. Again, authoring programs such as *EZ Pilot* and *Superpilot* (Apple Computers, Inc.) allow clinicians to develop language-learning programs for individual children.

Larson and Steiner (1985) described an intervention program with a 5-year-old language-delayed child using computer-based language instruction. They reported that during this instruction the child produced 28 communication behaviors in 15 minutes. More traditional language intervention tasks yielded nine communication behaviors per 15 minutes. They described the child as being more active when engaging with the computer.

Meyers (1985) describes the computer as a "unique language prosthesis" (p. 1) because it can provide access for the handicapped child through keyboards, interfaces, and switches. She has been using computers successfully with language-delayed preschoolers to facilitate comprehension and production skills. Meyers' programs are based on the language acquisition principals involving play, exploration, and meaningful context. Using her software system, *Programs for Early Acquisition of Language* (*PEAL*), individualized language-learning lessons can be developed. The *PEAL* system has a membrane keyboard. Symbols such as line drawings, photographs, and pictures can be displayed using an overlay covering the keyboard. When the keyboard is touched, graphics are displayed on the monitor in addition to the synthesized speech output. Meyers contends control of speech output and graphics is not only more motivating to children but also increases vocalizations. Meyers has found that in addition to facilitating language development, this technique increases attention span, develops fine motor and eye–hand coordination, and encourages scanning and play skills.

Goosens and Kratt (1985) state that "technological advances alone are not sufficient to ensure successful language intervention" (p. 58). They support a maximally interactive approach to language intervention. This involves modeling and expanding target communicative behaviors within naturalistic contexts. Such an approach may not be simulated by computer technology at present.

The mild to moderately cognitively handicapped child can use word processing software to facilitate expressive and written language skills. Word processing programs allow children to be more creative and efficient writers. Revisions do not require recopying. Editing of material is easy, rapid, and neat. The final document can be produced rapidly using an external printer connected to the computer. Word processing programs can help alleviate the frustration associated with writing experienced by many learning-disabled and physically handicapped children and adults.

The use of microcomputers for telecommunications has been found to be practical and efficient. It requires the use of a modem or an acoustic coupler connected to the microcomputer. This tool allows access to telephone lines, electronic mail, teleconferencing, electronic information access, and even shopping. Hagen (1984) has identified educational advantages to the use of microcomputers for telecommunications. She reported that the oral and written language skills of her congenitally deaf son Mark improved significantly within 2½ years with the use of a telecommunication system. Electronic bulletin boards and "CB" simulations on systems, such as Compu-Serve, provide the child with experiences outside of his immediate environment.

HOW TO CHOOSE SOFTWARE

Since more and more software is being marketed, educators are finding it necessary to critically evaluate the quality of these programs. Schwartz (1984) proposes that the initial selection criteria be based on the following questions: "What is the object of the program?" and "Is the object of the program worth it?" Lahm and Behrmann (1984) contend that software should be evaluated in the following areas prior to purchase: (1) descriptive information, such as the purpose of the software, (2) technical soundness, and (3) program flexibility.

To aid decision making, several evaluation tools have been developed such as the Council for Exceptional Children's *Software Search Evaluation Form* and the *Teacher's Guide to Educational Software, K-12* (Shanahan & Ryan, 1984). The Council for Exceptional Children now operates a Special Education Software Center that disseminates information about educational and administrative software for use in special education. The Center's data base can be accessed by calling an 800 telephone number (Baker, 1985b). The Trace Center has developed an International Computer Registry that lists, classifies, and describes software written for both disabled and nondisabled individuals. Swift's *1984–85 Educational Software Directory, Apple II Edition*, lists software by subject and publisher. In addition, periodicals such as *Byte, The Computing Teacher, Computer Classroom News*, and *Compute* are excellent resources for the application of microcomputer technology in education. A list of periodicals can be found at the conclusion of this chapter.

COMPUTER ACCESS BY THE DISABLED

Many moderate to severely physically disabled individuals cannot access the standard computer keyboard. Recent technological advances, however, allow the physically disabled user easy access. In general, these developments involve customizing standardized software and equipment or modifying and adapting standard equipment. Customization is usually cost prohibitive. Maintenance and repair may be difficult. Also, with the rapid increase in standard software programs, customization would be extremely time consuming (Vanderheiden, 1981). In contrast, electrical modifications such as detachable adaptations are becoming more available, more easily maintained, and less costly. These include special interfaces, key guards, expanded keyboards, voice input modules, touch sensitive screens, and nonstandard input control devices such as keyboard emulators.

Computers are often built by the manufacturer with great flexibility. The computer inside of the case will have slots or sites where additional circuit boards can be added. The circuit board and modification to the circuitry can be made with relative ease. Apple Computer was one of the first computer companies in the field to do this; they knew other inventors would add features to their computer, which would make the interest in it even greater. The Apple II+ computer has stood the test of time in terms of having accomplished this. Of course, it would be nice to be able to have the disabled individual use standard software without modifications. There are two hardware options, which are similar yet importantly different, that allow this in effect to happen.

The first option involves the use of another device or second computer to interact with the user. This is accomplished through a scanning mechanism or alternate direct-selection techniques that then communicate directly with the second computer with the appropriate American Standard Code for Information Interchange (ASCII) code that then communicates directly with the second computer using standard protocols. The second computer is interfacing with the user while the primary computer runs the standard software. The primary computer has no idea that it is controlled any differently than usual.

The second hardware option for interfacing with a primary computer is to use "add on" circuit boards that fit within the primary computer. Speech recognition units are available that interface with a number of commercially available computers. These have the advantage of providing multiple lists of vocabularies and a means of changing from one vocabulary list to another. Voice recognition input to a computer requires preprogramming of the computer to respond to the characteristic frequency patterns of an individual speaker. A significant drawback for this application in children is that young children are unable to consistently repeat a word with the same force and inflection. Also, children who have more severe language-production and breath-control problems are unable to repeat the same sound pattern consistently.

Another add-on option, developed by Schwejda and Vanderheiden (1982), involves what they call an adaptive firmware card. This card is inserted into the circuitry of the computer so that it sits between the keyboard and the master operating system of the computer. Activation of a switch immediately initiates a scanning sequence along the lower area of the screen. Through the appropriate tapping of a single or double switch, the user then inputs the particular character he or she wishes. If you will, the scanning feature is transparent to computer operation. The character input is passed on to the computer and the activity is carried out. This system is so effective that a child could play a game on the computer that was keyboard-controlled, going in and out of the scanning mode. Computer operation is halted during the scanning mode operation and then resumes at the next input. Touch screens represent an additional form of input. Computers are already able to use software developed for that. The concept of the "mouse" is another means of providing scanning and input without having to use the keyboard.

Computer usages for the deaf and the blind are fairly obvious. For deaf users there is the capability of speech production through the use of small, portable, programmed computers with speech production circuitry. Speech recognition is currently not to the point where the deaf are able to carry a translator of word to text that would be useful to them. For the blind and partially blind, software allows the use of the computer screen to generate large, bold text to facilitate reading of the material. Many innovative and fairly inexpensive techniques have been developed to allow a computer to generate Braille text.

The computer itself offers the ability to interface environmental control systems. Again, in thinking of the appropriate piece of equipment to purchase for a child, anticipated needs and environmental control should be considered at the time of purchase.

Butler, Okomoto, and McKay (1983) have shown that children as young as 20 months of age, given appropriate adaptive seating and a conventional motorized wheelchair, are able to have independent mobility. There are a number of wheelchair-control hardware options that allow the more physically compromised to use power mobility as well. Slot switch input, sip-and-puff control, and speech recognition using a computer become possible options for powered mobility.

The final computer prescription will weigh factors relevant to what the computer is to accomplish, the age of the child using it, the degree of sophistication of school and family in computers, add-on capabilities for future needs, availability of servicing, and dealer support. Most importantly, computers that are used in the future must allow the disabled to have access to the largest domain of software.

SYSTEM SELECTION

System selection involves five phases: (1) multidisciplinary evaluation, (2) system recommendations, (3) training, (4) follow-up, and (5) procurement and funding.

Multidisciplinary Evaluation

When prescribing equipment for a nonvocal, physically handicapped individual, the evaluation should focus on the needs and abilities of the user and determining the individual's method of learning. A thorough multidisciplinary assessment is needed, including review of past medical history; sensory abilities; cognitive and academic functioning; communication skills and interaction needs; seating, positioning, and control site; and nature and quality of supportive services. Initially, data is gathered from other professionals who have been working with the individual. Interviews are conducted with the individual and his or her family or primary caretaker(s) to determine their appraisal of the individual's current level of functioning and their expectations. Standardized testing is conducted when possible. Some individuals do not have a reliable mode of response. Thus, a variety of informal measures and observational data will be necessary.

The individual's visual and auditory acuity levels should be determined.

If standard testing cannot be conducted, the degree of impairment may be a clinical judgment based on how he or she responds to stimuli in his or her daily environment and during testing. Educators at the Non-Oral Communication Center of the Plavan School, Fountain Valley, California (Montgomery, 1980) contend that the sensory assessment should aim to provide information that can be applied. Useful information involves reporting, for example, that the child can see a certain type of drawing at a certain distance rather than that the child has 20/80 acuity. Psychologists, social workers, and educators should provide information about the individual's intellectual functioning, learning style, academic skills, and social–emotional behaviors as well as the caretaker's level of support, expectations, and reactions.

The speech/language pathologist should conduct an evaluation of communication skills to obtain information regarding the individual's (1) present communication mode, results of his/her communication attempts, where interactions break down, and response to failure (Bottorf & DePape, 1982); (2) prelanguage capabilities such as attention, matching, and nonverbal classification skills; (3) auditory comprehension; (4) semantic skills including an analysis of various types of symbol systems; (5) syntactic skills; (6) pragmatic skills such as eye contact and turn-taking and how the individual uses language in expressing feelings and needs, making requests, obtaining information, and sharing ideas and experiences; and (7) interaction factors and needs such as: What are his or her interests? Who are the people he or she interacts with most frequently? What situations does he or she need to communicate in? For example, if the child will be utilizing the aid in school, the aid should allow independent academic work. Thus, both vocal and printed output would be desirable.

A major goal of the motor control assessment is to determine optimal body positioning. Motor control is greatly influenced by positioning, and information should be gathered regarding how different positions and body-part movements affect the total body. Input from the physical and occupational therapist and physician are needed to determine the optimal switch placement. The wrong placement of a switch could influence symmetry of body position and lead to fixed deformity. This information will also be used when deciding where to place additional equipment. Specific motor abilities to be assessed include (1) force, or minimum and maximum pressure an individual can exert using a specific body part; (2) range of excursion—the maximum distance across which an individual can move a body part; (3) resolution of movement—the minimum movement that is reliably and accurately executed for a best-control site (the anatomic site that achieves the greatest accuracy and reliability); (4) endurance, (5) reaction time; and (6) response repetition—the average number of responses in a given period of time that the user is capable of making with specific control sites.

System Recommendations

Once information is accumulated in all the aforementioned areas, system election is pursued. An analysis of performance may be conducted on more than one system. Performance is systematically evaluated for accuracy. Lahm and McGregor (1984) have developed an assessment tool for analyzing the needs of a group of users or an individual user. The Handicapped User's Method for Analyzing Needs-Systems Development (HUMAN-SD) includes a useful error-analysis matrix to assist in analyzing and characterizing the user's error, such as performance out of sequence, nonrequired action, switch too far to reach, and forgotten sequence. When considering which system to select, user performance is among many critical factors. User satisfaction, support system satisfaction, safety, size, weight, portability, flexibility, memory capacity, length of time that the child is expected to use the system, market availability, and service requirements are among the other determining factors.

Training

Training objectives must ensure that the child is able to independently use the system. The design of a treatment program for the development of an unaided communication system, such as gestural codes, is based on results of the capabilities, needs, and interest assessment and the normal sequence of language development. For example, the functional sign language program developed by Rittenhouse and Myers (1985) for the severely disabled child teaches 250 functional signs in discreet steps. They suggest that the first 50 signs elected be concrete and taught by category. Rittenhouse and Myers propose demonstrating the sign and shaping the child's hand if imitation and close approximation are not achieved. They teach signs in naturally occurring contexts and provide consistent reinforcement.

Regarding communication board use and symbol training, Silverman (1980) suggests that the "smallest set of pictures should be selected initially by which necessary messages can be encoded" (p. 90). Schiefelbusch (1980) also suggests that the first communication board contain only a few lexical items. He contends that parents and significant others should participate in the development of the board. A child may have a series of boards, using each in different communicative situations. In general, as the user becomes more linguistically sophisticated, changes in the system will be necessary.

Beukelman, Yorkston, and Dowden (1985) suggest three phases of training for electronic devices: (1) control drills, which focus on learning how to operate the system's controls; (2) message preparation tasks, to simulate interaction such as letter writing and preparing memos; and (3) training in interaction, where information is received, exchanged, and analyzed. They suggest training "conversational control" (p. 17), referring to exchanges that involve initiating, turn-taking, and changing roles.

The communication system, regardless of the type selected, should incorporate the aforementioned functions of language. Unfortunately, training too often emphasizes the communication of basic needs, excluding many of the other forms of interaction. A training program should give a child the opportunity to obtain information; describe events; predict; express intentions, beliefs, and emotions; and to indicate a desire to continue or discontinue communication.

Follow-Up

Follow-up should be conducted after the first 3 to 6 months and as needed thereafter. User and caretaker satisfaction, efficiency, and effectiveness should be reevaluated. System modifications and additional training are provided as needed.

Procurement and Funding

To ensure success, the funding process should be approached in a systematic and organized manner. The steps involved in securing funding have been detailed by several clinicians, researchers, and educators (Blackstone, 1984; Depape & Krause, 1980; Montgomery, 1980; Ruggles, 1979). In general the following strategies are recommended:

1) A person should be selected to coordinate the funding effort. This person should be familiar with the terminology and interpretation of legislation regarding procurement and reimbursement.

2) The potential funding resources should be identified. These may include family–client resources such as employer contributions, savings bonds, trust funds, and inheritances; government programs including Medicare and Public Assistance, and those of the Office of Vocational Rehabilitation Services and Crippled Children's Services; private insurance; voluntary health organizations such as United Cerebral Palsy, American Cancer Society, Muscular Dystrophy Association; service organizations; religious organizations; labor unions; and grants.

3) Appropriate funding resources should be educated about the technology and the type of individual who needs it. This professional education can be offered to one person within the agency or to a group. A contact person within each agency should be identified. Funding applications may be submitted to more than one potential source simultaneously.

The agency or funding source should be given identifying information about the individual needing financial support, and should be provided with data regarding the nature of the individual's ability to successfully interact without the device. A medical prescription may be useful, particularly if the agency is medically oriented. A description of the system, its features, and functions should be explained. Most importantly, the agency must realize the changes in functional status that will be achieved with the device. The system's impact on the user's independence and educational and vocational opportunities should be emphasized. Should a claim be rejected, the reason(s) behind the decision should be investigated and the application resubmitted as appropriate.

Another option for securing equipment is by rental or leasing agreements. Manufacturers, distributors, assessment centers, and state agencies may provide equipment through loan, rental, or leasing programs.

Recently an 18-month study was conducted by Beukelman, Yorkston, and Smith (1985) to investigate third-party payment response to requests for purchase of augmentative communication systems in the state of Washington. Of the 53 requests returned, 70% were approved. In general, individuals with a diagnosis of cerebral palsy, traumatic brain injury, or degenerative neurological disease were granted funding between 68% to 80% of the time. In the category of adult onset of nontraumatic disease such as cerebral vascular accident and encephalitis, only 4% of the total requests were funded. Responses for funding were obtained within a 6-month period for all third-party payers. Regarding age, the highest proportion for approvals (80%) was given to young adults, ranging in age from 19 to 40 years. All seven systems that ranged between $800 and $1,500 were approved. Systems priced greater than $1,500 (10) were approved 40% of the time. It was noted that Medicaid approved between 83% and 100% of the 29 requests. Private insurance approved between 9% and 36% of the requests (15). Of the remaining nine requests, only one was rejected. Beukelman et al. (1985) urged the compilation of data from different regions of the United States to analyze the possibility of trends and assist in developing regulations and national policy decisions.

Funding for technical aids is possible. However, public education, perseverance, and an organized approach are necessary.

CONCLUSION

Through technology, cognitive–communicative skills in young children can be developed. Augmentative communication systems can be provided for the nonvocal individual. Technology can address computer access by the disabled, and, thus expand their academic, recreational, and vocational opportunities. However, quoting William L. Rush (1983), a cerebral-palsied and nonspeaking individual and Honors graduate of the University of

Nebraska, "scientists have not invented the machine to hug me warmly or give me a word of encouragement or make me feel needed."

Human interaction cannot be simulated. Meeting the psychosocial need: of the disabled can mean the difference between having a prescribed system sit in a closet and user independence. Thus, the challenge is not to answer the question, "What system can an individual use effectively?" Rather, the true challenge is to determine how we, as educators and health care professionals, can work together with the disabled and their support systems to help them build the self-confidence and self-esteem needed to fully utilize the technologies currently available.

MANUFACTURER ADDRESS LISTING

John Adair
P.O. Box 270115
Houston, TX 77217
713-960-9842
Control aids

Adaptive Communication Systems,
Inc.
994 Broadhead Road, Suite 202
Coraopolis, PA 15108
412-264-2288
Control aids & augmentative communication equipment

American Communication Corporation
180 Roberts Street
East Hartford, CT 06108
203-289-3491
Augmentative communication
equipment

Arroyo & Associates
88-45 79th Avenue
Glendale, NY 11385
718-849-9306
Control aids & augmentative communication equipment

Baggeboda Press
1128 Rhode Island Street
Lawrence, KS 66044
913-842-0490
Picsyms

Blissymbolics Communication Institute
350 Rumsey Road
Toronto, Ontario M4G 1R8
Canada
416-424-3806
Blissymbol material

Canon USA
One Canon Plaza
Lake Success, NY 11042
516-488-6700
Augmentative equipment

Cleo Living Aids
3957 Mayfield Road
Cleveland, OH
216-382-9700
Augmentative communication
equipment

Communication Research Corporation
1720 130th Avenue N.E.
Bellevue, WA 98005
206-881-9550
Augmentative communication
equipment

Computers for the Physically
Handicapped, Inc.
7602 Talbert Avenue, Suite 5
Huntington Beach, CA 92647
714-848-1122
Adapted microcomputer

Contemporary Artistic Technology
P.O. Box 58430, Station L
Vancouver, British Columbia
 V6P 6K2
Canada
604-324-8119
Expanded keyboards, augmentative
 communication equipment

Convaid LTD
2586 Holly Springs Drive
German Town, TN 38138
213-271-3649
Augmentative communication
 equipment

Crestwood Company
P.O. Box 04513
Milwaukee, WI 53204
414-351-0311
Augmentative communication
 equipment

Don Johston
Developmental Equipment
981 Winnetka Terrace
Lake Zurich, IL 60047
312-438-3476
Control aids, augmentative communication equipment

Help Me to Help Myself Communication Aids
824 Acre Avenue
Brownsburg, IN 46112
Augmentative communication
 equipment

Imaginart Press
P.O. Box 1868
Idyllwild, CA 92349
714-659-5905
Augmentative communication
 equipment

Innocomp
Innovative computer applications
33195 Wagon Wheel
Solon, OH 44139
216-248-6206
Augmentative communication
 equipment

Intex Micro Systems, Inc.
725 S. Adams Road, Suite L-8
Birmingham, MI 48011
313-540-7601
Augmentative communication
 equipment

Jim's Instrument Manufacturing
P.O. Box 5157
Coralville, IA 52241
319-351-3429
Control aids

Steve Konar
Toys for Special Children
8 Main Street
Hastings-on-Hudson, NY 10706

Krown Research, Inc.
6300 Arizona Circle
Los Angeles, CA 94005
213-641-4306 (Voice or TTY)
TTY

Laurente Learning Systems
1 Mill Street
Burlington, VT 05401
Educational software

Microwriter, Inc.
251 E. 61st Street
New York, NY 10021
212-319-8602
Augmentative communication
 equipment

Minnesota Educational Computing
 Consortium
2520 Broadway Drive
St. Paul, MN 55113
Software company

Palmetto Technologies, Inc.
P.O. Box 498
Duncan, SC 29334
803-439-4309 (Voice or TTY)
Augmentative communication
  equipment

Peca, Inc.
Extronix Division
592 Winks Lane
Bensalem, PA 19020
215-245-1550
Augmentative communication
  equipment

Phonic Ear, Inc.
250 Camino Alto
Mill Valley, CA 94941
415-383-4000
Augmentative communication
  equipment

Pitts Corporation
4260 N. 650 E.
Provo, UT 84604
801-225-6441
Augmentative communication
  equipment

Pleasure Endeavors
375 Laguna Honda Boulevard
San Francisco, CA 94116
415-864-5821
Augmentative communication
  equipment

P.M.V. Systems, B.V.
Postbox 16
4273 ZG HANK
The Netherlands
31/1622-2958
Augmentative communication
  equipment

Prentke-Romich Company
1022 Heyl Road
Wooster, OH 44691
216-262-1984
Control aids & augmentative communication equipment

Rushakoff, E.G.
Box 3W
New Mexico State University
Las Cruces, NM 8003
Talk II Program

Shea Products
235 Avon Industrial Drive
Auburn Hills, MI 48057
313-852-2163
Augmentative communication
  equipment

Si/Comm
7545 Whitlock Avenue
Playa Del Ray, CA 90291
213-823-1202
Augmentative communication
  equipment

Sontek Medical Inc.
Division of Sontek Industries, Inc.
31 Fletcher Avenue
Lexington, MA 02173
617-863-1410
Augmentative communication
  equipment

Specialized Systems, Inc.
6060 Corte del Cedro
Carlsbad, CA 92008
619-483-8800
TDD

TASH, Inc.
70 Gibson Drive
Markham, Ontario L3R 2Z3
Canada
416-475-2212
Adapted toys, training aids, & contro
  interfaces

Texas Instruments
Attention: Parts
P.O. Box 53
Lubbock, TX 79408
806-741-3064
Augmentative communication
  equipment

3M Company
Business Communication Products
  Division
3M Center
St. Paul, MN 55144
612-733-5454
TDD

Toby Churchill LTD
20 Panton Street
Cambridge, England CB2 1HP
Adapted typewriter

Typewriting Institute for the
  Handicapped
3102 W. Augusta Avenue
Phoenix, AZ 85021
602-939-5344
Adapted typewriters

Ultratec, Inc.
442 Normandy Lane
Madison, WI 53719
608-273-0707
Augmentative communication
  equipment

Unicom
297 Elmwood Avenue
Providence, RI 02907
Software company

Wayne County Intermediate School
  District
Attn: Greg Turner
33500 Van Born Road
P.O. Box 807
Wayne, MI 48184
313-467-1415
Augmentative communication
  equipment

Words+, Inc.
1125 Stewart Court, Suite D
Sunnyvale, CA 94086
408-730-9588
Control aids & augmentative communication equipment

Zygo Industries, Inc.
P.O. Box 1008
Portland, OR 97207
503-297-1724
Control aids & augmentative communi-
  cation equipment

COMPUTER JOURNALS, PERIODICALS, AND NEWSLETTERS

ACCESS: Microcomputers in Libraries. P.O. Box 764, Oakdridge, OR 97463

AEDS Journal. 1201 Sixteenth Street, N.W., Washington, DC 20036

AEDS Monitor. 1201 Sixteenth Street, N.W., Washington, DC 20036

Byte. McGraw-Hill, 70 Main Street, Peterborough, NH 03458.

Closing the Gap. Budd and Dolores Hagen, P.O. Box 68, Henderson, MN 56044.

Communication Outlook. Artificial Language Laboratory, Computer Science Department, Michigan State University, East Lansing, MI 48824.

Compute. P.O. Box 5406, Greensboro, NC 27403.

Computer Classroom News. Intentional Educations, Inc., 51 Spring Street, Watertown, MA 02172.

Computing Teacher, The. Department of Computer and Information Science, University of Oregon, Eugene, OR 97403.

Creative Computing. P.O. Box 789-M, Morristown, NJ 07960.

Curriculum Product Review. The Educators Guide to Instructional Materials. Pitman Learning, Inc., 530 University Avenue, Palo Alto, CA 94301.

Education Technology. 140 Sylvan Avenue, Englewood Cliffs, NJ 07632.

Educational Software Directory, Apple II Edition. Sterling Swift Publishing Co., 1600 Fortview Road, Austin, TX 78704.

Educator's Microdigest and Software Exchange. Educorp 21 Ltd., P.O. Box 162, Madison, WI 53791.

Educational Computer. P.O. Box 535, Cupertino, CA 95015.

80 Micro. P.O. Box 981, Farmingdale, NY 11737.

Electronic Education. Electronic Communications, Inc., Suite 220, 1311 Executive Center Drive, Tallahassee, FL 32301.

Electronic Learning. 902 Sylvan Avenue, Englewood Cliffs, NJ 07632.

Incider. 80 Pine Street, Peterborough, NH 03458.

Infoworld. Popular Computing, Inc., 375 Cochituate Road, Box 880, Framingham, MA 01701.

Journal of Computer-Based Instruction. Western Washington University, Bellingham, WA 98225.

Journal of Courseware Review. Apple Educational Foundation. 20525 Mariani, Cupertino, CA 95014.

LOGO and Educational Computing Journal. Krell Software Corporation, 1320 Stony Brook Road, Stony Brook, NY 11790.

MACUL Journal. Michigan Association for Computer Users in Learning, Wayne County ISD, 33500 Van Born Road, Wayne, MI 48184.

The Mathematics Teacher and The Arithmetic Teacher. National Council of Teachers of Mathematics. 1906 Association Drive, Reston, VA 22091.

Media and Methods. The Magazine of the Teaching Technologies. 1511 Walnut Street, Philadelphia, PA 19102.

Medical Computer Journal (MCJ). Aziz Ghaussy, M.D., 42 East High Street, East Hampton, CT 06424.

Microcomputers in Education Queue. 5 Chapel Hill Drive, Fairfield, CT 06432.

Microcomputing (formerly *Kolobaud Microcomputing*). 80 Pine Street, Peterborough, NH 03458.

Nibble. P.O. Box 325, Lincoln, MA 01773.

PC. 39 E. Hanover Avenue, Morrisplaines, NJ 07950.

Personal Computing. 1050 Commonwealth Avenue, Boston, MA 02215.

Popular Computing. McGraw-Hill, 70 Main Street, Peterborough, NH 03458.

Recreational Computing. P.O. Box E, Menlo Park, CA 94025.

chool Microwave Reviews. Dresden Associates, P.O. Box 246, Dresden, ME 04342.

Softalk. 11021 Magnolia Boulevard, North Hollywood, CA 91601.

Software Review. Microform Review, 520 Riverside Avenue, Westport, CT 06880.

T.H.E. Journal. P.O. Box 992, Acton, MA 01720.

TRS-80 Microcomputer News. P.O. Box 2910, Fort Worth, TX 76113.

REFERENCES

The Ad Hoc Committee on Communications Process and Non-Speaking Persons. (1980). Position statement on non-speech communication. *American Speech-Language-Hearing Association, 23* (8), 267–272.

Baker, B. (1982). Minspeak. *Byte, 7* (9), 186–202.

Baker, B. (1983). Communication disabilities—An overview. *Rehabilitation World, 7* (2), 3–7.

Baker, B. (1985a). The user of words and phrases on a minspeak communication system. *Communication Outlook, 7* (3), 8–11.

Baker, P. (1985b). Searching for the best software. *Classroom Computer Learning,* October, 53–58.

Beesley, M. (1981). *Toys help—A guide to choosing toys for handicapped children.* Toronto: Canadian Association of Toy Libraries.

Behrmann, M. (Ed.) (1984). *Handbook of microcomputers in special education.* San Diego, CA: College Hill Press.

Behrmann, M., & Lahm, E. (1984a). Using computers with young and cognitively low functioning children. In M. Behrmann, (Ed.), *Handbook of microcomputers in special education.* San Diego, CA: College Hill Press.

Behrmann, M., & Lahm, E. (1984b). Critical learning: Multiply handicapped babies get on-line. In M. Behrmann and E. Lahm, (Eds.), *Proceedings of the National Conference on the Use of Microcomputers in Special Education.* Reston, VA: Council for Exceptional Children.

Beukelman, D., Yorkston, K., & Dowden, P. (1985). *Communication augmentation: A casebook of clinical management.* San Diego, CA: College Press.

Beukelman, D., Yorkston, F., & Smith, K. (1985). Third-party payer responds to requests for purchase of communication augmentation systems: A study of Washington State. *Augmentative and Alternate Communication, 1,* 5–9.

Blackstone, S. (1984). Criteria for appropriate augmentative devices and systems for non-speaking children. Paper presented at the California Speech and Hearing Association Convention.

Blakely, D. (1985). Adapted toys and communication devices for special students. Paper presented at the Assistive Device Conference, Carlisle, Pennsylvania.

Bloom, B. S. (1964). *Stability and change in human character.* New York: Wiley.

Bloom, L., & Lahey, M. (1978). *Language development and disorders.* New York: Wiley.

Bottorf, L. & DePape, D. (1982). Initiating communication systems for severely speech-impaired persons. *Topics in Language Disorders, 2,* 55–71.

Bowe, F., & Little, N. (1984). Computer accessibility: A study. *Rehabilitatie Literature, 49* (9–10), 289–291.

Bricker, D. (1972). Imitative sign training as a facilitator of a work-object associa tion with low-functioning children. *American Journal of Mental Deficiency, 7* 509–516.

Brinker, R., & Lewis, M. (1982). Making the world work with microcomputers: learning prosthesis for handicapped infants. *Exceptional Children, 49* (2), 163 170.

Burkhart, L. J. (1980). Homemade Battery Powered Toys and Educational Device for Severely Handicapped Children. Catalog. (Available by writing to 850 Rhode Island Ave., College Park, MD 20740.)

Butler, C., Okamoto, G., & McKay, M. (1983). Powered mobility for very youn disabled children. *Developmental Medicine and Child Neurology, 24,* 472–47

Capozzi, N., & Mineo, B. (1984). Non-speech language and communication sy tems. In A. Holland (Ed.), *Language Disorders in Children.* San Diego, C/ College Hill Press.

Carlson, F. (1982). *Prattle and play: Equipment recipes for non-speech communicatio* Omaha: Meyer Children's Rehabilitation Institute, University of Nebrask Medical Center.

Carlson, F. (1985). *Picsyms categorical dictionary.* Lawrence, KS: Baggeboda Press

Chapman, R., & Miller, J. (1980). Analyzing language and communication in th child. In R. Schiefelbusch (Ed.), *Non-spoken language and communication: Acqu sition and intervention.* Baltimore: Maryland University Press.

Charlebois-Marois, C. (1985). *Everybody's technology.* Quebec, Canada: Charle coms.

Coker, W. (1984). Homemade switches and toy adaptations for early training wit non-speaking persons. *Language, Speech and Hearing Services in the Schools, 1* 32–36.

Council for Exceptional Children. (1983). Software Search Evaluation Form. Res ton, VA: Council for Exceptional Children.

DePape, D., & Krause, L. (1980). *Guidelines for seeking funding for communicatio aides.* Madison, WI: Trace Research Center and Development Center on Com munication Goals and Computer Access for Handicapped Individuals, Univer sity of Wisconsin-Madison.

Fishman, S., Timler, G., & Yoder, D. (1985). Strategies for the prevention an repair of communication breakdowns in interaction with communication boar users. *Augmentative and Alternate Communication, 1,* 38–51.

Foort, J. (1985). Comments for a new generation of rehabilitation engineers. *Journa of Rehabilitation Research and Development,* January, 2–8.

Goosens, C., & Kratt, A. (1985). Technology as a tool for conversation an language learning for the physically disabled. *Topics in Language Disorders, 6* (1) 56–70.

Hagen, D. (1984). *Microcomputer resource book for special education.* Reston, VA Reston Publishing.

Harris, D. (1982). Communicative interaction processes involving non-vocal physi cally handicapped children. *Topics in Language Disorders, 2,* 21–37.

Huber, L. (1985). Computer learning through Piaget's eyes. *Classroom Compute Learning,* October, 39–42.

Jeffrey, G. (1981). Why toys help. In M. Beesley (Ed.), *Toys help—A guide t choosing toys for the handicapped children.* Toronto: Canadian Advocates on Toy Libraries.

Karlan, G., Breen-White, B., Lentz, A., Hoder, P., Egger, P., & Frankoff, D. (1982). Establishing generalized productive verb-noun phrase usage in a manual communication system with moderately handicapped children. *Journal of Speech and Hearing Disorders, 47*, 31-42.

Lahm, E., & Behrmann, M. (1984). Software Evaluation. In M. Behrmann (Ed.), *Handbook of Microcomputers and Special Education.* San Diego, CA: College Hill Press.

Lahm, E., & McGregor, J. (1984). Hardware selection and evaluation. In M. Behrmann (Ed.), *Handbook of Microcomputers and Special Education.* San Diego, CA: College Hill Press.

Larson, M., & Steiner, O. (1985). Topics in language disorders. *High Technology and Language Disorders, 6* (1), 63-74.

McCormick, L., & Schiefelbusch, R. (1984). *Early language intervention.* Columbus, OH: Charles E. Merrill.

McWilliams, P. (1984). *Personal computers and the disabled.* Garden City, NY: Quantum Press.

Mahaffey, R. (1985). An overview of computer applications. *Topics in Language Disorder, 6* (1), 1-10.

Meyers, L. (1985). Using computers to facilitate oral and written language development in language disabled children. Paper presented at the University of Pittsburgh, Pittsburgh, Pennsylvania.

Montgomery, J. (1980). *Non-oral communication—Training guide.* Fountain Valley (California) School District. California State Department of Education.

Muma, J. (1978). *Language handbook: Concepts, assessment, and intervention.* Englewood Cliffs, NJ: Prentice-Hall.

Musselwhite, C., & St. Louis, K. (1982). *Communication programming for the severely handicapped: Vocal and non-vocal strategies.* Houston, TX: College Hill Press.

Office of Technology Assessment. (1983). Health technology case study 26: Assistive devices for severe speech impairments (p. 4-5). Washington, DC: Government Printing Office.

Papert, S. (1980). *Mind storms.* New York: Basic Books.

Poulton, K., & Algozzine, P. (1980). Manual communication and mental retardation: A review of research and implications. *The American Journal of Mental Deficiency, 85* (2), 145-152.

Proceedings of the Johns Hopkins First National Search for Applications of Personal Computing to Aid the Handicapped. (1981). Baltimore, MD: Johns Hopkins University Press.

Report and recommendations of the Professional Advisory Group on Augmentative Communication Systems and Service Needs for Non-Speaking Children in the Commonwealth of Pennsylvania (June, 1985). Harrisburg, PA: Pennsylvania Department of Health, Division of Rehabilitation.

Rittenhouse, R., & Meyers, J. (1985). Teaching functional sign language to severely disabled children. *Teaching Exceptional Chldren, 18* (2), 62-70.

Ruggles, V. (1979). *Funding of non-vocal communication aids: Current issues and strategies.* New York: Muscular Dystrophy Association of New York.

Rush, W. (1983). A personal view. *Rehabilitation World, (7)*, 2-39.

Rushakoff, G. E. (1981). Prescribing the microcomputer for non-vocal physically handicapped children. Department of Speech, University of Florida, Gainesville.

Scarr-Salapatek, S., & Williams, M. (1973). The effects of early stimulation on low birthweight. *Infants, 44* (1), 94-101.

Schanahan, D., & Ryan, A. (1984). A tool for evaluating software. *Teaching Exceptional Children*, Summer Issue, 242-247.

Schiefelbusch, R. (1980). *Non-speech, language and communication analysis and intervention.* Baltimore, MD: University Park Press.

Schiffman, G., Tobin, D., & Buchanan, B. (1982). Microcomputer instructions for the learning disabled. *Journal of Learning Disabilities, 15* (9), 557-559.

Schwartz, A. (Ed.), (1984). *Handbook of microcomputer applications in communication disorders.* San Diego, CA: College Hill Press.

Schweja, P., & Vanderheiden, G. (1982). Adaptive—firmware card for the Apple II. *Byte*, September, 276-314.

Shane, H., & Blau, J. (1981). Communication software selection for persons who are non-speaking. Paper presented at the Northeast Regional Conference of the American Speech-Language and Hearing Association.

Shane, H., Costello, J., & Davison, K. (1985). *Communication software selection for persons who are non-speaking.* Paper presented at the Annual American Speech Language and Hearing Association Convention, Washington, DC.

Shein, G., & Mandel, A. (1982). Large area flap switch to control battery operated toys. *The American Journal of Occupational Therapy, 36* (2), 107-110.

Silverman, F. (1980). *Communication for the speechless.* Englewood Cliffs, NJ: Prentice-Hall.

Stevens, J. (1982). From 3-20: The early training project. *Young Children, 37* (6), 57-64.

Thomas, W. (1984). Computers: How do they work and what do they do? In M. Behrmann (Ed.), *Handbook of microcomputer applications.* San Diego, CA: College Hill Press.

Vanderheiden, G. (1979). *Augmentative modes of communication for the severely speech and motor impaired.* Madison, WI: Trace Research and Development Center, University of Wisconsin.

Vanderheiden, G. (1981). *Practical applications of microcomputers to aid the handicapped.* Madison, WI: Trace Research and Development Center, University of Wisconsin.

Vanderheiden, G. (1982). Computers can play a dual role for disabled individuals. *Byte, 7* (9), 136-162.

Vanderheiden, G. (1985). *Non-vocal communication resource book.* Baltimore, MD: University Park Press.

Vanderheiden, G., & Grilley, K. (1984). *Non-vocal communication techniques and aids for the severely physically handicapped.* Austin, TX: Pro-Ed.

Weir, S., Russell, S., & Valente, J. (1982). Logo: An approach to educating disabled children. *Byte, 7* (9), 342-360.

5

Functional Electrical Stimulation and the Rehabilitation of the Spinal Cord-Injured Patient

Jerrold S. Petrofsky

Prior to World War II spinal cord injuries did not themselves present a long-term medical problem. Individuals with such injuries usually died soon after the initial trauma due either to neurogenic shock or to kidney or bladder infections (Guttman, 1976). With the advent of sulfa drugs and improved medical treatments, most persons with spinal cord injuries now not only survive the injury but live fairly long life spans. However, throughout their lives the spinal cord-injured remain predisposed to a variety of problems including atrophy of paralyzed muscle, demineralization of bone, reduced circulation and oxygen uptake in paralyzed portions of the body, and increased incidence of kidney and bladder infections. These problems, in turn, frequently lead to the development of other secondary medical problems including pressure sores, fractures (including spontaneous pathological fractures), thrombophlebitis, respiratory diseases, and other clinical disorders.

It is these secondary medical complications that pose the greatest problems for spinal cord-injured patients, both in terms of health care and lifetime medical costs. For example, recent studies published by the National Spinal Cord Injury Centers (Young, Burns, Bowen, & McCutcheon, 1982) indicate that the average cost for the initial rehabilitation of a person with a spinal cord injury is between $100,000 and $200,000. Throughout life, adjusting for inflation, the average spinal cord-injured person will

The author acknowledges the assistance of Ms. Debra Hendershot and Ms. Sue Stacy in the preparation of this manuscript.

spend another $4,000,000 in medical costs. Actual costs vary considerably according to a number of factors, including level and completeness of the lesion. All in all, however, health care costs as well as expenses associated with housing needs and personal assistance make spinal cord injury a costly medical problem. With an average incidence of 10,000 to 15,000 new cases a year, the overall health care costs borne by society amount to an additional $30 to $40 billion annually. Thus, while the number of people with spinal cord injuries is small, the high medical costs associated with their treatment make this disability a significant socioeconomic and medical problem.

A number of approaches have been taken to help people with spinal cord injuries and to reduce the health care and economic burden borne by them and society. The most effective way would be by repairing the lesion itself. While this avenue is being pursued through research into omentum transplants (Goldsmith, Stewart, Chen, & Duckett, 1982), tissue transplants for neural regeneration (Kao, Bunge, & Reier, 1982; Perkins, Aquayo, & Bray, 1981), electric fields for regeneration (Rowley, Roman, Strahlendorf, & Chung, 1985), and a variety of pharmaceutical interventions (Faden, Jacobs, Feuerstein, & Holiday, 1981; Naftchi, 1982), none offers an immediate solution to the problem. At present, the only existing technology that seems to offer hope for resolving some of the health care problems associated with spinal cord injury is the use of electrical stimulation for functional movement.

FUNCTIONAL ELECTRICAL STIMULATION

Functional electrical stimulation (FES) for the treatment of paralysis is not a new concept. In 1744 Kruger published a paper in which he stated that the best use of electricity would be to restore sensation and movement in paralyzed individuals. Based on Kruger's initial observations, Galvani found that electricity was conducted in the spinal cord in the form of an "action potential." From these experiments, electrical stimulation as a therapeutic modality for paralysis, stroke, rheumatism, arthritis, and heart disease gained a great deal of popularity in the 1800s and early 1900s (Hambrecht & Reswick, 1977). Unfortunately, electrical stimulation as a therapeutic modality lost favor almost universally because of its use by charlatans and quacks. Although mild electrical stimulation was used in the early and mid-1900s, it has only been during the last two to three decades that it has slowly regained popularity as a viable treatment option.

The simplest form of electrical stimulation is transcutaneous electrical nerve stimulation, or TENS. With TENS low-level stimulation at the threshold level is applied with surface electrodes through the skin. When applied properly this level of stimulation can be used to reduce pain.

Scoliosis is another type of disorder that can be successfully treated with electrical stimulation (Granek & Granek, 1985). By using multiple electrodes placed along the length of the spinal column, low-level electrical stimulation has been shown to be as effective in reducing scoliosis as is the use of braces. Low-level electrical stimulation also has been proven effective in retarding some muscle disuse atrophy following casting for some types of fractures (Basett & Becker, 1962).

Because it has proven to be useful in the treatment of some disorders, the TENS market has grown significantly in the last five years. Millions of dollars in TENS stimulators are being sold annually. However, like many types of stimulation, TENS is poorly understood. This may be related to the number of different TENS stimulators and types of electrodes available to the consumers. Incompatible matches between electrodes and stimulators are common. Further, no two stimulators offer identical stimulation parameters. Therefore, because of differences in electrode placement and variations in the characteristics of the electrodes and the stimulators themselves, it is difficult at best to obtain reliable and replicable results from those using TENS stimulation in treatment. However, in spite of these irregularities, TENS stimulation is slowly becoming an accepted therapeutic modality.

Electrical stimulation such as that utilized in TENS therapy involves a type of technology called open-loop stimulation. Open-loop control technology requires the placement of electrodes on a muscle. The muscle is then stimulated. Since sensation is intact, stimulation is kept at low enough levels to prevent overstimulation of the muscles and the resulting adverse torques in joints that could cause permanent bone damage from hyperextension.

Although conventional stimulators using open-loop control have been on the market for years, the literature indicates that these types of technologies offer only a small reversal of muscle atrophy and provide little help in reversing complications such as thrombophlebitis and pressure sores (Guttman, 1976; Hudlicka, Brown, Cotter, Smith, & Vrobova, 1977; Peckham, Mortimer, & Marsolais, 1976; Pette et al., 1975; Pette, Smith, Staudte, & Vrobova, 1973; Salmons & Vrobova, 1969). In some respects, this finding is not surprising because the activity generated with most types of electrical stimulation simply involves a muscle moving against a variable load. Experiments on nonparalyzed muscle demonstrate that it is not the number of muscle contractions that is the important variable in training. Rather, it is the metabolic load induced on the myofibrils. For example, slow contractions against a heavy load induce hypertrophy of fast-twitch motor units. Fast contractions against a light load (if the metabolic demand is high) induce hypertrophy of slow-twitch motor units. It is not surprising then that stimulating a muscle with no load has little effect on the paralyzed muscle.

Over the past two decades a second electrical stimulation technology has developed. This type of technology is called closed-loop control. In closed-loop control sensors on the joints provide information to the stimulator to report the movement in a given muscle. In other words, the stimulation itself is modified to make sure that joints do not become hyperextended.

ACTIVE PHYSICAL THERAPY AND FUNCTIONAL ELECTRICAL STIMULATION

The technology using computer-controlled exercise has been called "active physical therapy." Unlike conventional physical therapy, active physical therapy requires patients to actively participate in the therapeutic modality, be it lifting weights or bicycling under computer control. Active physical therapy is meant to complement and not to replace passive physical therapy.

The simplest form of active physical therapy is weightlifting. For example, to exercise the quadriceps muscle, a subject sits in a special chair with electrodes placed across the muscle. With this type of device, electrical stimulation is provided alternatively to the different heads of the muscle (Figure 5.1). This accomplishes two things: First, it minimizes the fatigue in the muscle; and, second, by stimulating the heads of the muscle in turn, contractions are smooth and even across the muscle, thus preventing any torques that might result from an imbalanced contraction across the joint (Lind & Petrofsky, 1979; Petrofsky, 1978, 1979; Petrofsky & Phillips, 1979; Rack & Westbury, 1969). A bracelet is placed around the ankle and connected to a steel cable that joins the ankle through a series of pulleys to a weight pan. Therefore, during contraction of the muscle, as the leg extends weights can be lifted. A sensor in series with the weight pan helps coordinate the computer to stimulate the muscles in a manner resulting in smooth, slow contractions and that prevents hyperextension of the knee (Hendershot, Petrofsky, Phillips, & Moore, 1985; Petrofsky, Heaton, & Phillips, 1984; Phillips & Petrofsky, 1985). This type of apparatus can be used for most major muscle groups accessible to surface stimulation. However, while weightlifting is a good way to build muscular strength, it is a poor way to build muscular endurance. Once muscles have sufficient strength, individuals can engage in aerobic exercise with active physical therapy through the use of a modified bicycle ergometer.

A typical bicycle ergometer widely used in rehabilitation centers throughout the United States is that developed by Therapeutic Technologies, Inc., of Fort Lauderdale, Florida (Figure 5.2). This bicycle ergometer uses sensors to measure the position of the pedals for a computer-controlled multichannel electrical stimulator, a high-back seat to provide postural support, and special shoes to protect the ankle while cycling. These features

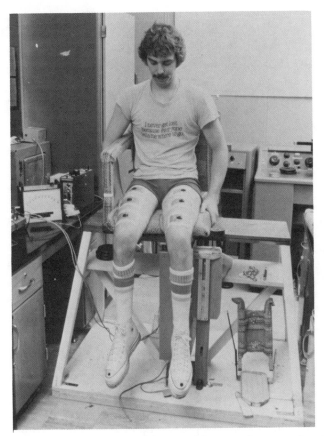

FIGURE 5.1 Isokinetic exerciser used for exercising muscles on paralyzed individuals.

help to provide smooth exercise and afford a good form of aerobic training (Petrofsky, Phillips, Heaton, & Glaser, 1984; Petrofsky, Phillips, & Hendershot, 1985).

An outdoor bicycle has been developed through research conducted by us. This particular bicycle (see Figure 5.3) incorporates many of the positive features of the indoor bicycle but uses a battery-operated computer and three wheels for balance (Petrofsky et al., 1983).

Biofeedback and Functional Electrical Stimulation

A final use of electrical stimulation for training purposes is the combined use of electrical stimulation with biofeedback techniques. Biofeedback has been used in treatment following stroke, partial spinal cord injury, and a number

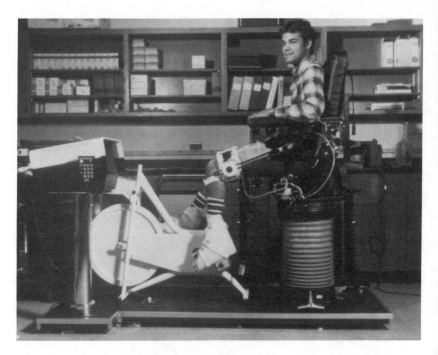

FIGURE 5.2 Bicycle ergometer manufactured by Therapeutic Technologies, Inc., being ridden by a T8-level complete paraplegic.

of other clinical disorders. The premise upon which the use of biofeedback with spinal cord-injured persons is predicated is based on the observation that some individuals with incomplete injuries can regain partial or complete function of the muscle through retraining the central nervous system and the spinal cord (Brucker, 1985; Petrofsky & Phillips, 1984). Biofeedback is obviously ineffective in 90% of the cases if there is permanent damage to the neural pathways. However, in about 10% of the cases it has proven effective in restoring some movement to the limbs. In addition, electrical stimulation, as cited above, offers the advantage of being a good way to build muscular strength. For an atrophied muscle in which no functional movement can be observed, biofeedback often results in an increase in electrical activity to the muscle with as little as a dozen training sessions. Functional movement, however, is not achieved via this method. Used together in treatment, electrical stimulation and biofeedback can result in strength and functional movement, and, in many cases, improved function. Subjects in the study described in Figure 5.4 had lesions at the C4, C5, and C6 levels.

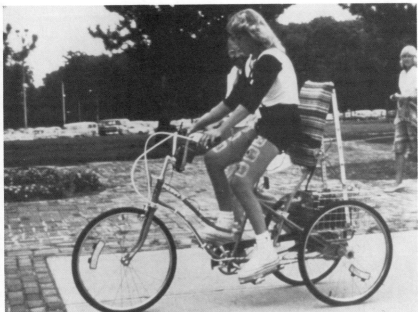

FIGURE 5.3 Outdoor bicycle with an onboard computer to elicit computer-controlled bicycling.

Physiological Effects of Active Physical Therapy

What are the physiological effects of active physical therapy? Obviously, muscles hypertrophy. With computer-controlled isokinetic weight lifting, weights are lifted at approximately 50% of the muscle's maximum strength, and muscle strength returns rapidly. Figure 5.5 illustrates the increase in strength in the quadriceps muscle achieved by four spinal cord-injured subjects. Figure 5.6 illustrates the increase of girth in the limb following 4 weeks of training during a 15-minute session conducted one, three, or five times per week. Four subjects were used in this study with lesions at the C6 to T10 levels. Exercise consisted of 6 seconds of slow contractions and 6 seconds of rest repeated for the 15-minute period. During such contractions, blood pressure increases. For example, Figure 5.7 presents the blood pressure response in 20 paraplegic and 20 quadriplegic subjects during electrically induced weight lifting. Both systolic and diastolic blood pressures increased throughout the exercise session. Heart rate, like blood pressure, also increased throughout computer-controlled exercise, as is shown for weight lifting in Figure 5.8. However, individual differences in

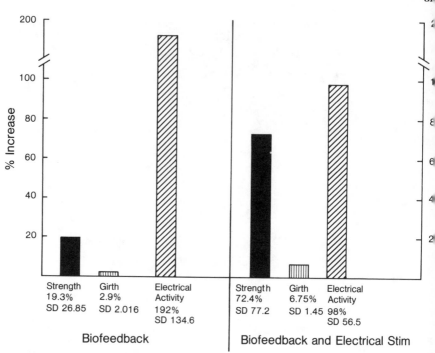

FIGURE 5.4 Increased forearm strength, forearm girth, and voluntary electrical activity with biofeedback alone compared with a combination of biofeedback and electrical stimulation. Change expressed as a percent of initial value.

heart rate and blood pressure are large. Generally, quadriplegics experience greater increases in blood pressure than paraplegics, while the reverse is true for heart rate during electrically induced exercise of the lower part of the body. Further, some individuals have a marked response to the exercise, while others respond modestly. Data presented in Figures 5.7 and 5.8 describe study outcomes where the percentage of duration was determined by normalizing the endurance time and where fatigue was determined when the muscle was unable to lift the weight in an arc of 60 degrees.

Benefits of Active Physical Therapy

Aside from physiological responses, such as increases in blood pressure and heart rate, what are the real, quantifiable health care benefits of active physical therapy? A study was recently conducted that included 51 subjects from the University of Miami; Wright State University; New Providence Hospital in Everett, Washington; the British Medical Council in London, England; and the Help Them Walk Again Foundation at the University of

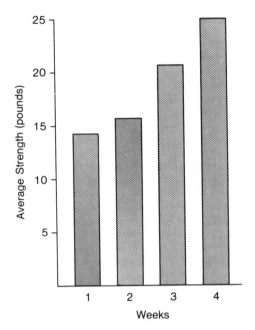

FIGURE 5.5 Increased quadricep strength associated with electrical stimulation of paralyzed muscle for a 15-minute session, once a day, three times a week.

Nevada—Las Vegas. Subjects underwent 1 year of bicycling, during which time they were carefully monitored for health care problems. Data obtained on them were then compared with those available on a group of 6,000 spinal cord-injured patients treated at the 17 national spinal cord injury centers (Young et al., 1982). Results of this study indicate that the incidence of pressure sores, fractures, kidney and bladder infections, and thrombophlebitis was reduced in subjects who maintained 15 minutes of exercise on a 3-day-per-week basis on the aerobic exercise system described above and shown in Figure 5.2. In addition, the incidence of pressure sores in the test group was significantly reduced.

Participation in the active physical therapy program also impacted health care costs. For example, not a single subject in the experimental group required hospitalization during the year. In contrast, the average health care costs, in 1985 dollars, of spinal cord-injured patients not in this program exceeded $12,000 per year, approximately $7,000 of which represented costs associated with hospitalization. The result of the reduction in fractures, kidney and bladder infections, and thrombophlebitis was a 90% decrease in medical costs. Extending these savings across the patient's life expectancy, use of active physical therapy can result in lifetime medical

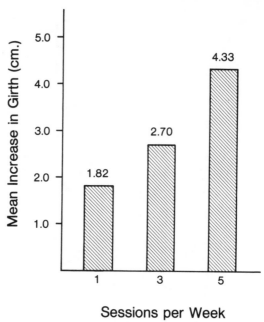

Sessions per Week

FIGURE 5.6 Increased girth of the quadriceps muscle with electrically induced exercise conducted for 15 minutes a day for either one, three, or five days per week.

savings that can exceed $2 million per patient. This also represents an annual savings of about $20 billion for the insurance industry over present medical costs.

Contraindications for Active Physical Therapy

Any type of technology or treatment, including active physical therapy, can have contraindications. For example, as shown in Figure 5.9, the maximum sweat rate (mean body sweat rate) during heat exposure and exercise (25 watts of work) at environmental temperatures of 30, 35, and 40°C resulted in significantly lower maximum sweat rates for quadriplegics than for paraplegics and control subjects (Petrofsky & Phillips, 1984). These lower sweat rates, which result from paralysis of the sweat glands, elicited a sharp rise in core temperature in paraplegic and quadriplegic subjects during these heat exposures at 25 watts of work (Figure 5.10). The overall result was that quadriplegics, when working at high temperatures and high humidities, became poikilothermic even during mild work. Therefore, these types of therapies must be avoided in hot, humid environments with individuals who have significantly impaired thermoregulatory systems.

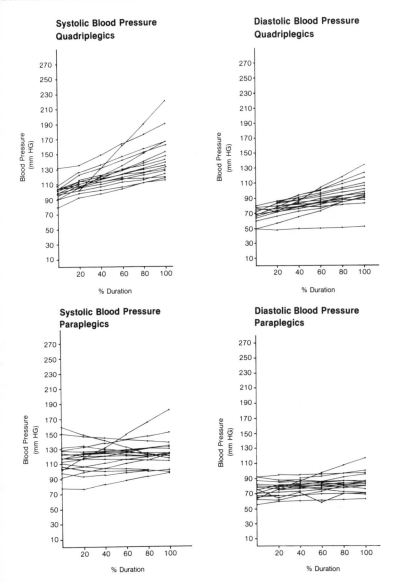

FIGURE 5.7 Blood pressure response in 20 paraplegic and 20 quadriplegic subjects associated with computer-controlled weight training of the quadriceps muscle. Work was set to fatigue the subject in 15 minutes.

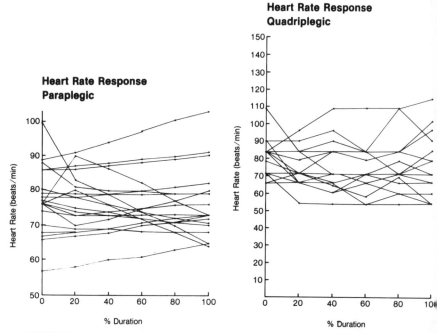

FIGURE 5.8 Heart rate response in 20 paraplegic and 20 quadriplegic subjects associated with computer-controlled weight training of the quadriceps muscle. Work was set to fatigue the subject in 15 minutes.

COMPUTER-CONTROLLED WALKING

Another application of electrical stimulation is the restoration of ambulation and movement in the hands in paralyzed individuals. Several laboratories have experimented with electrical stimulation in an attempt to restore a degree of primitive grasp and hand function in paralyzed individuals (Peckham et al., 1976; Peckham, Mortimer & Van der Meulen, 1973; Petrofsky & Phillips, 1984, 1985). However, the most exciting advances in electrical stimulation in terms of functional movement have been associated with walking.

The objectives of any research program working with functional electrical stimulation for ambulation should be to develop a system that is easy to use, cosmetic, and permits a number of different tasks to be completed that are difficult to perform from a wheelchair. Walking should be done at a speed that compares favorably to that achieved while using a wheelchair. The system should require low maintenance but be highly reliable, capable of protecting the user from falls in case of system failures, and provide good

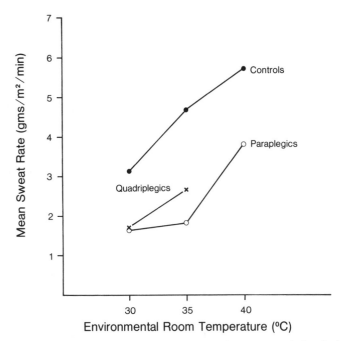

FIGURE 5.9 Mean body sweat rates (*top*: resting; *bottom*: exercise) calculated for typical paraplegic, quadriplegic, and normal subjects during work in heat. Work consisted of armcrank ergometry at a load of 25 watts with varying environmental room temperatures, and a relative humidity of 50%.

coordination and balance. Estimates based on data obtained from surveys conducted by us indicate that a practical system must be put on and taken off in less than 5 minutes and be cosmetically acceptable to the wearer. The walking speed must be a minimum of 1 mile an hour (preferably 2 miles an hour), and walking distance should exceed 1 mile with good energy efficiency.

While these criteria can be met by utilizing a number of different approaches, a primary issue confronting investigators is whether the system should be implantable or external. Implantable systems currently are being investigated by Marsolais (1985); Holle et al., (1984); and Petrofsky and associates (e.g., Petrofsky et al. 1984; Petrofsky, Phillips, Glaser, & Heaton, 1983; Petrofsky, Phillips, Larsen, & Douglas, 1985). External stimulation systems are being developed by Kralj and his colleagues (e.g., Kralj, Bajd, & Turk, 1980; Kralj & Jaeger, 1982); and Petrofsky and others (e.g., Petrofsky, 1978, 1979, in press; Petrofsky, Heaton, & Phillips, 1984; Petrofsky, Phillips & Hendershot, in press). An implantable system, by nature, would mask most of the wiring associated with activating muscles

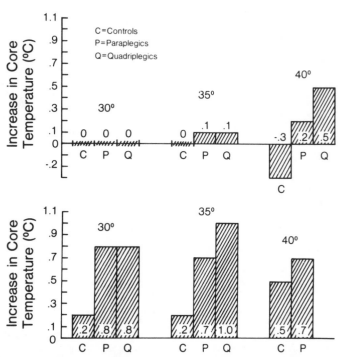

FIGURE 5.10 Increased core body temperature in typical paraplegic and quadriplegic subjects at rest and exercise during exposure to varying room temperatures at 50% relative humidity.

and presumably make the system more attractive. However, a problem for all implantable systems, be it a pacemaker or computer-controlled walking device, is the underdeveloped nature of the technology itself. In the last few years, the pacemaker industry has suffered a number of setbacks related to the fact that lead wires generally begin to malfunction after 3 to 5 years. For the average spinal cord-injured individual, who acquires his or her injury at age 17, a system must be practical and functional for at least 30 to 40 years if repeated surgeries to replace malfunctioning equipment are to be avoided. Stimulation of all the major muscle groups in the legs may require as many as 100 electrodes. This number of electrodes in an implantable system requires extensive surgery. Further, the high surface area of all the wiring increases the risk of cyst formation and lead-wire breakage. For example, Marsolais and his colleagues have published data that demonstrate that on the average 2.5% of their electrodes break per month, requiring surgical intervention to replace the electrodes at least every few years (E. B. Marsolais, personal communication, 1985; Marsolais, in press). This high incidence of electrode breakage and a mean electrode life of not greater than 3 years for the best electrode would require continuous extensive surgery if this type of package is to be used in a practical way (Phillips, in press). Thus, lead-wire breakage is a problem that must be resolved before an implantable system becomes a practical reality.

Walking with open-loop control systems always has required a very high level of energy consumption (Chizeck, 1985, Kralj & Jaeger, 1982; Marsolais, 1985). For example, Marsolais has presented data showing the energy consumption to be as high as 20 times above that for normal standing and walking when stimulating muscles with open-loop control (Marsolais, 1985). Their best subject has only been able to walk 20 feet with crutches and, at best, 700 or 800 feet with a walker prior to becoming totally fatigued. To avoid this problem, a closed-loop control system has been used in our own laboratory.

Some coordinated movement can be obtained with closed-loop control systems using either internal electrodes (e.g., Petrofsky & Phillips, 1984, 1985) or external stimulation (e.g., Petrofsky, 1979; Petrofsky et al., 1983). Closed-loop control systems use just enough activity in muscles to obtain the coordinated movement necessary for standing or walking. With this type of system, energy efficiency is high and walking is done with good posture over long distances. A closed-loop control system is under development by Marsolais and his colleagues (Chizeck, 1985). Using closed-loop control, however, even with an implantable system, requires external bracing to mount sensors (Chizeck, 1985). Currently there is no sensor available that can be placed inside the body and remain functional over an extended period without corroding from tissue fluids. Therefore, as a result of limitations in technology, even with an implantable system, part of the package must remain external.

In work conducted by us at the Wright State University's National Center for Rehabilitation Engineering (Dayton, Ohio), we have been developing systems using a combination of electrical stimulation and sensors for feedback control. Initially the system used a series of discreet electrodes on the surface of the body with as many as 36 electrodes being placed over the lower part of the body and as many as 100 wires leading to a small computer, which allowed subjects to walk under computer control (see Figure 5.11) (Petrofsky, Phillips, & Heaton, 1984). This type of closed-loop control proved to be efficient and allowed subjects to walk substantial distances. It was, however, unattractive and difficult to use. In an attempt to make it more reliable, a hybrid system was developed (see Figure 5.12).

A major component of this hybrid system is the Louisiana State University Reciprocating Gait Orthosis (LSU RGO) (Douglas, Larson, & D'Aubrosia, 1983). In their original form these braces were designed primarily to facilitate walking in children with spina bifida and cerebral palsy, as well as

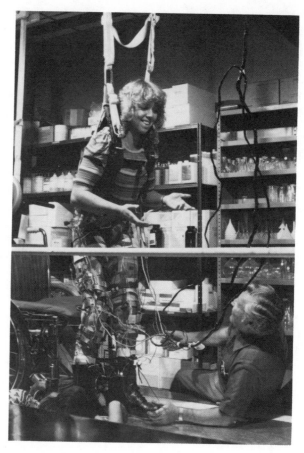

FIGURE 5.11 Early walking system using closed-loop system.

spinal cord-injured individuals. One might think that spinal cord-injured persons with high-level lesions, minimal energy, and poorly developed upper-body strength would be unable to ambulate in braces such as these. However, it was possible for them to do so for considerable distances.

A principal advantage of using the LSU RGO is the postural stability it provides. Postural stability is one of the highest energy-consuming components of a walking system. By using the LSU RGO for postural stability and the concomitant advantages of its reciprocating gait action, electrical stimulation can be added to form a hybrid system that works more efficiently (Petrofsky et al., in press; Petrofsky, Phillips, Larsen, & Douglas, 1985).

If the electrical system completely malfunctions while the subject is wearing the braces, he or she cannot fall because the braces provide postural

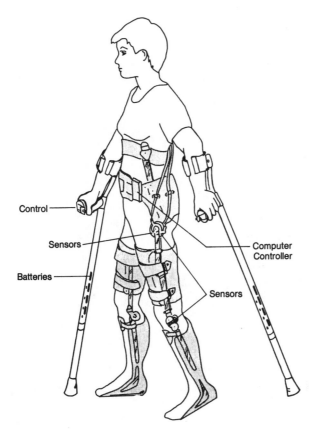

Control

Sensors

Batteries

Computer
Controller

Sensors

FIGURE 5.12 Hybrid walking system.

stability and serve as an emergency backup system. The subject still can walk to his or her car without stimulation and get home. This factor dramatically increases the system's reliability.

Further, with the LSU RGO joints are protected from adverse torques and turning. Since there are hundreds of muscles in the lower part of the body, it is impossible to stimulate enough of them to prevent torque and rotation in all the joints, thus increasing the potential for damage. With the RGO, the stability afforded by the brace itself makes walking safer and more efficient.

To eliminate the need for electrodes, a garment was developed by Bio-Stimu Trend Corporation of Opa Locka, Florida (Granek & Granek, 1985) that subjects could wear to electrically stimulate their muscles (Figure 5.13). This garment uses conductive threads connected to electrodes that are sewn in the garment and placed over the major muscle groups in the

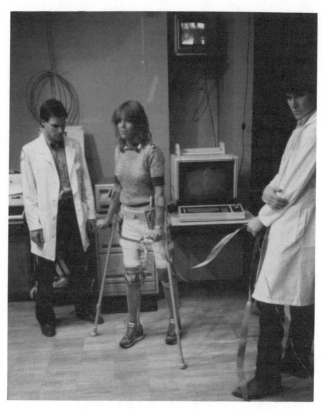

FIGURE 5.13 Paraplegic walking with Lofstrand canes in the combined RGO-FES walking system.

lower part of the body. The garment is elastic, and individuals simply slip it on like tightfitting underwear. One plug connects the garment to a small computer controller and the muscles are then activated. Sensors are placed on the braces to provide a full closed-loop control system. Walking speeds in excess of 2 miles an hour have been achieved by most of the subjects using the combined system (Petrofsky et al., in press). Further, since the power for walking is supplied by stimulating the lower leg muscles, very little weight is carried on the arms during steps. With the combined system and computer-controlled electrical stimulation, paralyzed individuals are able to accomplish tasks like going up and down ramps and steps, walking on uneven surfaces or wet surfaces such as snow, and engaging in many types of recreational activities such as golf. Recently, a paralyzed female in the project (T4 paraplegic, complete injury) used the system to walk the first 7 miles in the Honolulu Marathon (see Figure 5.14).

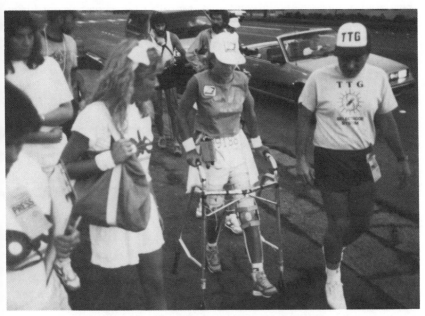

FIGURE 5.14 Paraplegic with hybrid walking system participating in the Honolulu Marathon (a total of 7 miles walked in 5 hours).

The hybrid walking system being experimented with in our Laboratory can be put on and taken off (complete with the electrically conductive clothing) in less than 5 minutes and be worn under clothing without being seen. It affords smooth, coordinated walking with a minimum of maintenance, high reliability, and an emergency backup in case of computer failure. Further, energy consumption levels are similar to those recorded in walking able-bodied individuals (Petrofsky, in press; Petrofsky, Phillips, & Hendershot, 1985).

Obviously, a great deal of additional work must be done to make the hybrid LSU RGO developed by us wholly functional. For example, with the electronics package, the present weight of the braces is approximately 8 pounds. We are attempting to reduce the system's weight by at least 50% by changing the structure of the orthosis. At least one half to two thirds of the existing structure of the brace can be removed and customized for a computer-controlled walking system. With continued development an initial commercial product should be available within the next 5 years.

In summary, electrical stimulation has come a long way in the last 30 years. It offers a wide range of health care applications from pain management, treatment of scoliosis, and reversal of muscle atrophy to more complex applications involving computer-controlled bicycling, weight lifting, and walking by spinal cord-injured individuals. However, only additional development of this technology will determine if such systems can become sufficiently practical for use by the consumer. Hopefully, that future is near.

REFERENCES

Basett, C. A. L., & Becker, R. A. (1962). Generation of electrical potential by bone in response to mechanical stress. *Science, 137*, 1063–1064.

Brucker, B. (1985). Biofeedback and FES to improve function. *Paraplegia News, 39*(12), 32–35.

Chizeck, H. J. (1985). Helping paraplegics walk: Looking beyond the media blitz. *Technology Review, 88*, 54–63.

Douglas, R., Larson, D., & D'Aubrosia, R. (1983). LSU reciprocating gait orthosis. *Orthopedics, 6*, 834–839.

Faden, A. I., Jacobs, T. P., Feuerstein, G., & Holiday, J. W. (1981). Dopamine partially mediated the cardiovascular effects of noloxone after spinal injury. *Brain Research, 213*, 415–421.

Goldsmith, H., Stewart, E., Chen, W. F., & Duckett, S. (1982). Application of intact omentum to the normal and traumatized spinal cord. In C. Rao (Ed.), *Spinal cord reconstruction.* New York: Raven Press.

Granek, H., & Granek, M. (1985). Transcutaneous transducer garments: Current mammalian usage and future applications. *Journal of Neurological and Orthopaedic Medicine and Surgery, 6*, 271–278.

Guttman, L. (1976). *Spinal cord injuries: Comprehensive management and research* (2nd ed.). Oxford, England: Blackwell Scientific.

Hambrecht, F. T., & Reswick, J. (1977). *Functional electrical stimulation.* New York: Marcel Decker.

Hendershot, D., Petrofsky, J. S., Phillips, C. A., & Moore, M. (1985). Blood pressure and heart responses in paralyzed and non-paralyzed man during isokinetic leg training. *Journal of Neurological and Orthopaedic Medicine and Surgery, 6*, 259–264.

Holle, J., Gruber, H., Frey, M., Kern, H., Stohn, H., & Thoma, H. (1984). Functional electrical stimulation in paraplegics. *Orthopedics, 7*, 1145–1160.

Hudlicka, O., Brown, M., Cotter, M., Smith, M., & Vrobova, G. (1977). The effect of long-term stimulation of fast muscles on their blood flow, metabolism and ability to withstand fatigue. *Pflugers Archives: European Journal of Physiology, 37*, 141.

Kao, C., Bunge, R., & Reier, P. (1982). *Spinal cord reconstruction.* New York: Raven Press.

Kralj, A., Bajd, T., & Turk, R. (1980). Electrical stimulation providing functional use of paraplegic patient muscles. *Medical Progress and Technology, 7*, 3–15.

Kralj, A., & Jaeger, R. J. (1982). Posture switching enables prolonged standing in paraplegic subjects functionally electrically stimulated. *Proceedings of the Fifth Annual Conference on Rehabilitation Engineering*, Houston, Texas.

Lind, A. R., & Petrofsky, J. S. (1979). The amplitude of the surface electromyogram during fatiguing isometric contractions. *Muscle and Nerve, 2*, 257–264.

Marsolais, E. B. (in press). Letter to the editor. *Journal of Neurological and Orthopaedic Medicine and Surgery.*

Naftchi, N. F. (1982). Functional restoration of the traumatically injured spinal cord in cuts by clonidine. *Science, 217,* 1042–1044.

Peckham, P. H., Mortimer, J. T., & Van der Meulen, J. P. (1973). Physiologic and metabolic changes in shite muscle of cat following induced exercise. *Brain Research, 50,* 524.

Peckham, P. H., Mortimer, J. T., & Marsolais, E. B. (1976). Alteration in the force and fatiguability of skeletal muscle in quadriplegic humans following exercise induced by chronic electrical stimulation. *Clinical Orthopedics, 114,* 326.

Perkins, C. S., Aquayo, A. J., & Bray, C. M. (1981). Behavior of schwann cells from trembler mouse unmyelinated fibers transplanted into myelinated nerves. *Experimental Neurology, 71,* 515–526.

Petrofsky, J. S. (1978). Control of the recruitment and firing frequencies of motor units in electrically stimulated muscles in the cat. *Medical and Biological Engineering and Computing, 16,* 302–308.

Petrofsky, J. S. (1979). Sequential motor unit stimulation through peripheral motor nerves in the cat. *Medical and Biological Engineering and Computing, 17,* 87–93.

Petrofsky, J. S. (in press). Functional electrical stimulation (FES) and its application to the rehabilitation of neurologically injured individuals. In R. Finger (Ed.), *Theoretical and controversial issues in recovery after brain damage.* New York: Plenum Press.

Petrofsky, J. S., & Phillips, C. A. (1979). Constant velocity contractions in skeletal muscle by sequential stimulation of muscle efferents. *Medical and Biological Engineering and Computing, 17,* 583–592.

Petrofsky, J. S., & Phillips, C. A. (1984). Closed-loop control for restoration of movement in paralyzed muscle. *Orthopaedics, 7,* 1289–1302.

Petrofsky, J. S., & Phillips, C. A. (1985). Feedback control stimulation to achieve movement in man. *Electronika, 14,* 53–60.

Petrofsky, J. S., Heaton, H. H., & Phillips, C. A. (1983). Outdoor bicycle for exercise in paraplegics and quadriplegics. *Journal of Biomedical Engineering, 5,* 296–297.

Petrofsky, J. S., & Phillips, C. A., Glaser, R. M., & Heaton, H. (1983). Application of the Apple as a microprocessor-controlled stimulator. *Collegiate Microcomputer, 1,* 97–104.

Petrofsky, J. S., Heaton, H. H., & Phillips, C. A. (1984). Leg exerciser for training of paralyzed muscle by closed-loop control. *Medical and Biological Engineering and Computing, 22,* 298–303.

Petrofsky, J. S., & Phillips, C. A., & Heaton, H. H. (1984). Feedback control system for walking in man. *Computing in Biology and Medicine, 14,* 135–149.

Petrofsky, J. S., & Phillips, C. A., Heaton, H. H., & Glaser, R. M. (1984). Bicycle ergometer for paralyzed muscle. *Journal Clinical Engineering, 9,* 13–19.

Petrofsky, J. S., & Phillips, C. A. & Hendershot, D. (1985). The cardiovascular stresses which occur during dynamic exercise in paraplegics and quadriplegics. *Journal of Neurological and Orthopaedic Medicine and Surgery, 6,* 252–258.

Petrofsky, J. S., & Phillips, C. A., & Hendershot, D. (in press). Cardiovascular responses of paralyzed individuals during electrically induced isokinetic exercise. *European Journal of Applied Physiology.*

Petrofsky, J. S., & Phillips, C. A., Larson, P., & Douglas, R. (1985). Computer synthesized walking: An application of orthosis and functional electrical stimulation (FES). *Journal of Neurological and Orthopaedic Medicine and Surgery, 6,* 219–230.

Pette, D., Smith, M. E., Staudte, H. W., & Vrobova, G. (1973). Effects of long-term

electrical stimulation on some contractile and metabolic characteristics of fa
rabbit muscle. *Pfleugers Archives: European Journal of Physiology, 338*, 257–27.

Pette, D., Ramirez, B., Müller, W., Simon, R., Exner, G. U., & Hildebrand, R
(1975). Influence of the intermittent long-term stimulation on contractile
histochemical and metabolic properties of fibre population in fast and slow
rabbit muscles. *Pflugers Archives: European Journal of Physiology, 361*, 1–7.

Phillips, C. A. (in press). Reply to a Letter to the Editor. *Journal of Neurology an
Orthopedic Medicine and Surgery.*

Phillips, C. A., & Petrofsky, J. S. (1985). A review of fracture cases in spinal cor
injured individuals participating in closed-loop functional electrical stimulatio
(FES) experiments. *Journal of Neurological and Orthopaedic Medicine and Surger,
6*, 247–251.

Rack, P. M. H., & Westbury, D. R. (1969). The effects of length and stimulus rat
on tension in the isometric cat soleus muscle. *Journal of Physiology, 204*, 443
460.

Rowley, B., Roman, G. C., Strahlendorf, H. K., & Chung, W. F. (1985). Electrica
resistance in low level direct current enhancement of sciatic nerve regeneration
Journal of Neurological and Orthopaedic Medicine and Surgery, 6, 279–281.

Salmons, S., & Vrobova, C. (1969). The influence of activity on some contractil
characteristics of mammalian fast and slow muscles. *Journal of Physiology, 201*
535.

Young, J. S., Burns, P. E., Bowen, A. M., & McCutcheon, R. (1982). *Spinal cor
injury statistics: Experience of regional spinal cord injury systems.* Phoenix, AZ
Good Samaritan Medical Center.

6

Advances in Electromyographic Monitoring and Biofeedback in the Treatment of Chronic Cervical and Low Back Pain

Susan J. Middaugh
William G. Kee

Electromyographic (EMG) biofeedback procedures are currently well recognized and routinely employed as useful treatment components in many rehabilitation programs, and both clinical experience and the research literature are rapidly expanding (Middaugh, 1982a, b, c; Basmajian, 1983). Most of the clinical applications involve relatively simple treatment procedures in two major areas of application. One major area is therapeutic exercise. EMG feedback procedures are primarily used to increase motor unit recruitment or improve muscle relaxation in an individual muscle or muscle group, and a series of well-controlled experimental studies carried out in our laboratory support this use (Middaugh, 1978; Middaugh & Miller, 1980; Middaugh, Miller, & Foster, 1982a; Middaugh, Miller, Foster, & Ferndon, 1982b; Middaugh, Miller, Foster, & Pien, 1982c; Middaugh, Miller, Foster, & Murphy, 1981). The second major area is treatment of musculoskeletal pain. In these applications EMG biofeedback

This research was supported in part by the General Clinical Research Center at the Medical University of South Carolina and N. I. H. Grant #RR1070.

procedures are often directed toward teaching generalized relaxation for stress reduction and pain management. Such biofeedback procedures have become a standard treatment component of behaviorally oriented pain management programs (DeGood, 1979; Libo & Arnold, 1983) as well as multidisciplinary chronic pain rehabilitation programs (Gottlieb, Alperson, Koller, & Hockersmith, 1979; Gottlieb et al., 1977; Jessup, 1984; Keefe, 1981; NIDA, 1981).

These basic clinical EMG biofeedback procedures can be carried out with relatively simple equipment. Typically, a commercially available, single channel EMG biofeedback device is employed to electronically record, filter, amplify, and integrate the EMG signal. This processed EMG signal is converted to an auditory signal or visual display that provides the patient with immediate and continuous information to guide voluntary, trial and error attempts to increase or decrease muscle contractions.

At present, biofeedback instrumentation, biofeedback treatment techniques, and clinical research are rapidly advancing well beyond these initial, basic, and very useful biofeedback procedures. This chapter will present recent work in the clinical research and patient treatment programs of the Biofeedback Laboratory in the Department of Physical Medicine and Rehabilitation at the Medical University of South Carolina (MUSC). This work is in an area that holds particular promise for widespread clinical application—EMG monitoring and EMG biofeedback for dynamic evaluation and treatment of muscles at the site of pain in patients with chronic cervical and low back pain.

MUSCLE SPASM AND THE PAIN CYCLE

Since the earliest days of biofeedback there has been considerable interest in the use of EMG biofeedback procedures in treatment of musculoskeletal pain syndromes (Budzynski, Stoyva, & Adler, 1970; Fowler & Kraft, 1974; Grabel, 1973; Jacobs & Felton, 1969). The underlying assumption is that sustained muscle contraction is a causative or contributory factor that initiates or perpetuates the pain. Based on this assumption, EMG biofeedback treatment procedures are designed to teach voluntary muscle relaxation and, by so doing, reduce or eliminate the muscle contraction and ameliorate the pain.

This assumption, and this treatment approach, are based on a widely held theory in which muscle spasm plays a prominant role. Pain, often from an initial trauma, is thought to trigger reflexive muscle contraction or "spasm." The muscle spasm, in turn, produces further pain to initiate a pain/spasm/ pain cycle (Calliett, 1981; Cobb, de Vries, Urban, Luekens, & Bagg, 1975; Simons, 1975, 1976; Travell, 1960). According to this theory the pain cycle may begin with acute trauma to the muscle, its connective tissue, or nearby skeletal structures. A more gradual onset of pain may come with musculo-skeletal strain caused by poor posture or repeated muscle overload during daily activities at home or on the job. Psychological stress is also regarded as an important initiating factor. Stress is thought to increase generalized physiological arousal, and this then leads to an increase in muscle tension, which, at a certain point, triggers episodes of sustained muscle spasm and pain (AMA, 1962; Holmes & Wolff, 1952; Jessup, 1984; Loeser, 1980; Whatmore & Kohli, 1974).

Once initiated, the pain cycle is thought to be further fueled and perpetu-ated by these same factors. Sustained muscle contractions are known to impair circulation, and reduced circulation within the painful muscle is thought to be an important contributor to chronic pain (Barcroft & Millen, 1939; Dorpat & Holmes, 1955; Mills, Newham, & Edwards, 1984; Rohter & Hyman, 1962). Microtrauma to muscle fibers has been found with chronic myalgia and has been attributed to localized ischemia (Fassbender, 1975). Posture typically worsens as the patient "gives in" to the pain and attempts to avoid movement of painful areas by adopting an antalgic posture while sitting, standing, and walking. Muscle overload and fatigue become prominent factors as muscles become weaker because of reduced activity levels. Psychological stress can increase as pain and physical debility disrupt the individual's daily activities and interpersonal relationships. These per-petuating factors are thought to play an important role in chronic pain syndromes.

EMG BIOFEEDBACK INTERVENTION IN THE PAIN CYCLE

Biofeedback procedures can be designed to intervene in this pain cycle in several different ways. Biofeedback procedures can be directed primarily toward stress management and related psychological factors such as percep-tion of self-control and the ability to cope. This is perhaps the most frequently offered rationale for the widespread use of EMG feedback proce-dures using frontalis muscle electrode placements in pain programs today (Jessup, 1984; Phillips, 1978).

Biofeedback procedures can also be designed to intervene more directly in the pain cycle by teaching relaxation of the specific painful muscles that are presumed to be in sustained contraction. Until recently this has also been a frequent rationale for EMG biofeedback procedures using frontalis place-ments. The muscles of facial expression were thought to reflect the general level of muscle activity throughout the body. Therefore, procedures that trained relaxation of these key muscles were thought to effectively train relaxation of all other muscles as well, including the muscles assumed to be in spasm in the neck or low back areas. Experimental studies and clinical observations have thoroughly discredited this notion (Carlson, Basilo, & Heaukulani, 1983; Cotton & Lawson, 1982; Whatmore, Whatmore, & Fisher, 1981). Frontalis biofeedback effectively produces relaxation only in scalp, facial, and jaw muscles (with perhaps some limited effect on cervical muscles as well) since these are all within the actual area of surface EMG recording (Basmajian, 1976). It is now recognized that there is no one muscle that reflects general muscle tension; and, in fact, there is quite probably no such thing as general muscle tension (Cotton & Lawson, 1982). Recent clinical and research interest has shifted emphatically toward the use of site-specific electrode placements and EMG biofeedback procedures that directly train relaxation of muscles within the areas of pain.

Biofeedback procedures can theoretically intervene in the pain cycle in two additional ways that are just beginning to attract clinical and experimental attention. Thermal biofeedback, using site-specific thermister placements, is a potentially useful tool in improving circulation in areas of noninflammatory musculoskeletal pain (Rouleau & Denver, 1980). Travell and Simons (1983) have emphasized the autonomic nervous system components of pain syndromes, which include vasoconstriction, yet few studies have addressed this aspect of chronic musculoskeletal pain. There is also considerable promise in the use of EMG biofeedback, using site-specific electrode placements, as a method for postural retraining to correct antalgic posture and gait. This is one of the more promising new uses of EMG biofeedback in use in our Chronic Pain Rehabilitation Program (Middaugh & Kee, 1984 a,b).

EMG biofeedback procedures that are based on the concept of intervention in a pain/spasm/pain cycle have met with substantial success in the treatment of muscle contraction headache (Blanchard, Jaccard, Andrasik, Guarieri, & Jurish, 1985; Jessup, 1984; Sharpley & Rogers, 1984). These procedures, which typically use forehead or posterior cervical electrode placements, are currently in wide use and are considered by many to be the treatment of choice for this condition, in the hands of an experienced clinician. There is considerable debate as to whether these EMG biofeedback procedures do, as assumed, teach relaxation of the specific facial, cervical, and scalp muscles thought to be responsible for triggering tension headaches or whether they primarily teach stress management; however, there is good agreement that clinical efficacy has been well demonstrated. Reviews of this extensive literature and current issues can be found in Holmes & Burish (1983), Phillips (1978), and Turner & Chapman (1982).

EMG biofeedback procedures based on the concept of interruption of a pain/spasm/pain cycle have met with considerably less success in treatment of chronic cervical and low back pain. In these treatment applications EMG biofeedback procedures are designed to directly intervene by training relaxation of muscles presumed to be in spasm in the areas of pain. However, clinical and experimental biofeedback studies have been surprisingly few in number, and the results of these studies have been problematical.

Two major impediments can account for the retarded development of effective, site-specific EMG biofeedback procedures for treatment of chronic cervical and low back pain. One major problem is that specialized clinical knowledge, specialized EMG recording equipment, and specialized biofeedback treatment techniques are required. Many different muscle groups are located within the relevant areas of pain, and considerable anatomical "know how" is required for selection of appropriate electrode placements. Clinical time constraints have dictated that equipment with two or more independent EMG recording channels or equipment with a capacity for muscle scanning (Cram & Steger, 1983) be used, and these equipment options are just beginning to be commercially available at accessible cost. Appropriate clinical treatment techniques also have been slow to develop. Most attempts at site-specific EMG biofeedback training for lumbar muscle relaxation, for example, have been carried out with the patient sitting still in a recliner because this has been the usual method for frontalis relaxation training. This position, in and of itself, greatly minimizes muscle activity in these postural low back muscles and leaves the patient with little to learn. Obviously, new treatment procedures that are more appropriate for cervical and low back pain patients need to be developed.

The second major impediment to progress has been the muscle spasm itself. This presumed culprit, which site-specific EMG biofeedback procedures are intended to eliminate, has proven to be quite elusive. The term "muscle spasm" usually implies a reflex contraction of muscles surrounding an area of injury (Mills, Newham, & Edwards, 1984). This is very evident, and can be very useful, in an acute injury when reflexive muscle spasm acts to immobilize the painful area to prevent further damage (Morris, Gasteiger, & Chatfield, 1957). However, there is little evidence that acute muscle spasm becomes chronic or that sustained; reflexive muscle contractions are actually present in patients with chronic cervical or low back pain. In multiple studies EMG measures of lumbar muscle activity in patients with low back pain have been compared with normal nonpatient control subjects. The results of these studies indicate that there are no consistent differences in mean quantitative EMG values in back pain patients as compared with normal controls, either at rest or during test movements. From this rapidly growing literature, it is apparent that EMG activity in chronic low back pain patients can be elevated, equal to, or below normal levels (Collins, Cohen, Naliboff, & Shandler, 1982; Hoyt, Hunt, et al., 1981; Miller, 1985; Sherman, 1985; Wolf, Basmajian, Russe, & Kutchner, 1979; Wolf, Nacht, & Kelly, 1982). Nouwen and Bush (1984), in an excellent review of current research on the relationship between paraspinal EMG and chronic low back pain, concluded that "the most striking point about this research is its lack of consensus." They further concluded that "were there consistent differences in absolute EMG levels these would by now have become apparent." It is not surprising, then, that the results of published studies on the use of EMG biofeedback procedures in treatment of patients with chronic low back pain, based on the presumption of muscle spasm, are also conflicting and inconclusive.

Clinical Case Reports

Published clinical case reports have been promising (Belar & Cohen, 1979; Jones & Wolf, 1980; Nigl & Fischer-Williams, 1980). In these studies, patients with chronic back pain have been taught to relax the relevant back muscles, typically the lumbar paraspinous muscles, using EMG biofeedback procedures. These patients (six in the three reports) have reported reductions in pain that appear to be well-correlated with learned muscle relaxation. The clinical value of these gains has been verified by concurrent reductions in pain medication and improvements in physical function. These reports are interesting but little can be concluded, if only because failures are seldom published (although one unsuccessful case has been reported by Todd & Belar, 1980). It is also relevant that these individual patients were selected as being particularly appropriate for a trial of EMG training by history and/or examination. Quite likely because of such selection, EMG values were found to be high prior to treatment in five of the six reported cases, and substantial reductions in EMG levels were obtained with relaxation training. These case reports do suggest that there are individual patients with elevated EMG, and for these patients EMG feedback procedures may be appropriate and effective.

Experimental Studies

Experimental studies of groups of patients provide a substantially different picture. In a number of studies EMG biofeedback has been used to directly train relaxation of lumbar paraspinous muscles in groups of patients with chronic low back pain in multiple sessions (8 to 20), conducted over a period of weeks (2 to 5) (Bush, Ditto, & Feuerstein, 1985; Flor, Haag, Turk, & Koehler, 1983; Freeman, Calsyn, Paige, & Halar, 1980; Nouwen, 1983; Nouwen & Solinger, 1979; Peck & Kraft, 1977). Two of these studies also included an unspecified number of patients with cervical/shoulder girdle pain for whom an upper trapezius training site was used (Flor et al., 1983; Peck & Kraft, 1977).

It is clear from these experimental studies that EMG biofeedback is highly effective in training relaxation of target muscles. In each of these studies EMG feedback groups showed EMG evidence of acquired muscle relaxation (or bidirectional muscle control, Bush et al., 1985), even in one study that trained reductions in lumbar muscle EMG during prolonged, and painful, standing (Nouwen, 1983). At the same time, EMG levels remained unchanged in untreated control groups (Nouwen, 1983; Nouwen & Solinger, 1979) as well as in pseudotherapy and medically treated groups (Flor et al., 1983). The exception is a single study in which the EMG biofeedback group, a placebo treatment group, and even a waiting list control group showed reductions in sitting and standing EMG measures from pre-test to post-test (Bush et al., 1985). This unusual finding suggests that repeated measurement, spontaneous improvement over time, or self-treatment stimulated by entry into a research protocol were the primary operative factors. Such factors are most likely to affect outcome in subjects with comparatively mild back problems such as those selected for the Bush et al. study.

It is also evident from these studies that elevated EMG levels are not a universal problem in chronic pain patients during quiet sitting, prone lying, or standing. In three studies (Flor et al., 1983; Freeman et al., 1980; Nouwen, 1983) subjects were selected for elevated EMG, indicating that above-normal EMG levels were not consistently found, and, in fact, had to be sought out. Freeman et al. (1980) observed that many potential patients referred for their study were not included because of "lack of significant EMG readings." Bush et al. (1985) noted that " . . . fewer than 10 subjects appeared to have abnormally high levels of EMG at the pretreatment assessment." This is only 15% of the 66 subjects in their study. In all but one study (Nouwen, 1983) training was carried out in a sitting or prone lying position. As far as can be determined, based on information provided concerning electrode placements and amplifier characteristics, EMG levels in these positions were relatively low, and learned reductions in EMG were necessarily small.

It is not surprising, then, that the outcomes of these studies primarily indicate that learned reductions in EMG levels during static training in a sitting, prone lying, or standing position are neither necessary nor sufficient for reducing pain or achieving clinical gains. In two studies (Nouwen, 1983; Peck & Kraft, 1977) EMG reductions were obtained without concomitant reductions in reported pain or other clinical change (Peck & Kraft noted reduced pain in 1 of their 8 subjects). In the one study that provides outcome data for individual subjects, Freeman et al. (1980) reported pain reductions and substantial clinical gains (increased activity, return to work or school) in 6 of 8 low back pain patients trained in relaxation of lumbosacral paraspinous muscles. However, two of their improved patients had very low EMG levels prior to training and did not achieve appreciable

EMG reductions. This suggests that learned alterations in lumbar EMG may have had little to do with the favorable clinical outcome. The role of acquired muscle relaxation is also questioned by Nouwen and Solinger (1970). They reported reductions in lumbar paraspinous EMG levels, decreases in low back pain, and functional gains in a single group of 18 EMG feedback subjects, while 7 waiting-list control subjects showed no change. At 3-month follow-up, however, EMG levels had increased to pretraining levels, while pain reductions and concomitant clinical gains were generally well maintained and even improved for some subjects.

Two studies with placebo or alternative treatment control groups also provide little evidence for a specific EMG feedback effect. Bush et al. (1985) found that subjects with low back pain who received EMG feedback treatment, who were assigned to a pseudotherapy control treatment, or who were simply placed on a waiting list all showed small but significant reductions in pain, anxiety and depression, and lumbar EMG. As noted above, the changes in the waiting-list control group poses a serious problem for this study, particularly since improvements in untreated control groups have not been found in other studies (Large & Lamb, 1983; Nouwen, 1983; Nouwen & Solinger, 1979; Turner, 1982). This finding may be due to the fact that the subjects in the Bush et al. study were not typical of pain clinic patients. However, this study does illustrate that nonspecific factors are likely to be present and contributory in the EMG biofeedback treatment situation.

In a more definitive study, Flor et al. (1983) compared EMG biofeedback with an equally credible pseudotherapy and conventional medical treatment in three groups of patients who were undergoing a 4-week inpatient stay in a rheumatology clinic. Patients were selected for elevated EMG in the area of pain, and training was carried out in two different postures (prone and sitting or standing) to encourage generalization and transfer of training. EMG levels decreased only with EMG biofeedback treatment, but, unfortunately, EMG was not reassessed at 4-month follow-up. Only the EMG biofeedback group showed significant reductions in pain at the end of treatment and at follow-up; however, a pain questionnaire indicated that these reductions in pain were largely a result of altered affective and cognitive components of pain. There was also a large reduction in negative cognitions for the biofeedback group. Number of physician visits was significantly reduced for both the biofeedback and pseudotherapy groups at follow-up, but more so for the biofeedback patients. Disability from pain was reported decreased for all groups at the end of treatment, but only for the biofeedback group at follow-up. In addition, the biofeedback patients were most satisfied with their treatment, more convinced they could relax and control the pain, and more optimistic about maintaining their improvenents. Based on these data, the authors concluded that psychological factors, particularly those related to affect and cognition, may be important mediators of beneficial biofeedback effects in chronic pain patients, and that these factors were probably more important than the reduction of muscle tension per se.

Clearly the process by which current, static EMG feedback procedures alter subjective pain and stimulate clinical gains is not as simple as initially proposed. There appears to be little demonstrable specific effect from muscle relaxation in and of itself. Based on their data and their observations of patients, formal and informal, several investigators (Flor et al., 1983; Freeman et al., 1980; Nouwen, 1983) suggest that clinical improvements were due, at least in part, to nonspecific factors related to reduction of anxiety, recognition of the relationship between stress and pain, enhanced feelings of self-control, and perceived ability to cope with pain. Cognitive coping skills and stress management principles are well recognized as important in self-regulation of chronic pain (Keefe, 1981; Turner & Chapman, 1982), and there are strong indications that these factors were operative in the studies discussed above.

NEW DIRECTIONS IN EMG BIOFEEDBACK

This body of work has erased the heretofore automatic assumptions of a one-to-one causal relationship between muscle tension and pain. It has also stimulated a good deal of creative and productive rethinking of theoretical and clinical approaches in the area of EMG biofeedback (Faltin, Sungaila, Hershman, & Dickinson, 1982; Kravitz, Moore, & Glaros, 1981; Middaugh,1982a,b; Sherman, 1985; Wolf et al., 1982). Premature and uncritical acceptance of muscle spasm as the universal cause of chronic musculoskeletal pain, and the resulting simplistic treatment procedures based on relaxation training at rest, have led to a state of confusion in the literature and some understandable, but highly premature, disillusionment about the usefulness of site-specific EMG biofeedback in treatment of patients with chronic cervical and low back pain. It is now evident that the problem is not EMG biofeedback, which is consistently highly effective in teaching muscle responses. Rather, the problem is one of discovering what muscle responses need to be changed. The solution requires suspending preconceptions concerning muscle spasm and pain; it requires developing good EMG evaluation procedures; and it requires going to the individual patient for answers about treatment needs and relevant EMG feedback procedures. In a number of laboratories, including ours, this process is leading to the development of appropriate theory, EMG evaluation procedures, and EMG feedback treatment procedures designed specifically for these patients. This new beginning is leading to rapid and exciting advances in our understanding of chronic pain syndromes and to new options for their treatment.

EMG EVALUATION AND TREATMENT OF PATIENTS WITH CHRONIC PAIN

Over the past 4 years the Biofeedback Laboratory at MUSC has participated in the development and implementation of the multidisciplinary Chronic Pain Rehabilitation Program. Patients referred to this program all have a history of daily pain for a minimum of 6 months that has not responded to standard medical or surgical intervention. Our work with these patients has led to systematic development, on both a research and clinical level, of procedures for using site-specific EMG recording for evaluation and biofeedback training of patients with chronic cervical and low back pain.

Our basic approach is based on extensive prior experience with EMG biofeedback in neuromuscular reeducation in this laboratory. As a result, EMG biofeedback training is individualized and is based on thorough, muscle-by-muscle EMG evaluation. Furthermore, EMG evaluation and biofeedback training are primarily dynamic rather than static, since most muscles do very little at rest; and as a result, static training may produce little change in muscle use during movement. In addition, posture is recognized as a major variable that can alter muscle activity and must, therefore, be considered during evaluation and treatment.

EMG recording techniques used in evaluation and treatment of patients with chronic cervical and low back pain are also based on our prior work with EMG biofeedback in neuromuscular reeducation. Two EMG channels are routinely used for evaluation using a TECA clinical electromyograph with an amplifier band-width of 20 Hz to 1,000 Hz and an oscilloscope, which permits monitoring of the raw (unprocessed) EMG signal. The signals are also stored on a built-in tape recorder for later verification and quantification. Through years of watching muscles with such equipment, it is evident that muscle contraction patterns are highly informative. The term "pattern" can refer to the time course of recruitment and relaxation of an individual target muscle during a test or training trial; it can refer to continuous variations in muscle contractions occurring during a complex movement or a functional task; or it can refer to the interaction between pairs of muscles with related actions. This information is often far more meaningful than absolute microvolt values, which can vary markedly from person to person, muscle to muscle, and with different electrode placements in normal individuals. Microvolt values are also altered by the filter characeristics of the amplifiers and the specific method of electronic processing for quantification. Patterns of muscle activity are particularly well obscured by quantitative EMG measurements that produce an integrated average for an entire trial or by measurement only at a designated end point such as the last minute of a 10-minute trial.

EVALUATION AND TREATMENT OF PATIENTS WITH CHRONIC CERVICAL PAIN

Subjects

Twenty consecutive patients with a diagnosis of chronic cervical and/or shoulder girdle pain were evaluated by surface-recorded EMG to assess muscle activity in the area(s) of pain. These patients typically reported pain in one or all of the following areas illustrated in Figure 6.1: the posterior cervical area, across the top of the shoulder, and between the shoulder blades. The pain was typically reported as more severe on one side but present bilaterally, particularly on the worst days. Dull occipital headache was a common symptom, which, in some patients, spread to include pain in the ear, jaw, temporal area, or eye. When severe, headache could include vascular symptoms with throbbing, visual disturbance, or nausea. Other common symptoms were pain, numbness, tingling, or subjective swelling in the arm and hand. The pain onset was traumatic in 10 patients, and auto accidents (4), and lifting injuries (4) were the most frequent causes. Pain onset was nontraumatic in the other 10 patients and caused by degenerative joint disease (5) or slowly developing muscle strain or fibromyalgia (5). Fourteen (70%) of these patients had no associated surgery. Other relevant subject characteristics are given in Table 6.1.

Evaluation Procedure and Results

EMG was recorded from two sites at a time, usually over the same muscle group on the right and left sides of the body. Beckman .8 mm diameter silver/silver chloride skin electrodes were placed over the target muscle group using a standard spacing of 2 inches center to center, after lightly abrading the skin using an abrasive soap (Brasivol™) or a teflon abrasive pad and then cleansing with alcohol. Skin resistance with this technique is reliably less than 10 kOhm. A ground electrode was placed equidistant from, and adjacent to, the two active electrodes of one recording site.

Two or four muscle sites were evaluated per patient according to the reported areas of pain. Even with unilateral pain the contralateral muscle group was always evaluated. For patients with cervical and shoulder girdle

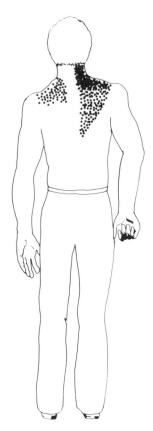

FIGURE 6.1 Common areas of reported pain in patients with chronic cervical and shoulder girdle pain.

TABLE 6.1. Characteristics of Patients with Chronic Pain in the Cervical/Shoulder Girdle and Low Back Area

Pain location	Sex		Age		Pain duration		Number of surgeries	
	Male	Female	$\bar{X}$ (yr)	Range (yr)	$\bar{X}$ (yr)	Range	$\bar{X}$	Range
Cervical/ shoulder girdle area (N = 20)	7	13	44.7	24–75	4.2	7 mo– 17 yr	.45	0–3
Chronic pain in low back area (N = 23)	13	10	42.9	29–68	5.2	7 mo– 19 yr	1.2	0–7

ymptoms, these sites were over the upper trapezius and levator scapulae muscles using a placement on the top of the shoulder, and over the midscapular muscles (the paraspinous, middle trapezius, and rhomboid muscles) using a placement parallel to the spine and between the shoulder blades. These electrode placements are shown in Figure 6.2. EMG was recorded during quiet sitting and also during repeated upper extremity movements designed to force contraction of the target muscles and permit assessment of muscle relaxation following use.

Table 6.2 presents EMG evaluation findings for the 20 patients. Results are presented in terms of the percentage of patients with above-normal levels of muscle activity under three standard conditions described below. The data are for the single site of greatest reported pain for each patient.

During the Quiet Sitting Test patients are asked to sit still in an armless straight back chair with hands in lap while muscle activity is observed for 2 minutes. The muscle groups tested normally relax completely in this position, and normal EMG levels will be at or very near the inherent noise level of the recording equipment with a comparable resistance in the circuit. This is $5\mu V$ peak-to-peak (pp) with our equipment. For the purposes of this evaluation, muscle activity is classified conservatively as above normal if it consistently meets or exceeds a criterion value of $25\mu V$ pp. By this

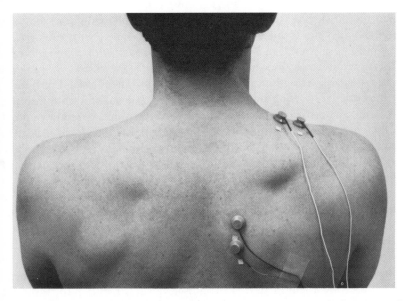

FIGURE 6.2 Electrode placements for evaluation of patients with chronic cervical and shoulder girdle pain.

TABLE 6.2. EMG Evaluation Findings in Patients with
Chronic Pain in the Cervical/Shoulder Girdle and
Low Back Area

	Cervical/shoulder girdle (N = 20)
Elevated sitting baseline	65%
Poor recovery of baseline after shoulder shrug	85%
Poor recovery of baseline after shoulder abduction	90%

	Low back (N = 23)
Elevated standing baseline	61%
Loss of reciprocal trunk rotation	87%
Poor recovery of baseline after trunk flexion	26%

criterion, EMG levels were elevated above normal during quiet sitting baseline in 65% of patients (Table 6.2).

During the Shrug/Return Test patients are asked to shrug both shoulders up, hold this position for 3 seconds, and then let the shoulders back down. The muscles are then observed for 1 minute to assess recovery of baseline. This procedure is repeated three times. Relaxation following brief shoulder shrug (shoulder elevation) is normally rapid and complete with good recovery of quiet sitting levels in 2 to 3 seconds. In this evaluation, the significant finding is a failure on the part of the individual patient to recover his own sitting baseline level within 30 seconds on two of three trials. This means that for patients showing muscle hyperactivity (elevated baseline) during quiet sitting, a positive finding on this second test requires an aggravation of this muscle symptom by movement and use. As seen in Table 6.2, such muscle "irritability" is a very frequent finding seen in 85% of our patients. Brief shoulder shrug provoked muscle contractions, which then persisted long after the movement had ended.

During the Abduct/Return Test the patient, still sitting, is asked to raise (abduct) the arms straight out to the side to a horizontal position, hold this position 3 seconds, and then lower the arms to resume baseline position with hands in lap. The muscles are then observed for 1 minute to assess recovery of baseline. This is repeated three times. In this test maneuver the patient is lifting the weight of the extended arm against gravity, and this movement requires a stronger contraction of the muscles than is required for shoulder shrug. Normal relaxation is rapid and complete after the movement has ended. A positive finding on this third test requires prolonged contraction above the patient's own quiet sitting baseline level on two of the three trials. As seen in Table 6.2, this maneuver produced signs of muscle irritability in 90% of patients.

Conclusions

The majority of patients with chronic cervical/shoulder girdle pain show objective evidence of muscle hyperactivity (elevated muscle activity) during quiet sitting, but a substantial number (35%) do not. Therefore, reliance on static, sitting evaluation alone may lead to a clinical impression (or experimental findings) of poor correspondence between EMG levels and musculoskeletal pain. However, dynamic evaluation reveals that a very high proportion of these patients show objective evidence of muscle irritability (poor relaxation of painful muscles following use) and this can be easily demonstrated with two simple shoulder/arm movements. The extent of muscle reaction can be marked, and these test movements often provoke contractions measuring $50\mu V$ to $250\mu V$ pp or more, which can continue for several minutes after return to the quiet sitting condition. Considering the many times each day the arms are used, it is apparent that the painful muscles are chronically contracting for extended periods of time. Muscle hyperactivity is strongly implicated as a major cause of continued pain in these patients.

Implications for Patient Treatment

This EMG evaluation procedure is a very useful one that permits categorization of the individual patient, muscle by muscle, in a manner that has direct application to subsequent treatment with EMG biofeedback procedures. Our EMG evaluation findings are consistent with the common patient complaint that pain is reduced with inactivity and increased by activities involving the upper extremities, particularly repetitive or nearly continuous activities such as writing or driving, and by activities requiring strong muscle use, such as picking up a child or carrying a bag of groceries. Typically, pain increases across the course of the day. Simple "muscle watching" (EMG monitoring) during patient interview will usually verify the formal evaluation findings and add additional information that is very useful for treatment planning. In some patients simply lifting an arm to briefly scratch the head can elevate EMG levels substantially for minutes. Using EMG feedback to show the patient that this is occurring and to teach him to relax quickly following movement is an obvious and effective treatment strategy. The relevance of site-specific and dynamic evaluation in treatment planning is illustrated in Figure 6.3. In Figures 6.3 through 6.13 the tape recorded, raw EMG signals have been converted to a graphic

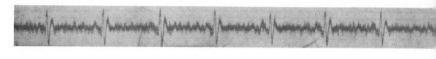

Left upper trapezius

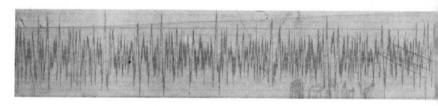

Left midscapular muscles

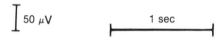

FIGURE 6.3 EMG recordings from two different sites of reported pain in a 42-year-old female patient. EKG artifact, top trace.

display by a Honeywell Visicorder oscillograph, a high-speed ultraviolet chart writer. EKG artifact is present in these figures because we record EMG at 20 to 1,000 Hz to avoid the loss of important low-frequency EMG components. The EKG signal is easily identified on the left in the cervical recordings and bilaterally in the low back recordings. In Figure 6.3 a 42-year-old woman with unilateral chronic pain reported at two sites (four years duration, traumatic onset, no surgery) demonstrated relatively complete, normal relaxation during quiet sitting at one site, the upper trapezius/levator scapulae recording site. At the same time the midscapular muscles at the second site show a strong, continuous contraction well above normal levels. Based on this test alone there appears to be an inconsistent relationship between pain report and EMG. Dynamic evaluation, however, reveals a different and more consistent picture. Figure 6.4 illustrates the EMG findings during abduct/return, second repetition. The tracing begins in the upper left hand corner with mild baseline elevation, just meeting the $25\mu V$ pp criterion, resulting from the first abduct/return trial. "Abduct" marks the beginning of the abduction movement, and "Return" marks the point at which the movement ends with the hands back in the lap. Although the patient has resumed quiet sitting, the muscle does not relax but continues to contract strongly. At "relax" the patient is instructed to "think about your left shoulder, let it drop and relax for the next minute or two."

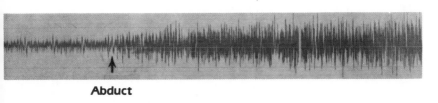

Abduct

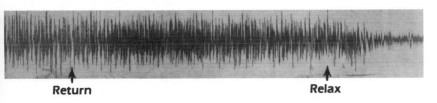

Return   **Relax**

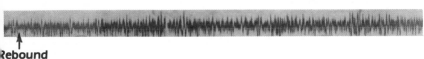

↑
Rebound

Left Upper Trapezius   ⎡50 μ V   **1 Sec**

FIGURE 6.4 EMG recording from the site of reported pain in the same patient shown in Figure 6.3 during the Abduct/Return Test. This irritable muscle contracts with the onset of movement (abduct) but does not relax when the movement ends (return). The muscle relaxes briefly with instruction (relax) but then resumes contracting (rebound) spontaneously.

With this instruction, which directs the patient's attention to the shoulder, relaxation is rapid and relatively complete (without EMG feedback). However, the muscle relaxes only briefly (1 to 2 seconds) and almost immediately ("rebound") resumes a continuous, and increasing, contraction in spite of the fact that the patient continues to concentrate on relaxing as instructed. In contrast, the patient could not relax the midscapular muscles voluntarily, even briefly (not shown).

For this patient the EMG feedback training procedure was different for the two sites. The patient practiced relaxing the upper trapezius muscle quickly, following brief, repeated cervical and upper extremity movements. She also learned to maintain relaxation, once achieved, to avoid the rebound noted in Figure 6.4. The patient was encouraged to develop an awareness of muscle tension and muscle relaxation while working with these tense/relax procedures. Once basic control was achieved, EMG feedback training with a portable unit was used to practice muscle relaxation while performing daily activities, particularly writing, simulated driving, and walking. For the midscapular site, EMG feedback was used to teach the patient to relax this muscle during quiet sitting and to maintain relaxation while shifting her attention away from the muscle. All training was to criterion, which was reliable performance without biofeedback, verified by EMG monitoring. This was achieved for both sites. Interestingly, training was carried out sequentially and began with the upper trapezius. The midscapular muscles did not improve until biofeedback training at this second site began.

The importance of extending EMG feedback training to include functional activity is illustrated in Figures 6.5 and 6.6. On initial evaluation (not shown) a 64-year-old man with pain in the right cervical area (traumatic origin, 17-year duration, one surgery) showed unilaterally elevated EMG levels in the right upper trapezius ms during quiet sitting, and increased EMG following shoulder shrug and abduction. EMG biofeedback training began with relaxation while sitting and following brief arm movements. Figure 6.5 shows the relatively complete muscle relaxation achieved after this phase. However, as illustrated in Figure 6.6, whenever the patient began talking, the right upper trapezius showed relatively strong, continuous contraction. When this was observed, biofeedback training was used to teach relaxation of this muscle while talking.

Since biofeedback training was carried out in the context of a multidisciplinary treatment program, the specific contribution of biofeedback training to clinical outcome in our patients cannot be stated at present. Two thirds of the patients participating in the Chronic Pain Rehabilitation Program are substantially benefited as measured by gains on seven objective success

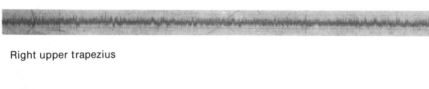

Right upper trapezius

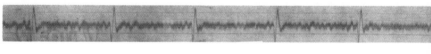

Left upper trapezius

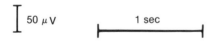

50 μV   1 sec

FIGURE 6.5 EMG recordings from the upper trapezius muscles of a 64-year-old male patient with right cervical pain during quiet sitting, after initial relaxation training. EKG artifact, bottom trace.

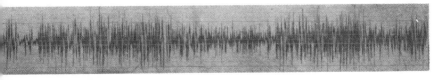

t Upper Trapezius

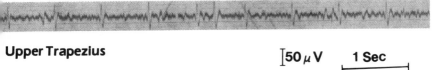

Upper Trapezius

$\rceil$50 μ V   1 Sec

FIGURE 6.6 EMG recordings from the upper trapezius muscles of the same patient shown in Figure 6.5 while talking. EKG artifact, bottom trace.

criteria that assess reductions in pain and medications and improvements in physical and psychological function at 1-year follow-up. Several relevant clinical observations can be made concerning the possible contribution of the biofeedback treatment component, and all of these observations are readily amenable to investigation within a multimodal treatment program.

One testable clinical observation is that for patients showing clear evidence of muscle hyperactivity in painful cervical and shoulder girdle areas, acquisition of good voluntary muscle relaxation skills does appear to be essential for good, lasting pain relief. Patients who achieve good reductions in pain, as did the two patients discussed above, also achieve good muscle control, and patients who show a recurrence in muscle hyperactivity at follow-up also report increased pain. Whether or not muscle hyperactivity was a causative factor originally, in many patients with cervical pain it does seem to be a strong perpetuating factor that must be dealt with.

A second testable observation is that learning to relax problem muscles during quiet sitting or while lying down is relatively easy and can often be achieved with a variety of methods, not just EMG biofeedback. This can be easily demonstrated if muscles are monitored by EMG during nonbiofeedback relaxation training. However, relaxation at rest does not readily translate into good muscle control during movement or performance of daily activities. Training must occur under active conditions, and EMG biofeedback is almost required for such training. Certainly EMG monitoring is invaluable for identifying problem muscles and determining appropriate training strategies. Muscle monitoring is also essential for determining whether or not muscle relaxation has actually been achieved, by whatever training method employed. Monitoring also permits continuous reevaluation, which encourages individualization of training and training to criterion.

A final testable observation is that acquisition of muscle relaxation is seldom sufficient for good alleviation of chronic pain. Most of these patients have, over time, developed substantial problems with posture, muscle tightness, and muscle weakness that must be dealt with. Simply teaching them to relax tight, weak muscles in a poor posture is not effective. Muscles simply cannot relax, for example, in some abnormal postures that force them to counter gravity. In addition, exercises that stretch tight muscles aid relaxation; for example, a flexible muscle is not constantly yanked with normal movement, so there is less need for protective muscle tensing. Many chronic pain patients also have problems with medication, depression, and anxiety. These are all perpetuating factors that must be reversed with appropriate physical and psychological measures for maximum clinical improvement.

EVALUATION AND TREATMENT OF PATIENTS WITH CHRONIC LOW BACK PAIN

Subjects

Twenty-three consecutive patients with a diagnosis of chronic low back pain were evaluated by surface-recorded EMG to assess muscle activity in the area of pain. These patients typically reported pain in the lower thoracic or lumbosacral area. The pain was often reported as being bilateral but more severe on one side, and in some patients was accompanied by pain, numbness, or tingling in the leg on one or both sides. The pain onset was traumatic in 15 patients with lifting injuries (7) and falls (6) the most frequent causes. Pain onset was nontraumatic in 8 patients because of degenerative joint disease (4) or slowly developing muscle strain or fibromyalgia (4). Fourteen (61%) had no surgery. Other relevant subject characteristics are given in Table 6.1.

Evaluation Procedure and Results

The equipment; the procedure for skin preparation; and the electrode type, size, and separation were the same as in the evaluation of cervical patients. Two or four muscle sites were evaluated per patient with the four possible sites being the right and left lumbar paraspinous muscles and the right and left lower thoracic paraspinous muscles. Electrodes were placed parallel to the spine, approximately 1 inch from the midline and 1 inch above and below L4. The thoracic placement was centered at T8 through T12 according to area of pain.

EMG evaluation findings for these 23 patients are presented in Table 6.2 in terms of the percent of patients with other-than-normal muscle activity under three standard test conditions described below. The data are for either the lumbar (21) or thoracic area (2), whichever was reported as most painful.

During *standing baseline* patients are asked to stand still, as straight as possible, with their weight equally distributed on the two legs. The muscles in the recording areas normally relax well during quiet standing with good posture, but the muscles may briefly contract and relax as the trunk sways slightly forward and back with normal postural sway. This normal in-and-out pattern and mild asymmetry in a normal, nonpainful back is illustrated in Figure 6.7. Muscle activity is classified as above normal if there is sustained activity above $25\mu V$ pp on one or both sides. By this criterion, 61% of our patients showed elevated EMG during quiet standing (Table 6.2). During *trunk rotation* patients are asked to continue standing with their arms relaxed and their hips stationary. They are directed to rotate the trunk to the right, hold for 3 seconds, and return to neutral. This is followed by rotation to the left. This is repeated three times or until a consistent pattern is established. The normal, reciprocal lumbar muscle contraction pattern is illustrated in Figure 6.8. With trunk rotation to the right, the left lumbar muscles contract more strongly; with trunk rotation to the left, the reverse is seen, and the right lumbar muscles are more active. For thoracic placements the increase is on the same side as the movement; that is, the muscles on the right contract with rotation to the right. Substantial deviation from this

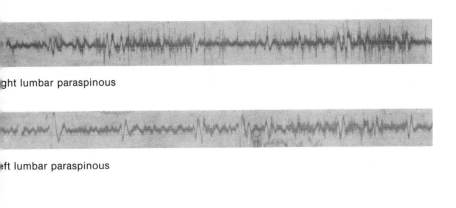

ght lumbar paraspinous

ft lumbar paraspinous

50 μV   1 sec

FIGURE 6.7 EMG recordings from the lumbar muscles in a pain-free, normal 40-year-old male. The muscles contract and relax as the trunk sways slightly forward and back during normal standing. EKG artifact, both traces.

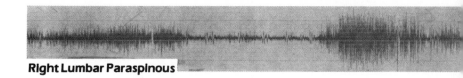

Right Lumbar Paraspinous

Left Lumbar Paraspinous

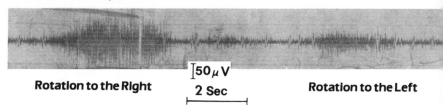

$\lceil$50 μ V

Rotation to the Right   **2 Sec**   **Rotation to the Left**

FIGURE 6.8 EMG recording of lumbar muscles in a normal, pain-free 40-year-old-male showing the normal reciprocal contraction of these muscles during standing trunk rotation. EKG artifact, both traces.

pattern is seen in 87% of our patients (Table 6.2). The most common deviation (seen in 65%) is illustrated in Figure 6.9. Trunk rotation to the right in this patient with low back pain is accomplished with bilateral contractions, which indicate mass action of the low back muscles. For this patient (and many patients) the movement and the muscle contraction is much slower than normal, and there is complete loss of the reciprocal pattern. Trunk rotation to the left (not shown) produced the same bilateral

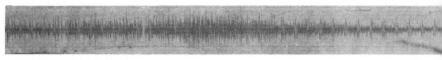

Left Lumbar Paraspinous

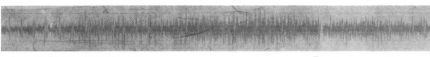

Right Lumbar Paraspinous $\lceil$50 μ V   **2 Sec**

FIGURE 6.9 EMG recordings from the lumbar muscles in a 42-year-old female patient with bilateral low back pain during trunk rotation to the right. EKG artifact, both traces.

contractions. In 13% of our patients there was underuse of the muscles on the most painful side, and in 9% there was little range of motion and little EMG change from standing baseline.

During *trunk flexion* patients were asked to bend forward from the waist as if attempting to touch their toes. This movement forces strong muscle contractions bilaterally even if there is very limited range of motion. In addition, the paraspinous muscles are stretched during trunk flexion, and this acts as an added provocation. Muscles on the right and left normally contract strongly and symmetrically during flexion, relax in the fully flexed position, and contract again during extension. On return to the upright position these muscles relax back to standing baseline levels almost immediately, within 2 to 3 seconds (Figure 6.10). In this evaluation procedure the most significant finding is poor recovery of the individual's own standing baseline EMG levels. That is, for patients showing muscle hyperactivity during quiet standing, a positive finding on this test requires an aggravation of this muscle symptom following movement requiring the muscle's use. Poor relaxation following contraction is a sign of muscle irritability or excessive reaction to normal use. Figure 6.11 shows the lumbar muscles in a patient with low back pain that is bilateral but more severe on the left. This patient showed normal relaxation during initial quiet standing (not shown), but showed asymmetrical contraction during flexion and extension, continued contraction in the fully flexed position, and incomplete recovery of baseline on return to the upright position. This maneuver produced signs of muscle irritability in only 26% of our low back pain patients (Table 6.2).

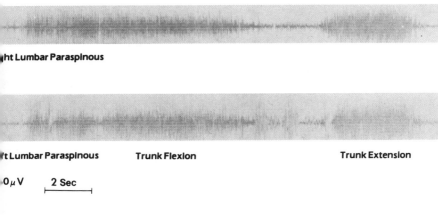

ht Lumbar Paraspinous

ft Lumbar Paraspinous   Trunk Flexion   Trunk Extension

0 μV   2 Sec

FIGURE 6.10 EMG recordings from the lumbar muscles of a 40-year-old, normal, pain-free male during trunk flexion and extension while standing. Movement artifact is present at full flexion, bottom trace, due to electrode slippage. EKG artifact both traces.

Right Lumbar Paraspinous

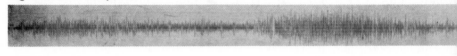

Left Lumbar Paraspinous

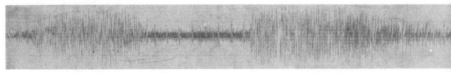

Trunk Flexion   **Trunk Extension**

⌐50 μV   2 Sec
         ├─────────┤

FIGURE 6.11 EMG recordings from the lumbar muscles of the same patient shown in Figure 6.9 during trunk flexion and extension standing. Pain is present bilaterally, but more severe on the left. EKG artifact, both traces.

Conclusions

The majority of low back pain patients show objective evidence of excessive muscle activity during quiet standing; however, many (39%) do not. In those patients who do have elevated muscle activity, poor standing posture appears to be the primary cause in many, if not most, instances. For example, many patients favored one side, shifting their weight away from a painful leg or hip, and this led to continuous contraction of the low back muscles, usually on one side, in an effort to stabilize the pelvis. Many patients with low back pain also stand with the trunk continuously flexed. Even slight trunk flexion shifts the center of gravity forward of the midline and forces the low back muscles to contract, often forcefully and bilaterally, to counteract gravity. In patients with long histories of chronic pain or multiple surgeries this posture can become relatively fixed, and the patient may not be able to assume a normally erect posture on request (and may never be able to). The elevated EMG during quiet standing could often be attributed to such postural factors, and posture must be considered when interpreting findings of elevated EMG while standing. Apparent "spasm" may readily disappear when the patient stands correctly (Figure 6.12). This interpretation is also supported by the observation that normal individuals standing in these poor postures show similar EMG profiles. Our conclusion is that elevated EMG during quiet standing most often represents inappropriate muscle use rather than muscle spasm.

In sharp contrast to our findings in cervical pain patients, only 26% of low back pain patients show evidence that the muscles are irritable; that is, are easily aggravated by movement and fail to relax rapidly and well following use. Disruption of the normal pattern of coordinated muscle use during trunk movement is our most frequent finding. Mass action of low back muscles, or avoidance of muscle contraction in the area of pain, were common (87% of patients).

Considered together, our findings on these three relatively simple but informative test maneuvers indicate substantial problems with inappropriate and inefficient use of low back muscles for posture and movement. Both overuse and underuse of the low back muscles are common. Muscle irritability is not a universal finding but does occur in a subset (26% in our series) of chronic low back pain patients.

Implications for Patient Treatment

Our findings are consistent with the clinical observation that most patients with chronic low back pain have major postural problems that develop in response to the pain, increase musculoskeletal strain, and contribute to pain chronicity (Calliett, 1979). As with cervical pain patients, EMG evaluation is highly informative and encourages individualization of EMG biofeedback treatment strategy. Our experience with these EMG evaluation procedures indicates that it is essential to simultaneously evaluate posture in order to interpret EMG findings. This is illustrated in Figure 6.12. A 37-year-old

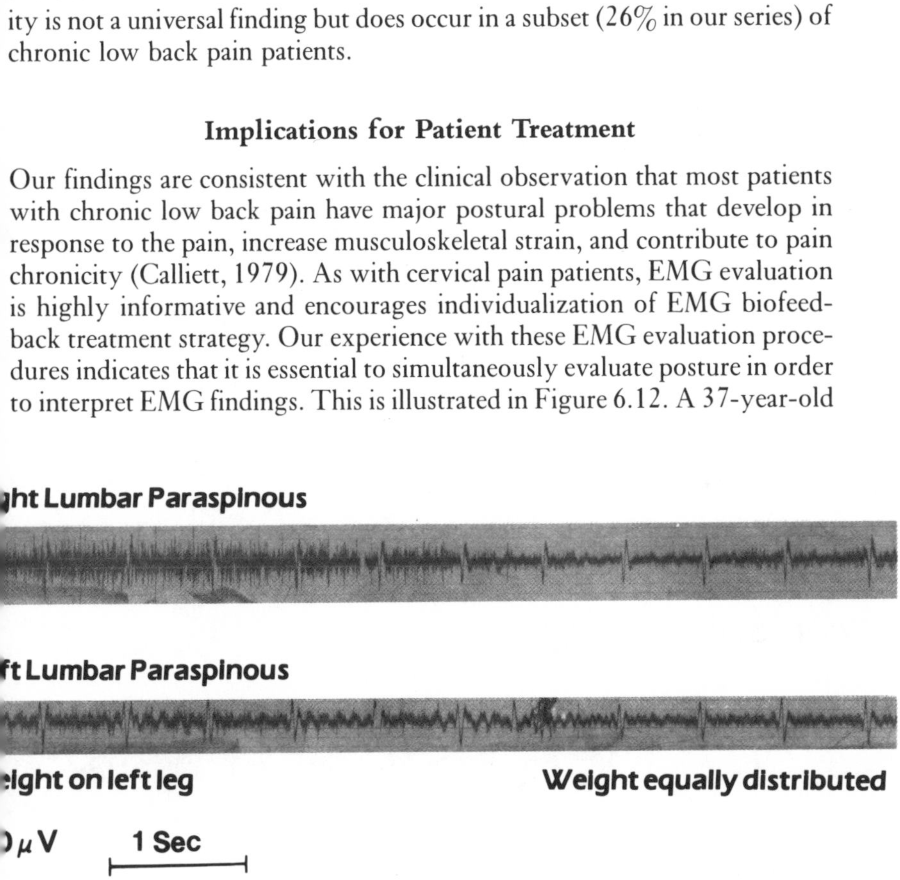

ght Lumbar Paraspinous

ft Lumbar Paraspinous

eight on left leg   **Weight equally distributed**

) μV   1 Sec

FIGURE 6.12 EMG recordings from the lumbar muscles of a 37-year-old male with right low back pain during quiet standing, first with the weight primarily on the left leg, then with the weight equal on both legs. EKG artifact, both traces.

male with low back pain (6-year duration, traumatic onset, no surgery) reported pain primarily in the right lumbar area. On evaluation he showed relatively strong, continuous contraction of the right lumbar muscles during quiet standing in his preferred mode with erect posture but with his weight carried predominantly on the left leg. When asked to shift his weight to the right to bear weight equally on both legs, the lumbar muscles relaxed almost completely.

Our experience with EMG evaluation procedures also points out the importance of independent monitoring of the right and left paraspinous muscles. Recording on a single channel with one electrode placed to the right and one to the left of the spine not only limits assessment (e.g., of reciprocal pattern during rotation) but can also lead to misinterpretation of findings. This is well illustrated in Figure 6.13.

A 37-year-old male with low back pain (3 years duration, traumatic onset, no surgery) reported pain predominantly on the right. On evaluation with dual-channel recording he showed strong, continuous muscle contraction on one side only, with good standing posture. Single-channel, bilateral recording would only indicate elevated EMG without revealing the side of occurrence. This would give a false impression of muscle spasm as a cause of pain when, in fact, the hyperactive muscles are on the nonpainful side. This is an example of protective bracing by muscles on the nonpainful left side. This was present while standing, but the muscles relaxed completely when sitting with the back supported. Further assessment also showed underuse of the painful right side during trunk rotation. This underuse was not due to surgery nor to demonstrable muscle weakness (compared with the nonpain-

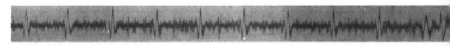

Right Lumbar Paraspinous

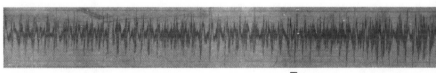

Left Lumbar Paraspinous   ⌉50 μV   1 Sec

FIGURE 6.13 EMG recordings from the lumbar muscles of a 37-year-old male with right low back pain during quiet standing, good posture. Elevated EMG is on the pain-free side. EKG artifact, both traces.

ful side) but to a reluctance to use the painful muscles. This conclusion was supported by a finding of good and comparable contractions bilaterally during trunk flexion, a movement that forced the patient to use the muscles on the painful side. We have found that trunk flexion is a valuable way to assess the ability of muscles to contract in an area of previous back surgery. The validity of surface EMG recording and EMG biofeedback in such patients has been questioned because there are often diagnostic signs (by needle EMG) of some degree of denervation in the paraspinous muscles on the operated side (Wolf et al., 1982). We have not found the paraspinous muscles on the side of surgery to be substantially different from those on the unoperated side in terms of surface EMG levels, nor did we observe major EMG differences between patients with and without surgery. Our informal observations have been confirmed in a recent study by Dolce, Doleys, Wolfe, & Crocker (in press).

We have not reported on EMG levels while sitting, although this is a standard part of our evaluation procedure. We have found that sitting EMG is markedly affected by the chair, and we were not initially consistent in the type of chair used. In the large majority of patients with low back pain, even those with large elevations in EMG while standing, the low back muscles relax easily and completely while sitting with the back supported in a cushioned chair. The cushioning permits the patient to lean back slightly, and this position reduces stretch on tight low back muscles and facilitates relaxation. When an elevated EMG is seen it can usually be attributed to the patient sitting on one hip and elevating the pelvis on the painful side. This finding highlights the inappropriateness of assessment and biofeedback training entirely while sitting, particularly in a recliner. There will be very little to train, other than sitting posture, for most back patients. For evaluation purposes we now use a straight-back chair with no arms, the seat slightly padded, and the back uncushioned. In this test position there is a small subset of patients who do show elevated EMG not attributable to hip hiking.

One of the most frequent uses of EMG feedback for low back pain patients in our laboratory is for postural retraining. Patients are shown the adverse effect of their habitual standing posture on their low back muscles using the oscilloscope. EMG feedback and instruction are then combined to teach correct standing and sitting posture. We find this to be a highly useful procedure. Although all low back pain patients are repeatedly told that posture is important, the feedback display reinforces this instruction in a way that is very concrete and effective. In addition, postural adjustments can be subtle, and the feedback display can coach the patient in a way that nonfeedback training cannot. The patient can often "relax" strong, bilateral muscle contractions with slight pelvic tilt and slight knee flexion. Alternation of feedback and nonfeedback practice is continued until the patient learns the "feel" of the correct posture and achieves reliable nonfeedback performance, which can be verified by EMG monitoring. Such training to criterion with verification is readily achievable with EMG feedback and very difficult without it. For the subset of patients who do show muscle irritability, EMG feedback training includes additional biofeedback training procedures. The patient practices achieving rapid and relatively complete relaxation following brief trunk and upper extremity movements in sitting and standing positions as warranted.

As with cervical pain patients, treatment was carried out as part of a multimodal chronic pain rehabilitation program with an overall two-thirds success rate at 1-year follow-up. As with cervical patients, we can offer several testable clinical observations on EMG biofeedback contribution to treatment outcome. The first testable observation is that muscle status is less clearly and directly related to the reported pain than in cervical pain patients, and acquisition of muscle relaxation per se appears to be less essential. Muscles that are overactive are not always sore, and good improvements can be obtained, at least in some patients, without change in muscle status, for example, in patients who are relatively fixed in slightly flexed trunk postures because of surgery or degenerative joint disease and cannot assume postures that make muscle relaxation feasible. For the subset of patients with muscle irritability, muscle tension may be more contributory to the pain, and muscle relaxation may be essential. This is a very interesting research question that could be answered. The second and third testable observations are essentially the same as those stated previously for cervical pain patients.

THE LITERATURE REVISITED

Our findings with regard to cervical pain patients are in agreement with recent research on tension headache patients. There is likely to be substantial overlap between these two patient groups, since many of our patients with cervical/shoulder girdle pain report posterior occipital headache as a major symptom and may seek treatment for this. We also find similar cervical muscle profiles in many of the patients referred to our biofeedback laboratory for treatment of tension headache. Haynes et al. (1983) measured both frontal and cervical EMG during resting baseline and in response to stressors in a single group of tension headache subjects under both headache and nonheadache conditions. There were no differences in resting level EMG for these two muscles, but 78% of patients showed significant EMG elevations in cervical, but not frontalis, muscles in response to stressors during headache. These investigators concluded that resting level EMG may not be an important factor in tension headache and also concluded that cervical electrode placements may be more appropriate for EMG biofeedback. Others have pointed to muscle reactivity as a possible contributing factor in tension headache (Phillips, 1978) and suggested that resting baseline EMG may be less relevant than recovery of baseline following contraction (Hobbs & Cox, 1982). These findings, and our own findings, indicate that cervical muscle evaluation, site-specific electrode placement, and dynamic EMG feedback treatment procedures should be systematically explored in tension headache patients.

There has been a single published experimental study of site-specific EMG feedback in cervical pain patients, an excellent, early study by Jacobs & Felton (1969). Interestingly, they reported significant elevations in upper trapezius EMG in response to repetitive shoulder abduction in their patients compared with normal controls. These results are very much in agreement with ours, 17 years later. There obviously needs to be more, far more, investigation of EMG biofeedback in treatment of cervical pain. By all indications these patients have a high incidence of demonstrable muscle involvement and are excellent candidates for EMG biofeedback treatment procedures.

Our findings in patients with low back pain pose problems for muscle spasm as a causative factor, and this conclusion is in agreement with the conclusions of others (Nouwen & Bush, 1984). We find that there is considerable muscle involvement in these patients, but that it is not attributable to reflexive spasm. Rather, we find a high incidence of muscle overuse and muscle abuse that stems from poor posture and protective bracing. Mass contraction of low back muscles during movement is common in our patients, and this finding has been reported by others over the years with some consistency (Fowler & Kraft, 1984; Holmes & Wolff, 1952; Kravitz et al., 1981). We also find protective underuse of painful muscles in some patients. Muscle irritability, our EMG finding that perhaps comes closest to muscle spasm both conceptually and physiologically, occurs in a minority of patients.

In spite of this lack of objective evidence of muscle spasm, our patients will often answer in the affirmative when asked, "Do you have muscle spasms?" Their descriptions of these muscle spasms tend to fall into two categories. In one category are descriptions of a quantitative increase in muscle pain or tightness without any special qualitative features. These patients seem to label any aggravation of their back symptoms as "muscle spasm." In the second category are reports of distinct episodes of painful muscle cramping that are clearly different, in the patient's mind, from their typical daily pain. These reports correspond more closely to the physiological characteristics of reflexive muscle spasm. By report, most chronic pain patients have long since learned to avoid these episodes by restricting their activity.

Based on our findings, most of the EMG biofeedback procedures used for treatment of chronic low back pain in the research studies discussed earlier in this chapter are marginally appropriate at best. Static training, or even contract/relax procedures, in sitting or prone positions is likely to have little specific effect on the muscle status of most back pain patients. This can account for the current difficulties in attributing clinical gains to the learned reductions in muscle tension per se in these studies.

There is excellent evidence in many studies that EMG feedback can teach muscle responses and do so very effectively, but we do have to know what we need to teach. Our findings and those of others (Sherman, 1985; Wolf et al., 1982) indicate that patients have very different muscle profiles; therefore, what we need to teach will be different for different patients. EMG monitoring and biofeedback procedures are ideally suited for the individualized approach that appears to be needed with these patients and provide for a continuous and accurate three-way interaction between clinician, patient, and instrumentation throughout the treatment process. Development of appropriate biofeedback procedures is just beginning, and it is far too soon to discount site-specific EMG feedback procedures in treatment of chronic musculoskeletal pain.

NEW DIRECTIONS IN CHRONIC PAIN

The body of work by ourselves and others presented in this chapter suggests several new directions for research and clinical application in the area of EMG monitoring and EMG biofeedback in chronic musculoskeletal pain. New evaluation and treatment methods that are appropriate for patients with chronic musculoskeletal pain need to be developed based on site-specific EMG recording, dynamic EMG evaluation, and dynamic EMG biofeedback training. These procedures should also include training to criterion, training during functional muscle use, and in vivo evaluation and training (LeVine, 1983).

EMG biofeedback procedures for patients with chronic benign pain should be combined as necessary (and appropriately integrated) with other treatment procedures that include physical rehabilitation. Programs that combine cognitive therapy and nonspecific biofeedback procedures without physical rehabilitation have reported excellent success rates for patients with headache and gastrointestinal pain (DeGood, 1979; Libo & Arnold, 1983). The success rates for chronic pain patients in these treatment programs have been relatively low (one third of patients improved at follow-up) and below the success rates (two thirds of patients improved) often achieved with multimodal rehabilitation programs.

Additional research is needed to directly compare the muscle status of normal individuals with that of pain patients. There is wide variation in quantitative EMG in both groups, with considerable overlap in distributions (Sherman, 1985). Posture certainly needs to be investigated as a variable in both groups. Many of the other-than-normal EMG findings in low back pain patients are related to posture, and it is certainly possible to have poor posture in pain-free controls. Rather than training to a "normal" value, which is an average of nonpain patients, many of whom have poor posture and poor muscular conditioning, EMG biofeedback training should probably be directed toward achieving, as far as possible, an ideal criterion or optimal condition, which may produce better posture and better relaxation or muscular control than that of some nonpain patients.

More attention should be directed toward muscle physiology and toward physiological mechanisms in muscle pain. This is not to downplay the importance of psychological and behavioral mechanisms in chronic pain. The research on psychological variables has led to the development of viable explanatory concepts, which have, in turn, led to important new treatment procedures. The same process needs to be applied to the investigation of musculoskeletal factors. There is a demonstrably high degree of muscle involvement in chronic pain patients, but the prevalent explanatory concept, the pain/spasm/pain cycle, is clearly deficient. Not surprisingly, EMG biofeedback treatment procedures based on this concept have largely led to a dead end. There are currently several relevant factors that should be explored in an effort to develop basic concepts and treatment rationales with more explanatory power than the spasm. Posture is one important factor, not simply because it places stress on the joints but also because it can impair circulation and tax the muscles (Calliett, 1979, 1981). Stretch reflex activity is likely to be an important factor since it is increased by muscle tension (Spirduso & Duncan, 1976) and is also likely to be affected by loss of muscle flexibility. Fatigue is a third relevant factor. Measurable muscle fatigue can occur after as little as 1 minute of continuous muscle contraction at 11% of maximum voluntary contraction (Hagberg, 1981). Not surprisingly, muscles have been found to fatigue more readily in patients with myofascial pain (Hagberg & Kvarnström, 1984). Circulatory factors should also receive more attention, since sustained muscle contractions reduce circulation within the muscle. Autonomically mediated vasoconstriction within an area of pain may also be important. All of these factors can interact, and all provide opportunities for developing new explanations and new interventions.

EMG biofeedback equipment needs to be designed more appropriately for muscle training, and significant advances are being made in this direction. The power spectrum of the EMG is such that the major portion of the signal lies below the 100 Hz low-frequency cut-off, which is often built in to the EMG amplifiers used for biofeedback. To compound the problem, the central frequency of the EMG decreases with relaxation and with fatigue (Petrofsky, 1981). It is not possible, therefore, to sample the EMG spectrum at 100 to 200 Hz and have this sample accurately represent th wideband EMG (van Boxtel, 1984). This amplifier limitation poses partic ular difficulties in patients with chronic cervical and low back pain fo whom muscle fatigue is likely to be a substantial factor. The use of wide band (20 to 1,000 Hz) EMG, however, does introduce an EKG artifact tha is very evident in cervical and low back recording. This EKG artifact is not major problem for biofeedback (the patient can easily recognize and dis count it), but EKG does interfere with EMG quantification by electroni averaging. This problem theoretically can, and should, be solved by elec tronic subtraction rather than by elimination of most of the relevant EMG signal. Oscilloscopic monitoring of the raw EMG signal by the clinician i highly informative and should be routine. Some of the more interesting anc thought-provoking events within the muscle are obscured by signal averag ing and processing. The rebound effect that is seen in many cervical pair patients is a case in point (Fig. 6.4). There is an appropriately strong current interest in the development and use of two- to four-channel EMG muscle-scanning units, telemetry, and equipment suitable for in vivo evalu ation and training. Such equipment options are either available now or wil become available in the very near future through biofeedback equipment manufacturers.

REFERENCES

American Medical Association. (1962). Report of the Ad Hoc Committee on the Classification of Headache. *Journal of American Medical Association, 179*, 717–718.

Barcroft, H., & Millen, J. L. E. (1939). The bloodflow through muscle during sustained contraction. *Journal of Physiology, 97*, 17–31.

Basmajian, J. V. (1976). Facts vs. myths in EMG biofeedback. *Biofeedback and Self-Regulation, 1*, 369–371.

Basmajian, J. V. (Ed.). (1983). *Biofeedback—principles and practice for clinicians* Baltimore, MD: Williams and Wilkins.

Belar, C. D., & Cohen, J. L. (1979). The use of EMG feedback and progressive relaxation in the treatment of a woman with chronic back pain. *Biofeedback and Self-Regulation, 4*, 345–353.

Blanchard, E. B., Jaccard, J., Andrasik, F., Guarnieri, P., & Jurish, S. E. (1985). Reduction in headache patients' medical expenses associated with biofeedback and relaxation treatments. *Biofeedback and Self-Regulation, 10*, 63–68.

Budzynski, T., Stoyva, J., & Adler, C. (1970). Feedback-induced muscle relaxation: Application to tension headache. *Journal of Behavior Therapy and Experimental Psychiatry, 1*, 205–211.

Bush, C., Ditto, B., & Feuerstein, M. (1985). A controlled evaluation of paraspinal EMG biofeedback in the treatment of chronic low back pain. *Health Psychology, 4*, 307–321.

Cailliet, R. (1979). Chronic pain: Is it necessary? *Archives of Physical Medicine and Rehabilitation, 60,* 4–7.

Cailliet, R. (1981). *Low back pain syndrome.* (3rd ed.). Philadelphia: F. A. Davis.

Carlson, J. G., Basilio, C. A., & Heaukulani, J. D. (1983). Transfer of EMG training: Another look at the general relaxation issue. *Psychophysiology, 20,* 530–536.

Cobb, C. R., deVries, H. A., Urban, R. T., Luekens, C. A., & Bagg, R. J. (1975). Electrical activity in muscle pain. *American Journal of Physical Medicine, 54,* 80–87.

Collins, G. A., Cohen, M. J., Naliboff, B. D., & Schandler, S. L. (1982). Comparative analysis of paraspinal and frontalis EMG, heart rate, and skin conductance in chronic low back pain patients and normals to various postures and stress. *Scandinavian Journal of Rehabilitation Medicine, 14,* 39–46.

Cotton, D. H. G., & Lawson, J. S. (1982). A factor analytic investigation of muscle tension: Implications for EMG biofeedback training. Paper presented at the 3rd Annual Meeting of the Society of Behavioral Medicine, Chicago, IL, March 3–5.

Cram, J. R., & Steger, J. C. (1983). EMG scanning in the diagnosis of chronic pain. *Biofeedback and Self-Regulation, 8,* 229–241.

Degood, D. E. (1979). A behavioral pain-management program: Expanding the psychologist's role in a medical setting. *Professional Psychology, 10*(4), 491–502.

Dolce, J. J., Doleys, D. M., Wolfe, S., & Crocker, M. F. (in press). Validity of paraspinal EMG assessment in post-surgical back pain patients.

Dorpat, T. L., & Holmes, T. H. (1955). Mechanisms of skeletal muscle pain and fatigue. *Archives of Neurology and Psychiatry, 74,* 628–640.

Faltin, R. J., Sungaila, P., Hershman, I., & Dickinson, M. V. (1982). The chronic lower back pain patient in motion: An EMG based treatment program which teaches control of motion-induced spasms. *Proceedings of the Biofeedback Society of America Thirteenth Annual Meeting* (pp. 79–81). Wheat Ridge, CO: Biofeedback Society of America.

Fassbender, H. G. (1975). *Pathology of rheumatic disease.* New York: Springer Verlag.

Flor, H., Haag, G., Turk, D. C., & Koehler, H. (1983). Efficacy of EMG biofeedback, pseudotherapy, and conventional medical treatment for chronic rheumatic back pain. *Pain, 17,* 21–31.

Fowler, R. S. Jr., & Kraft, G. H. (1974). Tension perception in patients having pain associated with chronic muscle tension. *Archives of Physical Medicine and Rehabilitation, 55,* 28–30.

Freeman, C. W., Calsyn, D. A., Paige, A. B., & Halar, E. M. (1980). Biofeedback with low back pain patients. *American Journal of Clinical Biofeedback, 3,* 118–122.

Gottlieb, H. J., Alperson, B. L., Koller, R., & Hockersmith, V. (1979). An innovative program for the restoration of patients with chronic back pain. *Physical Therapy, 59,* 996–999.

Gottlieb, H., Strite, L. C., Koller, R., Madorsky, A., Hockersmith, V., Kleeman, M., & Wagner, J. (1977). Comprehensive rehabilitation of patients having chronic low back pain. *Archives of Physical Medicine and Rehabilitation, 58,* 101–108.

Grabel, J. (1974). *Electromyographic study of low back muscle tension in subjects with and without chronic low back pain.* Doctoral dissertation, United States International University, San Diego, CA.

Hagberg, M. (1981). Electromyographic signs of shoulder muscular fatigue in two elevated arm positions. *American Journal of Physical Medicine, 60,* 111–121.

Hagberg, M., & Kvarnström, S. (1984). Muscular endurance and electromyographic fatigue in myofascial shoulder pain. *Archives of Physical Medicine and Rehabilitation, 65,* 522–525.

Haynes, S. N., Gannon, L. R., Cuevas, J., Heiser, P., Hamilton, J., & Katranides, M. (1983). The psychophysiological assessment of muscle-contraction headache subjects during headache and nonheadache conditions. *Psychophysiology, 20,* 393–399.

Hobbs, W., & Cox, D. (1982). Methodological and analytic procedures which differentiate tension headache from control subjects. Paper presented at the Third Annual Meeting of the Society of Behavioral Medicine, Chicago.

Holmes, D. S., & Burish, T. G. (1983). Effectiveness of biofeedback for treating migraine and tension headaches: A review of the evidence. *Journal of Psychosomatic Research, 27,* 515–532.

Holmes, T. H., & Wolff, H. G. (1952). Life situations, emotions, and backache. *Psychosomatic Medicine, 14,* 18–33.

Hoyt, W. H., Hunt, H. H., DePauw, M. A., Bard, D., Shaffer, F., Passias, J. N., Robbins, D. H., Runyon, D. G., Semrad, S. E., Symonds, J. T., & Watt, K. C. (1981). Electromyographic assessment of chronic low back pain syndrome. *Journal of American Osteopathic Association, 80,* 57–59.

Jacobs, A., & Felton, G. S. (1969). Visual feedback of myoelectric output to facilitate muscle relaxation in normal persons and patients with neck injuries. *Archives of Physical Medicine and Rehabilitation, 50,* 34–39.

Jessup, B. A. (1984). Biofeedback. In P. Wall and R. Melzack (Eds.), *Textbook of Pain.* New York: Churchill Livingstone.

Jones, A. L., & Wolff, S. L. (1980). Treating chronic low back pain, EMG biofeedback training during movement. *Physical Therapy, 60,* 58–63.

Keefe, J. (1981). Behavioral assessment and treatment of chronic pain: Current status and future directions. *Journal of Consulting and Clinical Psychology, 50,* 896–911.

Kravitz, E., Moore, M. E., & Glaros, A. (1981). Paralumbar muscle activity in chronic low back pain. *Archives of Physical Medicine and Rehabilitation, 62,* 172–176.

Large, R. G., & Lamb, A. M. (1983). Electromyographic (EMG) feedback in chronic musculoskeletal pain: A controlled trial. *Pain, 17,* 167–177.

LeVine, R. (1983). Behavioral and biofeedback therapy for a functionally impaired musician: A case report. *Biofeedback and Self-Regulation, 8,* 101–107.

Libo, L. M., & Arnold, G. E. (1983). Relaxation practice after biofeedback therapy: A long-term follow-up study of utilization and effectiveness. *Biofeedback and Self-Regulation, 8,* 217–227.

Loeser, D. (1980). Low back pain. In J. Bonica (Ed.), *Pain.* New York: Raven Press.

Middaugh, S. (1978). EMG feedback as a muscle reeducation technique: A controlled study. *Physical Therapy, 58,* 15–22.

Middaugh, S. (1982). Muscle training. In D. M. Doley, R. L. Meredith, & A. R. Ciminero (Eds.), *Behavioral medicine: Assessment and treatment strategies.* New York: Plenum.

Middaugh, S. J., & Kee, W. G. (1984a, March 23–28). Role of EMG evaluations in the multimodal treatment of chronic pain. In *Proceedings of the Fifteenth Annual Meeting of the Biofeedback Society of America,* Albuquerque, New Mexico.

Middaugh, S. J., & Kee, W. G. (1984b, May 23–26). EMG evaluation of chronic neck and back pain patients. Presented at the *Fifth Annual Meeting of the Society of Behavioral Medicine.* Philadelphia.

Middaugh, S. J., & Miller, M. C. (1980). Electromyographic feedback: Effect on voluntary muscle contractions in paretic subjects. *Archives of Physical Medicine and Rehabilitation, 61,* 24–29.

Middaugh, S., Miller, M. C., Foster, G., & Murphy, E. (1981). EMG feedback in neuromuscular reeducation: Effect on voluntary relaxation of spastic muscles. *Proceedings of the Biofeedback Society of America 12th Annual Meeting* (pp. 23–25). Wheat Ridge, CO: Biofeedback Society of America.

Middaugh, S., Miller, M. C., & Foster, G. (1982a). Voluntary relaxation of spastic muscles in stroke patients: Comparison of EMG feedback, non-feedback and baseline groups. *Proceedings of the Biofeedback Society of America 13th Annual Meeting* (pp. 127–129). Wheat Ridge, CO: Biofeedback Society of America.

Middaugh, S. J., Miller, M. C., Foster, G., & Ferdon, M. B. (1982b). Electromyographic feedback: Effects on voluntary muscle contractions in normal subjects. *Archives of Physical Medicine and Rehabilitation, 63,* 254–260.

Middaugh, S., Miller, M. C., Foster, G., & Pien, L. (1982c). EMG feedback: Effect on voluntary muscle contractions in stroke patients. *Proceedings of the Biofeedback Society of America Thirteenth Annual Meeting* (pp. 205–207). Wheat Ridge, CO: Biofeedback Society of America.

Miller, J. (1985). Comparison of electromyographic activity in the lumbar paraspinal muscles of subjects with and without chronic low back pain. *Physical Therapy, 65,* 1347–1354.

Mills, K. R., Newham, D. J., & Edwards, R. H. T. (1984). Muscle pain. In R. Melzack & P. Wall (Eds.), *Textbook of Pain* (pp. 319–330). New York: Churchill Livingstone.

Morris, F. H., Jr., Gasteiger, E. L., & Chatfield, P. O. (1957). An electromyographic study of induced and spontaneous muscle cramps. *Electroencephalogy and Clinical Neurophysiology, 9,* 139–147.

National Institute on Drug Abuse. (1981). *New approaches to treatment of chronic pain: A review of multidisciplinary pain clinics and pain centers* (Research monograph series, 36). Rockville, MD: Department of Health and Human Services, Public Health Service.

Nigl, A. J., & Fischer-Williams, M. (1980). Treatment of low back strain with electromyographic biofeedback and relaxation training. *Psychosomatics, 21,* 495–499.

Nouwen, A. (1983). EMG biofeedback used to reduce standing levels of paraspinal muscle tension in chronic low back pain. *Pain, 17,* 353–360.

Nouwen, A., & Bush, C. (1984). The relationship between paraspinal EMG and chronic low back pain. *Pain, 20,* 109–123.

Nouwen, A., & Solinger, J. W. (1979). The effectiveness of EMG biofeedback training in low back pain. *Biofeedback and Self-Regulation, 4,* 103–111.

Peck, C. L., & Kraft, G. H. (1977). Electromyographic biofeedback for pain related to muscle tension. *Archives of Surgery, 112,* 889–895.

Petrofsky, J. S. (1981). Quantification through the surface of EMG of muscle fatigue and recovery during successive isometric contractions. *Aviation, Space, and Environmental Medicine, 52,* 545–550.

Philips, C. (1978). Tension headache: Theoretical problems. *Behavior Research and Therapy, 16,* 249–261.

Rohter, F. D., & Hyman, C. (1962). Blood flow in arm and finger during muscle contraction and joint position changes. *Journal of Applied Physiology, 17,* 819–823.

Rouleau, J., & Denver, D. R. (1980). Electromyography (EMG) and temperature biofeedback of the "Pure Fibrositis Syndrome." *Proceedings of the Biofeedback Society of America 11th Annual Meeting* (p. 142–145). Colorado Springs, Colorado.

Sharpley, C. F., & Rogers, H. J. (1984). A meta-analysis of frontalis EMG levels with biofeedback and alternative procedures. *Biofeedback and Self-Regulation, 9,* 385–393.

Sherman, R. A. (1985). Relationships between strength of low back muscle contraction and reported intensity of chronic low back pain. *American Journal of Physical Medicine, 64,* 190–200.

Simons, D. G. (1975). Muscle pain syndromes - Part I. *American Journal of Physical Medicine, 54,* 289–311.

Simons, D. G. (1976). Muscle pain syndromes - Part II. *American Journal of Physical Medicine, 55,* 15–42.

Spirduso, W. W., & Duncan, A. M. (1976). Voluntary inhibition of the myotatic reflex and premotor response to joint angle displacement. *American Journal of Physical Medicine, 55,* 165–176.

Todd, J., & Belar, C. D. (1980). EMG biofeedback and chronic low back pain: Implications of treatment failure. *American Journal of Clinical Biofeedback, 3,* 114–117.

Travell, J. (1960). Temporomandibular joint pain referred from muscles of the head and neck. *Journal of Prosthetic Dentistry, 10,* 745–763.

Travell, J. G., & Simons, D. G. (1983). *Myofascial pain and dysfunction: The trigger point manual.* Baltimore, MD: Williams and Wilkins.

Turner, J. A., & Chapman, C. R. (1982). Psychological interventions for chronic pain: A critical review. I. Relaxation training and biofeedback. *Pain, 12,* 1–21.

Turner, J. A. (1982). Comparison of group progressive-relaxation training and cognitive-behavioral group therapy for chronic low back pain. *Journal of Consulting and Clinical Psychology, 50,* 757–765.

van Boxtel, A., Goudswaard, P., & Schomaker, L. R. B. (1984). Amplitude and bandwidth of the frontalis surface EMG: Effects of electrode parameters. *Psychophysiology, 21,* 699–707.

Whatmore, G. B., & Kohli, D. R. (1974). *The physiopathology and treatment of functional disorders.* New York: Grune and Stratton.

Whatmore, G. B., Whatmore, N. J., & Fisher, L. D. (1981). Is fortalis activity a reliable indicator of the activity in other skeletal muscles? *Biofeedback and Self-Regulation, 6,* 305–314.

Wolf, S. L. , Basmajian, J. V., Russe, T. C., & Kutner, M. (1979). Normative data on low back mobility and activity levels. *American Journal of Physical Medicine, 58,* 217–229.

Wolf, S. L., Nacht, M., & Kelly, J. L. (1982). EMG feedback training during dynamic movement for low pain patients. *Behavior Therapy, 13,* 395–406.

SECTION III
Selected Topics in Rehabilitation

Burn Rehabilitation

Myron G. Eisenberg

Section Editor

Cancer Rehabilitation

Roy C. Grzesiak

Section Editor

Burn Rehabilitation
Introduction

Myron G. Eisenberg

The sequelae of burn injuries are staggering in terms of their resulting human and economic costs. According to the National Institutes of Health and other reporting organizations, 2 million Americans experience a burn injury each year. Of these, 300,000 are seriously burned and 50,000 to 70,000 are hospitalized for a period ranging from 6 weeks to 2 years. Moreover, the National Commission on Fire Prevention reports that of those who suffer serious burns 12,000 die every year. In addition, there is evidence that 50% of these fatalities occur before arrival at the hospital emergency room.

A second measure of the burn problem is the cost of treatment. In 1972 the daily cost during intensive care in highly specialized facilities was between $250 and $400. By 1974 these figures had jumped to between $350 and $800, and by the end of 1976 patient charges for the same services were running between $500 and $1,100 per day. Currently, burn patients pay as much as $2,000 per day for treatment.

An equally important measure of this problem is the effect of burn injuries on the victims and their families. There are few if any injuries requiring long hospitalization that are more traumatic than severe burns. The frightening circumstances of the injury, the long isolation from the family, the continuous pain during recovery, the stigma of disfigurement— all these contribute to a deep despondency and, frequently, loss of the will to live. In addition, the toll taken by this tragedy also must be measured in terms of those who grieve the loss of loved ones, those who are left jobless or impoverished because of permanent disability, and those left to deal with the staggering cost of hospital bills.

During the last 20 years an increased emphasis on burn care has resulted in improved survival rates of patients with all levels of burn severity and a decreased length of hospitalization. Concomitant with the development of more effective life-support measures, antimicrobial therapy, and surgical techniques has been the evolution of a more positive and organized approach to rehabilitation of the thermally injured patient. It has been demonstrated that a meaningful and enthusiastic integration of efforts by the rehabilitation team is vital to competent and total care of thermally injured patients. It is from this perspective that this section was prepared.

This section is comprised of two chapters that attempt to present our current understanding of rehabilitation practice following burns. Chapter 7 "Rehabilitation Management of the Burn Patient," considers treatment strategies employed throughout the rehabilitation period. Its author discusses practical rehabilitation efforts that are designed to maintain joint and skin mobility and exercises to maintain strength and endurance. The psychosocial component of burn management also is addressed, including ways of helping to preserve patients' sexuality and recreational and social contacts.

Chapter 8, "Management of Pain After Thermal Injury," focuses on the physical and emotional management of pain following a burn injury. Emphasis is placed on pragmatic modalities that are designed to ameliorate pain and promote the patient's emotional and physical recovery.

7

Rehabilitation Management of the Burn Patient

Elizabeth A. Rivers

The medical literature contains a plethora of proposals for burn management. Such divergence of opinion is to be expected for an injury so varied. In the past, medical literature was concerned with emergency and life-saving interventions. Now articles are published dealing with the quality of the survivor's life and the role of burn team members. Successful recovery from a burn injury includes returning to a productive, satisfying life in the home, family, workplace or school, and community.

About 1% of the United States population sustains a burn injury annually. Not all of these are severe, but most are painful and interfere with the person's life activities while the injury heals. In a recent article Tollison, Still, and Tollison (1980) noted that to be extensively burned is to suffer one of the most devastating and dehumanizing injuries one can experience. Before the burn each person had a preburn, genetic set of attributes and a physical, emotional, intellectual, and spiritual history. These formed a relatively permanent personality. The maturity of each person in these areas depended on previous trials and errors and the rewards perceived for activities. Immediately after the burn the well-developed, old coping skills will be used. However, new coping skills may be needed. Preburn participation in physical fitness programs will probably speed healing. The athletic individual more readily understands rehabilitation management. When an appreciation of proper breathing, slow stretching, and frequent, graded exercise are a part of the patient's history, it reduces the frustrating hours spent learning these skills. The therapist and patient are then freed to concentrate on other important parts of rehabilitation.

The rehabilitation outcome, even for the severely burned victim treated in a burn center, has improved dramatically in the past 5 years. The four most important contributors to this change are new, safer, and more effective methods of surgical debridement, nutritional support, improved antibiotic dosage by pharmacokinetics, and early individualized rehabilitation.

Surgical debridement followed by autograft, hemograft, temporar biological dressings, or synthetic skin has decreased sepsis. In burns ove 50% of the body surface, skin may be cultured to cover the open wounc Very thin donor skin may be used, allowing the skin to be reharvested at 5 day intervals. Surgeons have known since ancient times that necrotic tissu must be removed for healing and survival. Recently technology has pro vided new dermatomes, improved skin meshers, microsurgical technique successful epithelial tissue culture, and topical hemostatics, all of whicl enhance safe surgical interventions. Grafting can confidently be initiated o the second or third day after injury (Heimbach & Engrav, 1984).

The ancients also knew the value of nutrition. Adequate and prope nourishment, documented by nitrogen balance studies, can now be adminis tered orally and parenterally. Nonirritating nasogastric tubes passed into the duodenum have the additional benefit of improved utilization of entera nourishment and fewer side effects, which might occur with intravenou nutrition. The ease of 24-hour-a-day tube feeding eliminates many staff-family–patient conflicts regarding eating when appetite is poor.

Bacterial adaptation in response to antibiotics and the need for individual ized dosing of medication has long been recognized as crucial for the survival of patients vulnerable to infections. Recent research and compute availability have simplified antibiotic administration. Pharmacokinetics as sist in determining the most effective drug, the safest, most effective dose and the administration interval that decreases both side effects and resistan bacteria.

Rehabilitation equipment has also become more sophisticated and effi-cient. Machines such as the Cybex®, Orthotron®, Nautilus®, and Baltimore Therapeutic Equipment Work Trainer give instant information about strength and endurance. Progress and change are recorded objectively. Continuous passive motion machines are used to avoid adhesions during healing. Furthermore, therapists have a better understanding of behavioral interventions. As a result of this understanding, patients are provided the opportunity to choose between a wide variety of rehabilitation techniques. This, in turn, facilitates patient responsibility and involvement in planning and implementing the therapy program. Patients take pride in planning their own rehabilitation. Individuals who feel influential in their own recov-ery benefit from improved self-esteem and self-confidence as well as func-tional recovery. Because the therapist is a professional, the patient is not allowed to deteriorate during the time it takes for him to choose appropriate and useful modalities.

The rehabilitation team (the physiatrist, the occupational therapist, the physical therapist, and the psychologist) brings insight and perspective to smooth the burn victim's road to recovery. The anonymous saying "Life is what happens to you while you are planning your future" characterizes burn victims. Some patients are caught up in their reaction to the severe trauma and find future independence difficult to imagine. The rehabilitation team contributes a frame of reference for doing it yourself. Patient participation both in the healing process and in independent living programs has long been encouraged by physiatrists. Pride in shared accomplishments encourages the person to expend greater energy, which in turn speeds the return of vigor and health.

Recovery after a severe burn injury is a process. The patient and family, familiar with time-limited events, such as healing broken bones, seek exact grafting or discharge dates. They are frustrated when the burn team cannot provide specifics. Burn recovery takes place on a continuum of several years. Individualized therapy must continue from the moment of injury until the healed wound is soft, supple, mobile, of proper color, and inactive. The skin that is severely burned will be permanently changed. It has a new texture, is less elastic, and has obvious color changes: hypopigmentation or hyperpigmentation.

Coping in a positive way with the changed body image often requires Olympian effort on the part of the patient, family, and community. Patients report that support and concern are the catalyst for successful coping during this prolonged adjustment period. Scars, contractures, residual pain, and disability are the physical problems the burn team endeavors to minimize. These were formerly believed to be normal sequelae of wound healing. Ugly, raised scars are not inevitable; they can be relatively flat. The areas that cannot be camouflaged or covered, if the patient chooses, are usually relatively small. Even patients who have amputations develop skill in making themselves resemble the able-bodied people who surround them. Therapists who work with burned people have noted tremendous emotional resilience that can be tapped. Patients may develop the increased ego strength and enhanced self-esteem that accompanies having successfully conquered an immense challenge. A small percentage of burned patients will never return to independent living and a few recover completely, by chance, without rehabilitation. However, for the majority rehabilitation professionals provide the tools for earlier return to independence with less emotional fallout.

Burn victims generally survive the initial injury and receive high-quality, on-the-scene care and emergency transportation to a burn center. Treatments vary depending on the geographical area in which the person is hospitalized. The medical literature contains a wide divergence of opinion regarding which treatments are optimal. However, there is agreement in general areas of management, and in centers using early surgical intervention, appropriate antibiotics, and conservative scar control, most severely burned patients return to work or school within 1 year. In 1985 the profile of the average patient injured on the job and treated at St. Paul-Ramsey Medical Center in St. Paul, Minnesota was as follows: A 23-year-old male sustaining 23% body surface burn, who needed one grafting, and spent 23 days in the hospital. This average burn victim returned to work in about 3 months.

This paper will examine treatment for severe burn injuries. Severe burns include electrical burns; any burn accompanied by inhalation injury; deep dermal burns of the face, hands, or genitalia, or of any body area involving more than 30% of the skin surface; and all full-thickness burns covering more than 10% of the body.

Burns can be caused by extremes of temperature (heat or cold), cutaneous contact with chemicals (acids, bases, or petroleum products), contact from high- or low-voltage electricity or lightning sources, and radiation (although this is rare). The severity of the burn depends on the duration of exposure to the burning agent or the temperature or both. It is important for professionals to be thoroughly familiar with each burned patient's history because the timing of appropriate intervention is crucial for high-quality, cost-effective rehabilitation. For instance, if meticulous hygiene is used, a person having a flash burn to the face can be treated as an outpatient. The injury will probably heal in less than 3 weeks with no complications. Healing in this case will occur by natural processes whether or not the person exercises, has a positive mental outlook, or resumes vocational activity as soon as possible. However, if the person with a facial flash burn also sustained an inhalation injury, was anoxic, or sustained associated closed-head injuries, impaired cognition should be considered. In this case the initial rehabilitation evaluation would include cognitive functions such as memory, perception, ability to concentrate, foresight, planning, and judgment. Cognitive retraining would commence based on this evaluation. The overall goal of therapy is the maximum, safe independence of the person burned with minimal contracture formation and disfigurement, achieved with the least expense.

BURN REHABILITATION IN THE EARLY POSTBURN PERIOD

The rehabilitation program can be divided into three overlapping phases to assist in prescribing effective treatments. The first phase of therapy begins with the burn incident. It continues through epithelial healing in partial-thickness injury or through debridement in full-thickness tissue destruction. This phase is commonly referred to as the "early phase" or "pregrafting period" of burn treatment. If the burn is all superficial and heals in 2 weeks, his is the only phase the patient will experience. The second phase of burn rehabilitation is commonly called the "immobilization for grafting period." This period begins in the operating room when the patient's skin is surgically transplanted and continues until the graft has vascularized or it necroses. After this time the surgeon will encourage free active motion and ambulation wearing vascular supports. The third or final healing phase begins with stable epithelium covering either the healed partial thickness or the grafted wound. At this time full active motion and ambulation as tolerated are appropriate. In this paper the final healing phase will be called the "postepithelial healing, wound maturation period."

The rehabilitation goals for each period are listed followed by the therapeutic modalities and patient approaches that can facilitate successful healing in each time period. Many patients do not pass through each period. Some heal quickly and need no further interventions or follow-up. The severely burned patient will progress through all three phases.

The goals of rehabilitation management during the early or pregrafting burn recovery period are the following:

1. To promote wound closure.
2. To control edema.
3. To maintain joint and skin mobility.
4. To maintain strength and endurance.
5. To facilitate family participation in wound healing and rehabilitation.
6. To teach self-feeding and independent personal hygiene.

Early Wound Closure by Primary Healing

Cleaning

There are a variety of rehabilitation modalities that will provide the meticulous hygiene required for early wound closure by primary healing. Since enteric bacteria are the most common wound-contaminating flora, many centers achieve cleansing by rinsing over a tub or washing using a basin of water. Whirlpool is another means of promoting good wound hygiene; it also applies heat. Carter (1983) suggests that simply soaking in a soap solution, which had been a time-honored tradition, is not adequate and may actually be deleterious, owing to maceration of the skin. In addition, he states that prolonged contact of delicate structures such as joint cartilage and tendon with the strong bactericidal soaps has been shown to cause cell necrosis. He suggests using sterile saline lavage under pressure, which decreases bacterial count and leads to lower wound infection rates. In the literature a great deal of controversy continues over the best means of cleaning the burn wound. Whatever means is used, adequate analgesia and a

skilled flexible technician are appreciated by the patient. The water shoul
be 100°F (38°C) and the duration of the bath limited to avoid chilling
which increases the already accelerated hypermetabolic load. The advantag
of transporting the patient by litter is that it helps to avoid dependent edem
when the elastic bandages are removed and reapplied. Using a lift for tul
entry is less painful and safer for the patient and attendant.

Debridement

Debridement is the act of removing dead and foreign matter from the
wound. When it is done with a daily bath, washing over the area with a
gauze will wipe away the topical ointment and any loose debris. Loosened
eschar can be cut away with sharp curved scissors. Picking up the edge o
the tissue with a forceps aids in removing the remaining nonvascularizec
material. Patients complain that this is the most painful part of recovering
from a burn injury. No analgesia provides enough pain relief at this time
Adequate anesthesia is not possible during tub baths, and therefore this is a
stressful procedure for the patient, nurse, physician (when involved), and
therapist. Heimbach and Engrav (1984) suggest one of the indications for
early excision is pain management.

Debridement by surgical excision is done in the operating room when the
patient is anesthetized. Heimbach and Engrav (1984) note that success with
this procedure requires an experienced surgeon. If dead tissue is left in the
wound, the graft will slough and the open area will have to be regrafted after
the granulation bed is clean. This prolongs hospitalization and time off
work and increases the donor area.

Controlling Edema

Antigravity positioning is universally used to decrease edema. Positioning is
defined as a proper arrangement of body parts. Patients are asked to assume
differing postures, which preserve the maximum length of the healed
wound and assist venous and lympathic circulation.

Edema control improves circulation and speeds healing by reducing venous and lympathic engorgement. Rapid blanch and return in the fingernail
bed may reflect good arterial circulation, even when cellular perfusion is
impaired from swelling inside the leathery burn eschar. Remensnyder
(1980) points out that secondary thrombosis or ischemia may convert a
partial-thickness burn to full-thickness epithelial destruction. Carter (1983)
notes the venous supply to the hand is much more interwoven and complex
than the arterial supply. In addition, most arteries have a pair of accompanying veins. Elevation of the part above the right atrium will give a "gravity
assist" to venous return. Some burn units use cotton batting and elastic

wrap dressings (Robert Jones, M.D., personal communication, 1985) and overhead suspension in the first 3 days to control swelling. The elastic wrap support, when the extremity is dependent, will also assist in edema control.

Covey (1985) reports successfully decreasing early hand edema by judicious use of the continuous passive motion machine. Elevated active motion during waking hours is also helpful for the alert patient.

Maintaining Joint and Skin Mobility

Exercise

Active range of motion is the only method of keeping the burned tissue elongated. Patients seeking pain relief are often seen lying in a flexed, adducted position. This is the position of withdrawal from pain. An extended position is equally comfortable once the tissue stretches. Immobility or rest does not relieve pain as well as analgesic medications, but, rather, increases pain because contractures will become resistant to being stretched. Walking is one of the more comfortable exercises. An overhead walker (see Figure 7.1) provides the patient with a graded method of elevation and exercise for the upper extremities. Additionally, squeezing the overhead bar facilitates the "pumping action," thereby reducing edema. Since the overhead bar is large, it tends to be less destructive to inflamed dorsal finger tendons than tight fist-making, which would endanger them. During the early treatment period ambulation three or four times a day using the overhead walker will maintain range of motion.

Passive range of motion or the therapist's moving the patient's joint through the free, painless motion is almost always contraindicated in the alert burn patient. All motion is at least uncomfortable, and past patients state that passive moving was very painful. The burned person must move the joints past the painful range to the extremes of motion. Gentle terminal stretch is the least painful method of achieving this mobility. Active assistive exercises with terminal stretching teach the patient how to move the body part and achieve the extremes of motion that are not used spontaneously. Prolonged, vigorous stretch, although appropriate with healed, contracted joints, is almost never appropriate with the early edematous burn.

The object of exercise is to speed healing by improving circulation, decreasing edema, and decreasing inflammatory response. Vigorous, agonizing stretching is not needed at this time. During the first week the patient, as expected, will believe all motion is severely painful until he or she has practiced frequent, slow moving to prevent stiffness. Establishing trust in the therapist early in the process will prevent many later power struggles.

Reciprocal pulleys, two-handed calisthenics, slow bicycling, and dowel exercises have been safe methods of providing passive motion. The patient

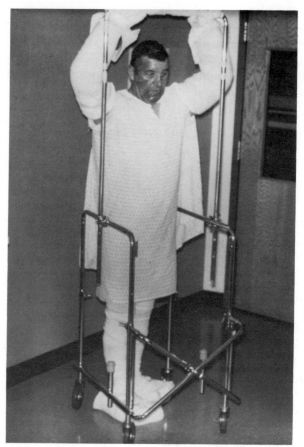

FIGURE 7.1 **Overhead walker gives constant reminder of arm elevation. Patient moves hands up to overhead bar as pain subsides during ambulation. Squeezing overhead bar pumps edema away.**

controls the speed and duration of passive stretch. The therapist is the coach. Multitudes of choices and written graded programs are helpful with the hostile, obstreperous patient. Since the patient cannot control whether or not the wound is cleaned, it is reassuring to be given as much control as possible in exercising.

There is some controversy about the best time to do exercises with the patient. If the bandages are dry and stuck or the xenograft has dried and will not bend, then pain will inhibit patient cooperation with full active range of motion. In this case, exercise during the bathing procedure will benefit the patient most; however, he or she may be distracted by pain and may not be able to do active motion or to remember the exercises. If there is topical medication under the gauze bandages, they are wrapped in a loose figure-of-eight method, and they slide easily, then exercise in the bandages is preferred by the patient. In all cases the therapist and prescribing physician should observe the tissue with bandages removed during the stretching exercises at least twice a week.

Splints

A splint or orthosis is a thin piece of metal, plastic, plaster, foam, reinforced cloth, or molded leather that holds a body part in a fixed position. An orthosis that has outriggers or attachments to provide stretching or to replace absent function is called a "dynamic splint." Static splints are fitted to individual body parts of the burned person who is unconscious or is unable to maintain full active range of motion by positioning and activity. The purpose of the splint in this stage of healing is to immobilize an unstable joint, to prevent formation of nonfunctional contractures, to keep ligaments in optimal position, or to assist with antigravity positioning.

To keep the cornea moist for the comatose, facially injured patient, transparent humidity domes can be fitted. These do not replace meticulous hygiene, eye drops, or lacrilube, but serve as a protective barrier until the blink reflex returns. The oral opening can be maintained with a Buckner microstomia-prevention appliance. If this appliance exacerbates lip eversion, then only active exercise should be used. A soft foam anterior collar can prevent early neck flexion contractures.

If the hand is edematous, a thermoplastic splint with 20° wrist extension, 50° to 70° metacarpal (MP) flexion, full interphalangeal (IP) extension, and thumb rotated into opposition with slight MP flexion can be secured with a gauze wrap. This can be worn 20 hours a day; however, it will not replace active motion. Another aid to hand edema control is the plastic air band, described by Barnett and Stafford (1984).

Elbows and shoulders can be splinted with foam pads until the tissue is healed. Some burn centers fit elbow extension splints or axillary abduction splints. When an elbow splint is used, careful observation must be exercised to avoid overextending the brachioradialis muscle and stimulating heterotopic ossification. Helm et al. (1982) suggested supination with elbow extension in the positioning splint to decrease the risk of calcium deposits. Foot drop can be prevented by the commercially available ankle–foot orthosis (AFO) or an individually fitted AFO. Knee extension splints are almost never used for the acute stage of burn care.

Maintaining Strength and Endurance

Daily, gently graded activity will diminish loss of strength. This is accomplished by every member of the rehabilitation team actively encouraging the patient and family to continue exercising despite the seriousness of the injury. Repeatedly stressing the value of activity, which improves circulation, thereby speeding healing, is motivating. Presenting numerous different types of activity helps the patient choose activity that is interesting. "Nerf" games, bicycling, stair-climbing, and calisthenics are good. Crafts, if the family is interested in joining the patient in these projects, will reinforce activity.

Family Education

Initiating clear, honest communication with family members at admission improves their ability to understand the expected course of wound healing. Relatives usually are well acquainted with the injured person and will be helpful in promoting rehabilitation. A family book containing a summary of expected treatments and terminology assists relatives to absorb complex information at an individual rate. Videotapes can also be helpful.

Fear that the patient may die or have intolerable pain often is the basis of family questions. After the initial phase of shock, other families or previously treated patients can provide helpful answers to questions and reassure the family of the recently admitted patient. When needed, family questions can be fielded by a specific team member. The primary nurse often fills this role, with other team members referring the family to this person for consistency. A family group meeting coordinated by a psychologist, counselor, psychiatric nurse, chaplain, or therapist is a useful way to communicate general information. Group discussions can develop a support system of friends who have experienced similar fears and triumphs in the burn center. Often, even though the families are geographically separated by hundreds of miles, these friendships continue for life; families exchange holiday greetings and write about memorable occasions.

Activities of Daily Living

Self-care activities improve morale and are an excellent distraction from pain. At first the patient can choose between several activities such as oral hygiene or self-feeding breakfast. Gradually, as able, he or she can resume responsibility for telephone use, hygiene, grooming, and toileting.

BURN REHABILITATION IN THE IMMOBILIZATION FOR GRAFTING PERIOD

Rehabilitation therapy goals during the immobilization phase of burn wound care include the following:

1. To consult with the surgeons to design splints and plan positioning, especially if the graft extends over a joint.
2. To provide an exercise program to prevent phlebitis, pneumonia, and contractures during the bed rest period, beginning one joint proximal and one joint distal to graft.
3. To decrease hallucinations and confusion by helping family and staff provide appropriate sensory stimulation, especially if the person is on a rotobed or clinitron bed or is sensory-deprived in other ways.
4. To reassure and educate the patient and family about graft appearance and the normal processes of wound healing.

Immobilizing Splints

The postoperative period, during which any joint underlying a skin graft must be immobilized, is dreaded by rehabilitation specialists. It is usually impossible to maintain ideal positioning at all joints. For the severely burned person, 3 to 7 days of immobility during skin graft vascularization causes severely limited active motion. When a severe inflammatory process surrounding a joint is noted preoperatively, the results of immobilization can be nearly disastrous. However, with early grafting procedures, early resumption of supervised, gentle active motion, and carefully designed immobilizing splints, satisfactory outcomes can be anticipated.

Widely varying materials and protocols have been suggested for postoperative skin graft dressings. All have the common purposes of immobilizing the grafted area, preventing edema, and speeding wound healing. Additional considerations are convenience, comfort, and cost.

In centers using the exposure method of graft healing, elevation, support, and protection of the grafted areas are accomplished with pillows, slings, open thermoplastic splints, or skeletal traction. Safely securing a thermoplastic splint without impairing circulation may be a challenge if the burn is circumferential and extends beyond the borders of the graft.

When the healed wound is expected to be especially fragile, as it is after artificial skin grafts, overhead suspension of the body part is indicated. The proper use of skeletal immobilization is reviewed by Parks, Caravajal, and Larson (1977), Harnar, Engrav, Heimbach, and Marvin (1985), and Johnson, O'Shaughnessy, and Ostergren (1981). Precautions noted include use of proper counterbalance weight for each individual, thoroughly investigating patient complaints, frequent observations to avoid weights resting on the floor or bed parts, lubricating pulleys with silicone spray before attaching traction, and protecting the weights from bumping by the passing visitors, children, and equipment.

A frequently used postoperative dressing is the bulky wrap. A single layer of nonadherent gauze is used in contact with the graft by many surgeons. Twenty-four completely opened gauze 4×4 sponges are then placed into the palm, between the interdigital webs, and into the thumb web space. One dozen fluffed gauzes are placed dorsally and the entire bandage is held in place with a snug Kling wrap. The entire wrap can be reinforced with a dorsal or a palmar plaster splint or both. The plaster should not contact the skin. A single layer of Webril interface makes removal of the plaster simpler. The splint can be secured with an elastic wrap.

When thermoplastic splints (Figure 7.2) are used, they may be fitted over a single layer of nonadherent gauze, over a bulky wrap, over a stent-dressing, or over a wet fine-mesh gauze dressing. Any plastic splint can be cut open so drainage can escape. Very wet dressings can cause maceration and superficial infection if not changed frequently. When the patient is fitted with the splint under anesthesia, it is important for the body parts to be anatomically aligned. It is often easier for the patient to adjust to wearing a splint during the time he is receiving maximum pain medication after surgery. Later, the splint often feels comfortable, which increases compliance.

The wrist extension (20°), MP flexion (70°), IP extension (0°), and thumb abduction–rotation hand splint is conveniently secured with a gauze wrap and elevated on a foam wedge. An elbow extension splint is another simple-to-use splint, combined with a foam wedge. Shoulders are more difficult and require team consultation to achieve maximum ease of wound care with minimum trauma or shearing to the healing tissue.

Another type of immobilizing splint is prosthetic foam/elastomer/elastic wrap (Figure 7.3A and 7.3B); the liquid silicone combined with stannous

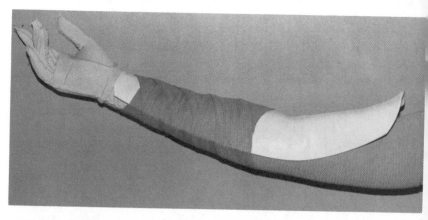

FIGURE 7.2 Thermoplastic splint blocks elbow flexion. Drop-out elastic wrapping encourages active extension. Glove support prevents hand edema.

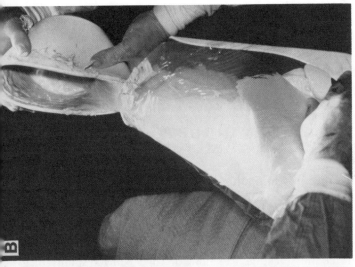

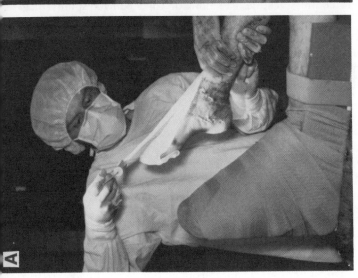

FIGURE 7.3 Prosthetic foam/elastomer/elastic wrap postoperative dressing. A: Left foot in finished gradient pressure elastic wrapped prosthetic foam/elastomer/elastic wrap (PFEEW). Right foot being prepared with single layer of xeroform gauze longitudinally over draft. B: 1:1 prosthetic foam/elastomer mixed with stannous octoate catalyst poured into closed cylinder around foot and ankle.

octoate catalyst is poured into a cylinder surrounding the grafted area and allowed to expand, forming an exact, total contact splint. The advantages of this splint include preventing graft dessication, allowing for perfect distribution of external pressure and internal lymphatic support, controlling edema and seroma formation by gradient elastic wrap pressure, and immobilizing the restless patient because of weight and relative rigidity in the total bandage. The likelihood of tissue maceration, the unsupervised patient pulling out of the bandage, and the inability to visualize the graft are serious disadvantages of this postoperative orthosis.

The rehabilitation goals 2, 3, and 4 are self-explanatory.

REHABILITATION IN THE POSTEPITHELIAL HEALING, WOUND MATURATION PERIOD

Rehabilitation therapy during this phase is a challenge to the burn victim, the rehabilitation team, and the family. The patient may see hospital discharge as a welcome termination of burn care and pain. He eagerly anticipates what he believes is a well deserved rest. Even the most recalcitrant patient may endure scar control at the hospital, but once safe at home, custom-made elastic stockings, traction, or total contact splints may be abandoned. The patient's firmly held dream is that returning home will magically bring back his previous physical and emotional status. However, it quickly becomes obvious that achieving epithelial healing to allow safe return home is only the beginning.

The goals of rehabilitation during the wound maturation phase of burn healing include the following:

1. To assist the patient in initiating discussion of sexuality.
2. To provide antigravity positioning.
3. To fit total contact, stretching orthoses.
4. To assist in regaining full active range of joint motion.
5. To promote return of normal strength and endurance.
6. To improve dexterity and coordination.
7. To successfully control edema.
8. To minimize hypertrophic scar formation.
9. To teach compensation techniques for exposure to friction or trauma, to ultraviolet light, to chemical irritants, and exposure to extremes of weather and temperature.
10. To make the patient aware of sensory changes, especially in the case of denervation.
11. To teach independent living skills.
12. To encourage taking part in recreational activities.

13. To successfully return to full-time participation in all school activities except contact sports.
14. To plan return to vocational duties.

Over the years this author has observed that many recovering burned patients find it difficult to get on with their lives because they are unable to regain the satisfying, relaxing intimacy they experienced before the injury. They have suddenly and traumatically been shocked into realizing their vulnerability and fragility in this industrialized society. Now, partially recovered, they want to deepen and strengthen relationships with a domestic partner and are afraid of rejection. Patients complain that professionals rarely initiate discussions of sexuality. The medical literature contains a paucity of studies or guidelines for sexual counseling of burned patients. Since patients nearly universally indicate that one of their least attended needs is recovering healthy sexuality, and they believe this is a crucial problematic issue, it has been placed first in the wound maturation period.

Sexuality

Resuming a sexual relationship is one of the first interests a patient voices. They find it reassuring when their doctor initiates matter-of-fact discussion of sex and birth control in the same way he discusses appetite or pain. It is important for the burned person to discuss his new family role as well as physical changes. Feeling secure in the family despite physical changes will facilitate reintegration of the person's changed body image. With emotional support he can assume responsibility for initiating communication with a domestic partner. Appearance, behavior, and personal hygiene reflect how the patient feels about himself. His new self-image influences his attitude toward sex. This quickly communicates to the spouse. The partner will appreciate openness. He or she will often be fearful of hurting the burned partner but will also be interested in finding ways to resume mutually satisfying, pleasurable sexual activity. Understanding, communication, trust, imagination, and experimentation can open opportunities to resume an exciting, loving relationship. The burned person can tell the partner which things are pleasurable and what hurts. A lubricant decreases friction blisters. However, blisters are only a nuisance; they will heal in a week and are not dangerous. Unburned parts will be helpful in sexual activity.

Arousal is more difficult when the mind is overloaded with frustrations. Unspoken doubts and fears undermine confidence and the ability of the burned person to be an inventive and satisfying sexual partner. Talking together, kissing, and caressing each other in a tender, caring, sensuous way can be arousing. Having mutually enjoyable goals and accepting, even enjoying, slow progress will increase excitement. As Mooney, Cole, and

Chilgren (1975) suggest, letting the mind enjoy itself, taking plenty of time, holding, gently stroking, and discussing mutual desires will enhance sexual intimacy.

For the sexually active female, birth control should be considered before menstruation resumes; the hormones produced during pregnancy increase the size and density of burn scars. Mature scars rarely interfere with pregnancy, and the growing baby will overcome scar resistance; however, scarred or lost mammary tissue may interfere with nursing a baby.

Direct injury to the penis or female genitalia is rare. When scars are present remodeling can be assisted by compression with elastic supports and bikini-type garments. These do not tent away from scars when the patient sits down. Commercially available scrotal supports with wide leg and waist bands, foam inserts, and frequent erections aid in reducing penile contractures. Vigorous stretching will help soften contracted soft tissue. Frequent massage with a nonviscous moisturizer will increase comfort.

Cooper-Fraps and Yerxa (1984) noted in a study of 10 adults that sexual competence was strongly correlated with activity level. In addition they found surprisingly high sexual activity levels reported by subjects who were greatly disfigured. It was speculated that denial may have affected the results of their study. As a result of this study, the authors postulate that denial may be important in achieving adjustment for the burned person. Constable, Bernstein, and Sheehy (1979) report similar findings.

Interested professionals may find Erickson's sexual counseling approach helpful. This approach, as described by Haley (1973), was to avoid pointing out or interpreting patient's fears. He did not emphasize insight. His approach was based on action to bring about change and he emphasized the positive. His focus was on expanding the person's world, not educating him about his inadequacies. When working with couples, Erickson often relabeled what they were doing in a positive way. He attempted to gain a small response and build upon that. In this way, positive forces were freed to allow the couple's further development. Couples who had worked out an amiable way of living together before a stressful event, with positive support and commitment to each other, resolved sexual difficulties. One of Erickson's basic premises was that the art of marriage included achieving independence while simultaneously remaining emotionally involved with one's relatives. This type of adjustment is crucial for the burned person, whose full recovery is dependent on his or her ability to capitalize on family resources.

Antigravity Positioning

Outpatient antigravity positioning is one of the first concerns of the therapist. Varying the burned person's position at rest can correct deformities and prevent blisters, decubitus ulcers, phlebitis, and pneumonia. As a burn victim holds his healed extremities in habitually flexed positions, they slowly contract. Any position of a burned part becomes "bad" if it is maintained too long, that is, more than several hours. Sinking into a soft bed causes shoulder and chest tightness. Patients rarely consider the tightly flexed elbow, held below the waist, when following the medical direction to keep the hand above the heart. Phone books on a table, sitting on a low stool, or using the back of a davenport or car seat can keep the arm at shoulder level. A triangular foam wedge is often used in the hospital. The hands must be kept above the elbows and the elbows above the heart to avoid swelling. For edema control as well as for mobility, position change must be frequent. Initially, dependent positions of both the arms and legs are painful, which instantly reminds the person to change positions. Later, setting a kitchen timer to ring every hour helps the patient take responsibility for varied positioning. If the ankles are edematous, foot elevation must also be above the heart, with the hip and knee extended.

A hospital bed is rarely needed to attach traction. Community nurses or carpenters can assist in creatively adapting a regular bed with pulleys or varied-height mattresses when needed. Initially the patient should expect to awaken frequently during the night to change position and return to sleep.

Orthotics

A variety of orthotic materials are available to assist in regaining functional mobility of contracted joints. Splints allow painless maintenance of exercise gains and are greatly appreciated by the patient. Daily half-hour periods of painful, prolonged aggressive stretching by a therapist to achieve elongated connective tissue are usually ineffective by themselves; the splint blocks undesirable motion and encourages active motion away from the restrictive orthosis (see Figures 7.2, 7.7, 7.11). The patient controls the speed and number of repetitions of stretch. The tissue is warm and moist under the total contact orthosis. Skin softened in this way is more comfortable to stretch.

Thermoplastic splints such as those described by Wright (1984) can save gains in horizontal or vertical lip stretching. Rivers et al. (1985) recommended an acrylic splint formed by a dental laboratory to a dentist's positive cast of the patient's teeth. This orthosis is an effective method of stretching the commisure distance. Cain and Greasley (1985) and Gay (1984) presented very similar commisure expanders. These splints have the additional advantage of preserving dental alignment when the patient is wearing a transparent or elastic facial scar-modifying orthosis.

Hartford, Kealey, Lavelle, and Buckner (1979) authored an article on the Buckner microstomia prevention appliance. This commercially available, adjustable appliance is another alternative.

Transparent plastic splints have been used to assist the remodeling of face and neck scars since 1974 (Figure 7.4). Rivers (1985) outlined the four-step process of taking a negative facial impression, forming a positive plaster cast, fabricating a transparent plastic total contact orthosis, and fitting the orthosis to flatten the scar tissue against the underlying skeletal structure.

Placement of the elastic straps to avoid mandibular retraction is important. Children look up much of the time and should not have a strap at the neckline. The safest system is to secure all straps toward the occipital area (Figure 7.5).

In a nine-year study, Feldman and MacMillan (1980) noted that there was a declining need for reconstructive procedures related to the increased use of transparent and molded polyvinyl chloride neck orthoses. Initially a soft foam neck splint is an adequate reminder to extend the neck. When numerous bulky, unnecessarily strong scars appear, the foam will compress, allowing neck flexion, scar growth, and contraction during wound maturation. Then a hard plastic splint will be needed 23 hours a day. This splint must not trap the anterior border of the mandible; that might cause mandibular retraction and limit neck rotation. Separate chin and neck splints will be needed if the mandibular area needs compression.

Total contact splints for axillary contractures are worn when the patient is

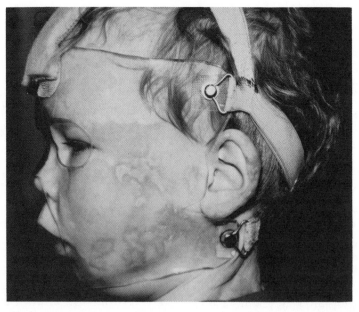

FIGURE 7.4 Total contact transparent facial orthosis. Note scar blanching in cheek area and lightweight elastic strapping, which avoids back of neck.

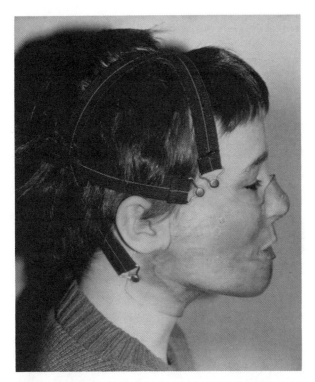

FIGURE 7.5 Safe strapping of transparent mask to occipital area. Mask contours spread tissue over underlying skeletal structure. Overly forceful elastic straps could change skeletal growth.

inactive, preferably during sleep. All splints and compression garments the patient will be wearing must be checked to avoid pinching or discomfort (Figure 7.6). During the day the figure-of-eight clavicle strap provides compression to the anterior and posterior axillary folds without decreasing active shoulder motion.

Splinting to soften anticubital scars improves elbow flexion and extension. A thermoplastic splint, secured wrist to elbow, may be used as a "fallout" splint to block flexion and increase active extention (Figure 7.2). A plaster fall-out splint can improve supination as well as elbow extension (Figure 7.7).

When the inflammatory process is active, splints must be removed daily for active exercise.

Wrist and hand contractures are often improved by overnight plaster splinting (Figure 7.8) away from the direction of the most severe contractures. Interested professionals are referred to Bell (1985) for an excellent overview of plaster casting of hand patients. A severe dorsal and palmar

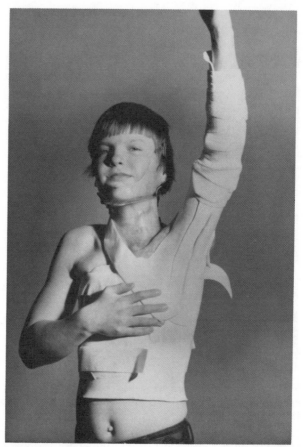

FIGURE 7.6 **Transparent chin and cheek orthosis, transparent neck compression orthosis, left elbow extension night splint, and total contact night axillary splint. Would be worn over elastic compression garment to relieve pinching. Check in lying position for best compliance.**

burn usually needs stretching in both flexion and extension. Advantages of plaster splinting are low cost and prevention of slippage. The cast is removed, prolonged stretching is followed by active exercise for several hours, and the cast can be reapplied, stretching the tissue away from the tightest residual contractures.

This modality is appropriate to begin as soon as the skin is healed, instead of waiting for a plateau of progress. Last resort serial casting is helpful. However, early use as an adjunct to active motion and prolonged stretch will prevent many contractures. Casts are usually fitted over wrinkle-free elastic gloves or garments. This avoids slippage, which may cause the patient to remove a positioning orthosis.

Elastomer silicone has been used in a similar way. The disadvantages are blisters, maceration, and difficulty keeping the elastomer odor-free. Having the patient remove and reapply splints increases the risk of pinching or misplacement. Silicone mitts can be boiled for cleanliness. Skin can be dried with corn starch to decrease moisture accumulation. Otoform K, silicone, elastomer, felt, Betapile™, Webril™, or any soft material may successfully stretch thumb web and interdigital web spaces. The spacer is usually inserted under an isotoner glove or between two pairs of gloves. When the tissue is fragile the spacers may be applied first. Then individual cloth fingers are stretched over a cylinder for comfortable donning of the entire elastic glove. Finally the pulmar part is folded toward the wrist (Figure 7.9). Finger web spacers work best when attached to a button on the "tubigrip" sleeve. This avoids use of a tight, edema-causing wrist band to secure the spacers.

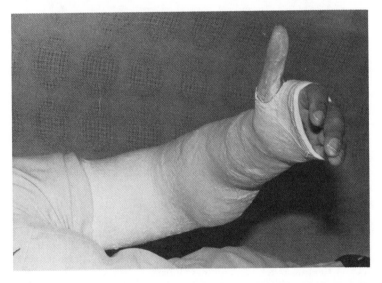

FIGURE 7.7 Serial drop-out plaster night cast stretches supination and elbow extension. Worn over compression sleeve or Webril wrap. Isotoner glove worn over cast.

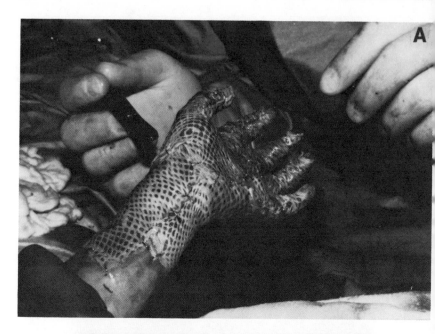

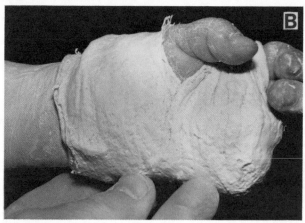

FIGURE 7.8 Full-thickness circumferential hand grafts need serial casting into flexion and extension. A: A deep circumferential burn on day 10, 4 days after graft. Postoperative PFEEW replaced with night flexion splint. If active motion decreases, begin serial casts. B: Sixty-five days after injury patient wears plaster flexion splint to therapy. C: Flexion cast removed for prolonged manual terminal extension and flexion stretch for 1 hour with breaks. D: Active exercise and play activity for strength and desensitization done 2 to 8 hours a day. E: Serial extension-abduction cast worn over elastic glove or coban wrap until next therapy.

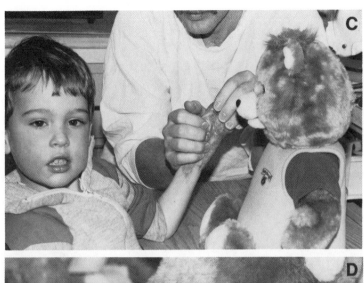

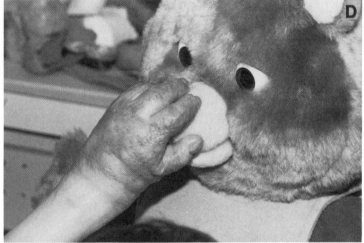

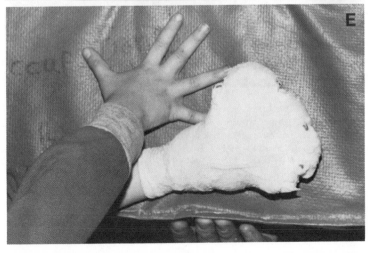

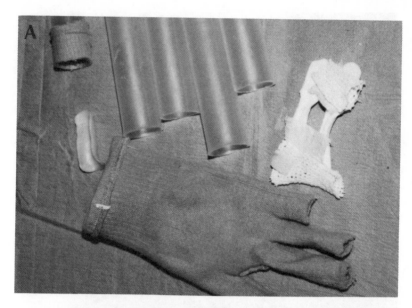

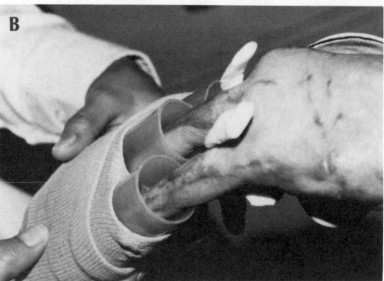

FIGURE 7.9 Donning gloves when fingers are edematous or draining. A: Clean compression glove, finger trough, and dressings for open areas and interdigital syndactyly orthoses. B: Syringe cylinders open glove fingers. Palmar area folded back over fingers. C: Patient places dressed fingers into cylinders. The palmar glove is folded down to wrist. D: Cylinders are gently removed. Glove comfortably applies gentle compression to fingers.

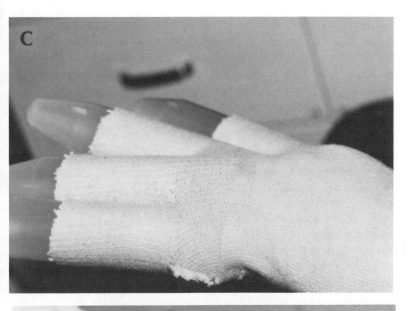

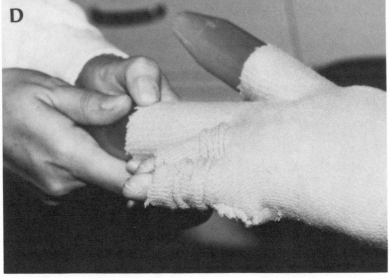

Single-finger trough splints of silicone or thermoplastic are helpful i stretching flexion contractures (Figure 7.10). These are often worn i addition to night casts or splints (see Figure 7.11) but do not replace activ motion.

If scoliosis or other trunk contractures resistant to active exercise develor an orthotist can fit a Milwaukee brace, which will remind the patient to pu away from the shortened tissue. Hip orthoses are rarely successful in reduc ing contractures, although spica serial casting during an immobile perio will improve hip motion.

The knee is treated in the same way as the elbow. However, wit ambulation begun as soon as the patient is medically stable, few kne contractures are noted. Night ankle–foot orthoses or high-top orthopedi shoes to stretch the toes into flexion are satisfactory to prevent foot contrac tures. During the day high-top shoes are lined to flex the toes or ankle a needed. A steel shank prevents a prolonged curled-toe positioning. Wher the burned foot, resistant to stretching, is casted into ankle flexion and to flexion, a temporary lift on the opposite shoe will prevent hip and kne strain during ambulation. Usually the cast is applied for 1 to 4 weeks, unti active motion can be maintained by the patient. Active children need fiberglass cast reinforcement for durability.

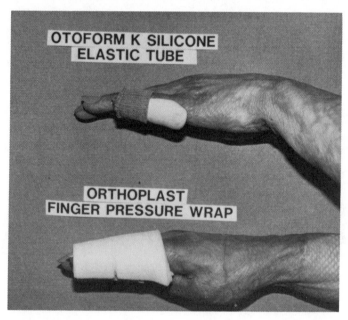

FIGURE 7.10 Individual little finger extension gutter. LMB finger pressure wrap secures orthoplast splint.

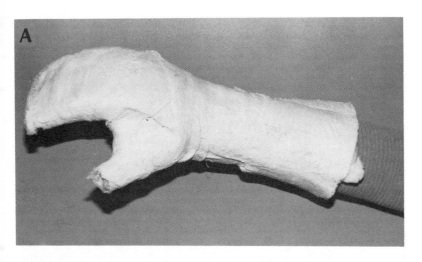

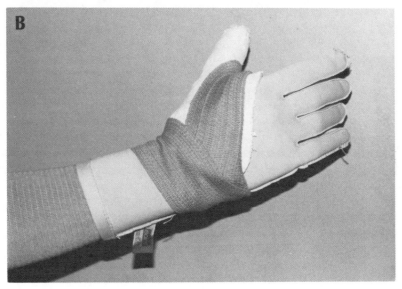

FIGURE 7.11 Serial plaster casts maintain gains of motion. A: Plaster MP flexion cast applied at night over individual coban syndactyly spacers, otoform K thumb insert, and finger extension troughs. B: Thumb web spacer worn at night, over double isotoner gloves, to stretch thumb metacarpal away from index metacarpal bone.

Healed tissue on the sole of the foot may remain fragile. A varied density soft orthotic shoe insert, made to a plaster model of the patient's foot by an orthotist, is the most satisfactory solution. The patient may need several inserts to keep the tissue dry and comfortable. Taking time to change the orthotic, stocking, and shoe may prevent pain and prolonged time off work for healing blistered skin.

Exercise and Activity

Full active range of motion returns most quickly when minimal inflammatory processes occur and when the patient continues hourly elevated active motion during waking hours. With reminders, the patient can move through the extremes of motion, which will prevent loss of joint function and will also better nourish the contracting joint soft tissue. The eyelids, mouth, neck, axilla, elbow, wrist, thumb, and hip are particularly vulnerable to contracture from unconscious positioning and from normal wound contraction. Co-contraction of muscles in preparation of anticipated pain slowly exacerbates progressive joint contractures. In the severely burned hand, tendons in the carpal tunnel area, the finger extensor mechanism, the oblique retinacular ligament, and the deep flexors may fibrose. Similarly, the anterior tibialis and Achilles tendons are susceptible to this problem in the lower extremities. Active motion and gentle terminal stretch are continued despite open tendons, except for the proximal interphalangeal (PIP) joint. It is rested in extension until skin coverage is complete.

Patients often need terminal stretch after active motion to understand that the joint will slowly move further. As the patient avoids taking the joint off stretch, discomfort also decreases. Each person can learn to do his own terminal stretch with his other hand or with environmental surfaces, such as stretching the Achilles tendon by wall push-ups with the heels flat on the floor. Prolonged manual or mechanical stretching is needed to reduce severe contractures. Microscopic tears in the connective tissue will increase the inflammatory process and will slow ultimate healing. Therefore the force must be gentle but progress daily as tolerance increases.

Strength and Endurance, Dexterity and Coordination

Manual resistive exercise, progressive resistive exercises, Cybex™, bicycle riding, and other therapy modalities done daily keep the patient from losing strength and endurance. They have an additional advantage in that patients keep the habit of leaving the house for productive work every day. Objectively documented improvement is encouraging. Attending a health club increases social contacts, and, at the same time, strength and endurance improves. It also establishes a habit of leaving home daily and may increase self-esteem.

Edema Control

Elevated positioning combined with external vascular support usually provides adequate control of swelling. However, for the severe circumferential burn, lymphatic return may become progressively worse. Chronic poor circulation accompanied by decubitus ulcers can be protected using Dr. Una's zinc oxide dressing under an elastic bandage. A Jobst Pump® worn at night with the extremity elevated is helpful for chronic edema. For severe unresponsive swelling a Wright Linear Compression Pump® may be necessary. The patient without severely impaired lymphatics may gradually decrease the frequency of night pumping.

Some patients will need lifelong vascular support. The least expensive commercially available support is usually successful. Moisturizing the underlying tissue several times daily will help avoid slipping and wrinkles in the elastic garment. At night, when the extremities are elevated, light support is adequate.

Whirlpool, a modality often requested by patients and physicians for its soothing heat, is deceptive. Interstitial edema can increase during whirlpool. The hand or foot is usually in a dependent position in the warm water, which exacerbates edema. In addition, rebound stiffness often occurs several hours after cooling. Heat can be applied by paraffin dips, as described by Head and Helm (1978) and Gross and Stafford (1984). In this case, the part is well elevated during the vasodilation period, which will prevent swelling.

Hypertrophic Scar Control

Fourteen factors that influence the formulation of unusually bulky, hard, unnecessarily strong raised scars are the following:

1. Familial predilection.
2. Growth hormones of pregnancy, puberty, and the growing child.
3. Tension on the healing wound from skin elasticity.
4. Burns that cross the lines of relaxed skin tension.
5. The presence of bacteria in the wound.
6. Increased wound tension from tight grafts, contractures, or activity.
7. Inflammatory response to suture materials.
8. Topical antibiotics that increase vascularity in the healing wound.
9. Poor microvascular circulation.

10. Crushing or irritating the wound.
11. Lack of systemic steroid hormones.
12. Poor cell nourishment.
13. Spontaneous healing of injury through the reticular dermis.
14. Collagen overgrowth during debridement and primary healing of full-thickness injuries.

A hypertrophic scar is a hard, red, collagenous bundle of connective tissue raised above the surface of the burn wound. Myofibroblasts remain active in this hyperemic, dynamically remodeling wound 24 hours a day until some currently unknown factor causes their regression some 18 months after healing. The patient, family, and burn team must accept the challenge of continuing and prolonged 23-hour-a-day diligence to achieve flat, soft, mobile, supple, light-color, durable scars. Good outcomes can be expected if the people involved can maintain intensity, tenacity, and persistence greater than the scar tissue. A sense of humor is helpful to defuse anger during this rigorous period.

Conservative hypertrophic scar control by splinting was originally described by Willis in 1969. External tissue compression and edema control are also important. Frequent exercise, meticulous hygiene, massage to improve venous return (but not to increase inflammation), and topical or intradermal steroids also help control scars.

When external tissue support is being used, figure-of-eight elastic bandage wrapping is the most supportive and least shearing to use on fragile, newly healed epithelium. Dr. Unna's zinc oxide dressing, xeroform, or fine-mesh gauze can protect blistered skin from shearing. Severely damaged, edematous fingers may tolerate individual spiral elset wraps over Unna's dressing when the figure-of-eight wrap, Coban, or an elastic glove are too abrasive. As the skin becomes more durable, soft elastic cloth such as isotoner gloves can be donned without damage. As healing progresses, cylinders or garments of rubber and cotton such as tubigrip, as outlined by Bruster and Pullium (1983), will be tolerated. If needed, patients may be fitted with more expensive, definitive, custom-made elastic garments. Jobst, Medi, Bioconcepts, and Gottfried are some companies supplying these garments.

Precautions

Custom-fitted compression garments will decrease the density of hypertrophic scar if the perpendicular fit is accurate. The patient who dons his garment and returns in 3 months wearing a deteriorated, sagging outfit will probably have unnecessarily heavy scarring. Expending the time, emotional investment, and expense to use custom-fitted garments should be rewarded by flat scar tissue. In this author's experience, healed burn epithelium stays flattest when plaster casts have been used for scar control. Elastic is not magic. The fit, as well as decreasing nourishment and oxygen supply to the scar, may account for the scar's coming to maturity earlier when compression is used, but this is undocumented.

Leung, Cheng, Ma, Clark, and Leung (1984) alert the burn team to complications of wearing elastic pressure garments over a long period. This author has not noted similar delayed growth that did not return to normal once the elastic garment was discontinued. However, it is important to observe for skeletal changes as part of the prolonged burn team follow-up.

Robertson, Zuker, Dabrowski, and Levison (1985) also alert us to another serious complication, that of compression of the neck area with elastic garments or splints. They caution regarding potential problems with sleep apnea, noted in patients wearing elastic chin straps or neck splints. Day wear of compression garments was recommended if this problem occurred.

Compensation Techniques for Exposure to Friction or Trauma, Ultraviolet Light, Chemical Irritants, and Extremes of Temperature

Blisters

Primary epithelial regeneration will close a wound that was injured into the superficial dermis. A split-thickness sheet graft or a split-thickness mesh graft is usually used to close a full-thickness wound or a wound into the deep reticular dermis. Up to a 3 × 5 mm sized full-thickness injury can be excised and closed primarily if the wound does not cross the body's natural tension lines. In all cases, the healed epithelium never regains its previous durability, elasticity, or pigmentation. In addition, many seriously burned individuals lose considerable subcutaneous fat, especially if the injury is to the palm or the sole of the foot. The subcutaneous tissue acts as a shock absorber in the unburned person. It protects the underlying nerves and blood vessels. In its absence, a slight blow may cause severe pain. The radial aspect of the thumb, the elbow, the anterior tibia, the heel, and the ball of the foot are areas especially vulnerable to this phenomenon. A thin pad such as Lois M. Barber™ (LMB) finger-pressure wraps or padded tubigrips under the vascular support garment will improve comfort. Spenco dermal pads or bikers' gloves can substitute for lost skin durability during activities such as lawn mowing or snow blower operation. Custom orthotics are needed to cushion the feet.

Besides not having adequate underlying padding, the skin may remain unusually fragile for a prolonged time. Friction or trauma of scratching, rubbing by bandages, swelling of a dependent part, chemical irritation, tape contact, or excessive heat can all cause blisters. Brand and Yancy (1984) cal a blister a dramatic, temporary miracle. A blister separates the epithelia layers, forms a perfectly round dome, cools the injured area, cushions shock perfectly disperses external stresses, and increases the sensitivity of the are; so further injury will be avoided. A burned person views blisters as ; frustrating nuisance. However, the blistering stage is temporary. If smal blisters are left intact, the protein fluid will speed healing and the driec epithelial cells will be protective. Large blisters that spread or trap infection should be drained and dead matter removed to speed healing.

Ultraviolet Light

Pigment cells travel along the basilar layer of the dermis. After a burn, o; when donor skin has been removed, the rate and density of pigment regen- eration is generally determined by the amount of inflammation during healing and by the person's heredity. When pigment cells are absent, ultra- violet rays can penetrate and damage the tissue under the thinned skin Protecting the body by using a 15- to 18-rated para-aminobenzoic acic (PABA) sunscreen when exposed to the sun is recommended. Burn patients often perspire when they are exposed to the sun, so they should alsc consider ultraviolet blocking lotions that do not wash off easily when ir contact with water. The Consumer's Guide (1983) is one excellent refer- ence, written in language a lay person can easily understand.

Chemical Irritants

Exposing thinned, fragile healed grafts or donors to irritants must be undertaken with care. Vapors from cleaning solvents, strong animal urine or other irritants that may be found at work sometimes cause severe derma- titis. Extra protection of the hands, feet, and legs is needed by concrete workers if they develop dermatitis or burns from the wet concrete o; concrete dust. Some healed workers view physical contact with irritants such as paint stripper or petroleum products as "macho." They may need counseling to accept their vulnerability to skin damage without lowering their self-esteem. Some persons will prefer to take a different job rather thar wear the cumbersome, hot, protective gloves over scar compression gar- ments. If coordination is impaired, the worker may in fact be safer in a new job.

Temperature Control

The tough outer layer of healed burn or donor tissue does not allow sweat glands to force perspiration through the pores to the skin surface. Sweat glands rarely survive in skin needing grafting. When the environmental temperature is above 80°F (27°C), former patients have reported feeling ill. They are unable to cool by evaporating perspiration. Perspiration stays in their sealed pores until the body reabsorbs it, only causing itching, not cooling. Scar tissue surrounding surface blood vessels prevents them from dilating or constricting properly. The newly formed blood vessels have poor tone. Persons having had severe burn injuries report exposure to temperatures below 30°F (−1°C) as very uncomfortable. Appropriate clothing improves the burned person's comfort. Avoiding constricting bands is also helpful. Proper air-conditioning, heating, and humidity may be crucial to the comfort of the healed severely burned person. Patients who valued peer recognition during unprotected exposure to the weather may reject suggestions of professionals regarding care. Suggestions regarding care from burn support-group members are often more easily accepted by the burned person who risks such injury.

Sensory Changes

Even without peripheral nerve damage, severely burned patients almost universally experience sensory changes. Itching is one of the healed person's more distressing phenomena. This author would postulate that besides the normal itching of healing, these severely injured people experience added and prolonged discomfort from the skin because the reticular formation and cerebral system have not integrated the new information transmitted from the healing nerve endings. Pain endings do not undergo adaptation. When pain centers are overstimulated, fatigue occurs, and the patient still has an awareness of itching.

At the moment of injury it is important for the person to reflexly recognize the injury and the need for emergency treatment and cooling. Later, when the tissue is healed, messages continue to arrive at the brain. In the past, the person would not have been aware of this information. Now, however, it is a central, compelling part of the awareness. The patient finds it difficult to tune it out, even if he was once skilled at single-minded concentration. Desensitization techniques will very slowly aid in normalizing attention to the healed tissue. Benson's relaxation (Bernstein & Borkovec, 1973) procedure, when practiced regularly, is also helpful.

Independent Activities of Daily Living

By the time the patient returns home, he has practiced phone use, eating, oral hygiene, bathing, shaving, and toileting, supervised by the nurses and therapy staff. Self-dressing is initiated close to the time of discharge, when wound drainage is minimal. Soft items such as jogging suits and tennis shoes are recommended for ease of donning and laundering. An additional benefi of soft fabric is the reduction of friction blisters.

Discharge of severely burned patients often occurs before they are independent in wound care or shampooing. These activities are learned with the help of family members. Tepid water is recommended for bathing or showering as an outpatient. Hot water increases the blood supply at the skin surface, pruritus, and the skin's vulnerability to breakdown from scratching Bathing in clear water is recommended. Soaking in a detergent, although time-honored, is harmful. It removes sebum, the body's natural lubricant and bacteriostatic agent, and has no effect in removing bacteria. Washing wounds with a clean, soaped cloth or gauze and rinsing well effectively removes debris. For the unusually pruritic patient, using superfatted soaps for personal hygiene may decrease dry skin. Others may use the body soap of their choice but observe for contact dermatitis if the soap contains perfume, since the recently healed tissue is sometimes sensitized to irritants.

Patients often worry about infections. Using a clean set of washcloths and towels daily and normal tub care is adequate protection from pathogens. It is difficult for patients to wean themselves from bathing with gauze squares because the texture of a washcloth feels rough. This is an excellent patient-controlled early desensitization exercise.

When a scalp burn or donor is present, careful attention to meticulous lubrication, moisturization, and washing is important. Brushing the hair with a soft, natural bristle brush will improve circulation and remove tough crusts, allowing hair growth. Trimming hair from open areas must be done often. Scalp massage feels good to the patient, improves venous return, and prevents selective tethering of the healing epithelium. Teaching the patient to do these tasks independently has the added benefit of upper-extremity exercise.

Safe meal preparation, shopping, laundering, cleaning, and independent transportation are also tasks relearned at home. Nurses, family, and therapists provide the tools for patient independence. If the patient has never done his own cleaning, it is probably inappropriate to plan on this as an endurance exercise. Flexibility, with the final goal of independence and enjoying life, will bring success most quickly.

Patients are very interested in resuming driving; they should be reminded to discontinue attention-altering medications before operating a motor vehicle. Also, many rehabilitation centers have automobile adaptations that the patient can try before choosing modifications for his or her own car. Insurance companies or state regulations may require relicensing if a major change in function, either physically or cognitively, has taken place. The injured person is responsible for inquiring about licensing rules, which vary in each state.

Recreational and Social Contacts

Patients are often reluctant to be seen in public. When therapists or doctors prescribe therapy at a health club, the patient more readily initiates new social contacts. Additionally, the patient may notice that stress reduction is a benefit of continuing frequent physical recreation. Participation in avocational activities with friends is a nonstressful way to prepare for return to work. Recreation is fun and doing things at a subcortical level decreases attention to pain and brings to awareness the benefits of keeping contractures stretched out. When the patient begins to do things for others, he has successfully overcome the narcissistic need for attention based on the injury. It is rewarding when the person is proud of real-world achievements, more than incidents during the hospital stay. Often, at this point, the ordeal they have survived becomes a source of wisdom, empathy, and concern for others. Sharing gives increased meaning to the now-recovered person's life.

Return to School or Work

If the patient was enrolled in school, he or she is encouraged to return soon after discharge. The ability to concentrate returns slowly, and it will be helpful if the teachers are made aware of this. Often a school nurse or physical education instructor will rewrap elastic bandages, lotion and massage dry, itchy skin, and give the child antipruritic medications if prescribed by the doctor. Frequent physical exercise prevents pain and stiffness and improves the student's attention span. When children are returning to school these ideas may be helpful:

1. A frame of reference in which authority figures communicate seeing burn injury survival and the child's return to school as heroic.
2. Have the child teach others about skin, scars, burns, exercises, and his hospital stay.
3. Let the child share with a friend feelings, wants, and thoughts.
4. Have students take turns in school telling the other children what they like about each other.
5. Let the students do a project defining how each child is different from the others and how each is special.
6. Let the students volunteer to do physical exercise or games with the burned child to make stretching more fun.
7. Use several friends to help the child catch up with homework to vary social contacts.

The child should participate in all physical education programs except contact sports. However, it may be necessary for him to shower at home because of the need for superfatted soaps, lotions, and pressure garments. Group swimming should be delayed until open areas are healed and cultures reveal no drug-resistant pathogens.

For the adult returning to work, the supervisor and employee must evaluate the employee's remaining open wounds; skin blisterability; heat, cold, and ultraviolet light intolerances; chemical and dust sensitivity; pain; edema; inability to concentrate; distractability; loss of joint motion; decreased coordination and endurance; visual impairment; changed ability to interpret sensations; and continued need for vascular and hypertrophic scar-compression dressings. It is the employee's responsibility to discuss return to work with his doctor. Food handlers must remain off-duty until open areas are closed and cultures reveal no pathogens. Heavy laborers may need job modification. Often a transition period of half-day work progressing slowly to full-time work is needed. Rehabilitation counselors or nurses can assist with changes in the work setting if these are needed.

In addition, psychological adjustment for returning to work in an area where the injury occurred must be considered. Few people will return easily to the injury site. Referral to a psychologist is appropriate. Return to work at the earliest possible time is important to maximize the benefits of routine and work. Strength and coordination improve much sooner from work than from therapy. Ego strength and social interaction are also improved on the job. Burns and Steger (1983) studied work-related burn victims. Early ongoing contact between the employer and the employee was one of the suggestions for successful reintegration into the work setting. This author's experience suggests that the injured person wants to be contacted by his direct supervisor, not a representative. The supervisor may be afraid of the employee's hostility or just be busy, but the burned person, with time on his hands, ruminates that "they don't like me" or "it was their fault I got burned, and now they are trying to get out of it." Whatever the facts may be, supporting contact as early as possible by the supervisor can facilitate all further attempts to reintegrate the employee into the work setting.

When attorneys and pending litigation are keeping the patient from returning to work, the patient must be made aware of the dangers of spending long periods of nonproductive time. Habits such as watching late-night TV, arising late, decreased physical activity, changed eating habits, and use of street drugs or alcohol gradually become entrenched. The patient's anger, fear, financial worry, concern of safety coupled with irritation, and depression and shrinking social contacts may be overwhelming. The patient may then be unable to initiate enough rewarding activity to resume a satisfying, enjoyable life-style. Before injury the person's occupation was one of the primary factors determining his income, his prestige, and his place in society. Work exerted an influence the person may not have recognized. Postinjury it is important for the attorney to be part of the team searching for choices that can maximize the employee's satisfaction and independence. There may have been a disparity between what the person was and what he dreamed of becoming before the accident. Now he may be forced to accept lowered standards; psychologists or vocational counselors can assist in dealing with these changes.

Sometimes return to the same job is inappropriate or impossible. Then it will be necessary for the person to find a new job. If jobs are plentiful, state job service agencies may be helpful. The former employer may make a new job available. However, if these options are unavailable, working with a vocational counselor to discover appropriate training programs is indicated. The vocational counselor will evaluate the patient's previous occupation, work history, and skills, as well as other parameters to make recommendations for optimal employment.

REFERENCES

Barnett, P. H., & Stafford, F. S. (1984). Use of plastic air bands for edema and scar contracture. *Journal of Burn Care Rehabilitation, 5*, 469–473.

Brand, P., & Yancy, G. (1984). *In his image.* New York: Zondervan.

Bell, J. (1985). Plaster of paris. *Hand splinting, principles and methods* (2nd ed.). St. Louis, MO: Mosby.

Bernstein, D. A., & Borkovec, P. D. (1973). *Relaxation training: A manual for the helping professions.* Champaign, IL: Research Press.

Bruster, J. M., & Pullium, G. (1983). Gradient pressure. *American Journal of Occupational Therapy, 37*, 485–488.

Burns, A. C., & Steger, H. G. (1983). Intervention strategies for victims of work-related burn injuries. *Occupational Health Nursing, 7*, 29–32.

Cain, J. R., & Greasley, J. W. (1985). Prosthetic management of electrical burns to the oral commissure. *Quintessence of Dental Technology, 9*, 249–252.

Carter, P. R. (1983). *Common hand injuries and infections.* Philadephia: Saunders.

Constable, J. D., Bernstein, N. R., & Sheehy, E. (1979). Unreasonable expectations of reconstructive patients affecting rehabilitation. *Scandinavian Journal of Plastic Reconstructive Surgery, 13*, 177–179.

Consumers Union of the United States. (1983). Sunscreens. *Consumer Reports, 48* (6), 275–278.

Cooper-Fraps, C., & Yerxa, E. J. (1984). Denial: Implications of a pilot study on activity level related to sexual competence in burned adults. *American Journal of Occupational Therapy, 38*, 529–534.

Covey, M. (1985). Special interest group, P.T./O.T. Round Table, American Burn Association 17th Annual Meeting, Orlando, Florida.

Feldman, A. E., & MacMillan, B. G. (1980). Burn injury in children: Declining need for reconstructive surgery as related to use of neck orthoses. *Archives of Physical Medicine and Rehabilitation, 61*, 441–449.

Gay, W. D. (1984). Prostheses for oral burn patients. *The Journal of Prosthetic Dentistry, 52*, 564–566.

Gross, J. D., & Stafford, F. S. (1984). Modified method for application of paraffin wax for treatment of burn scar. *Journal of Burn Care Rehabilitation, 5*, 394.

Haley, J. (1973). *Uncommon therapy.* New York: Norton.

Harnar, T., Engrav, L., Heimbach, D., & Marvin, J. A. (1985). Experience with skeletal immobilization after excision and grafting of severely burned hands *Journal of Trauma, 25*, 299–302.

Hartford, C., Kealey, G., Lavelle, W. E., & Buchner, H. (1975). An appliance to prevent and treat microstomia from burns. *Journal of Trauma, 15*, 356–360.

Heimbach, D. M., & Engrav, L. H. (1984). *Surgical management of the burn wound.* New York: Raven Press.

Head, M. D., & Helm, P. A. (1977). Paraffin and sustained stretching in the treatment of burn contractures. *Burns, 4*, 136–139.

Helm, P. A., Kevorkian, C. G., Lushbaugh, M., Pullium, G., Head, M. D., & Cromes, G. F. (1982). Burn injury: Rehabilitation management in 1982. *Archives of Physical Medicine and Rehabilitation, 63*, 6–16.

Johnson, C., O'Shaughnessy, E., & Ostergren, B. (1981). *Burn management.* New York: Raven Press.

Leung, K. S., Cheng, J. C. Y., Ma, G. F. Y., Clark, J. A., & Leung, P. C. (1984). Complications of pressure therapy for post-burn hypertrophic scars. *Burns, 10*, 434–438.

Mooney, T. O., Cole, T. M., & Chilgren, R. A. (1975). *Sexual options for paraplegics and quadriplegics.* Boston: Little, Brown & Company.

Parks, D. H., Caravajal, H. F., & Larson, D. L. (1977). Management of burns. *Surgical Clinics of North America, 57*, 875–895.

Remensnyder, J. P. (1980). Management of the burned hand. In Wolfert, F. G. (Ed.). *Acute hand injuries—A multispecialty approach.* Boston: Little, Brown.

Rivers, E., Collin, T., Solem, L. D., Ahrenholz, D., Fisher, S., & Macfarlane, J. (1985). Use of a custom maxillary night splint with lateral projections in the treatment of microstomia. *Proceedings of American Burn Association's 17th Annual Meeting,* Orlando, Florida.

Rivers, E. (1985). Management of hypertrophic scars. In S. Fisher & P. Helm (Eds.), *Comprehensive rehabilitation of burns.* Baltimore, MD: Williams & Wilkins.

Robertson, C. F., Zuker, R., Dabrowski, B., & Levison, H. (1985). Obstructive sleep apnes: A complication of burns to the head and neck in children. *Journal of Burn Care Rehabilitation, 6*, 353–357.

Tollison, C. D., Still, J. M., & Tollison, J. W. (1980). The seriously burned adult: Psychologic reactions, recovery and management. *Georgia Medical Association Journal, 69*, 121–124.

Willis, B. (1969). The use of orthoplast isoprene splints in the treatment of the acutely burned child: Preliminary report. *American Journal of Occupational Therapy, 23*, 57–61.

Wright, P. C. (1984). Fundamentals of acute burn care and physical therapy management. *Physical Therapy, 64*, 1217–1231.

8

Management of Pain after Thermal Injury

David H. Ahrenholz
Lynn D. Solem

Of all the sensations perceived by living organisms, perhaps the most important are the noxious stimuli commonly referred to as acute pain (Katz, Varni, & Jay, 1984). The negative reinforcement value of painful stimuli cannot be overestimated. An individual quickly learns to avoid activities that produce pain, thus preventing serious or even lethal injury. Not all deleterious acts have immediate painful consequences (e.g., cigarette smoking) but those that do are quickly avoided. In the absence of pain, devastating effects are seen in man. Denervated extremities develop ulcers and infections: in leprosy the anesthetic fingers are destroyed by unsensed trauma, not bacterial activity.

It is not easy to define the concept of pain, although virtually everyone has experienced the sensation. Wall (1979) describes pain as a need state similar to hunger rather than a distinct sense like taste or smell. Pain has two components, the *physical perception* of pain and the *emotional reaction* to this unpleasant experience (Katz et al., 1984). Social embarrassment may be recalled as a painful experience, although pain receptors are not involved. Loud noises may be painful. Pain may be sensed internally, as with colic or acute appendicitis, but visceral pain is dull, diffuse, and poorly localized compared with cutaneous sensations.

It is difficult to appreciate how subjective the sensation of pain is. Pain does not exist at the site of nerve stimulation—irritating stimuli do. These trigger electrical activity in the afferent nerves, which are interpreted in the brain as pain. Patients who have an exaggerated response to pain are told, "It's all in your head" (Goodman, 1983). Pain is not an objectively quantifiable entity (Torgerson, 1984). It cannot be isolated and purified, although some chemical substances evoke marked responses from pain receptors in the tissue. There is no available instrument that can be used to detect pain or, conversely, to prove its absence. We are entirely dependent upon the patient to define the intensity, quality, and location of pain. Phantom pain— pain in an amputated body part—is real, even though the subjective site of the pain is surgically absent.

NEUROPHYSIOLOGY OF PAIN PERCEPTION

Scattered throughout the body tissues are a variety of tactile sense organs. Cutaneous pain is largely mediated by the nocioceptive receptors in the skin, supplemented by input from pressure, heat, and cold receptors, with lesser contributions from proprioceptive or vibratory receptors (Casey, 1980). Of these, the pain receptor appears the least specialized. Grossly, it appears as a multiply branching fine nerve fiber without specialized modifications (Melzack & Taenzer, 1977).

Many sense organs respond only to rapid changes in stimulus frequency or intensity. Vibratory sense organs can respond to very rapid changes in stimulus intensity but quickly adapt to a constant stimulus so that the sensation is lost. In contrast, pain receptors show little or no adaptation to stimuli of constant intensity (Guyton, 1968).

Many peripheral sensory receptors show a logarithmic response effect. That is, a 10-fold increase in stimulus intensity is perceived subjectively as a two-fold increase. In the ear this gives a hearing range extending over a several million-fold range of intensities. No similar logarithmic response has been found with pain receptors. Instead, as there is an increase in the intensity of painful stimuli at a given site, it is perceived as pain increasing in intensity and extending to encompass a much larger area (Guyton, 1968).

It is apparent that pain fibers respond most strongly to stimuli that actually damage tissue (Livingston, 1943). Mediators may be chemical ions, polypeptides, or other factors such as histamine, serotonin, or bradykinin released in response to injury (Goodman, 1983). The result is an electrical action potential that is propagated centrally along the peripheral nerve. No pain is appreciated if this action potential fails to reach the cerebral cortex. Pain fibers transmit their action potential centrally via fine myelinated (A, delta) or unmyelinated (C) sensory fibers (Casey, 1980). For the most part these enter the spinal cord via the dorsal horn and ascend several segments before crossing to the lateral spinothalamic tract.

A considerably greater number of afferent neurons enter the dorsal horns than are found in the lateral spinothalamic tract. Several factors allow relatively precise localization of peripheral painful stimuli (Guyton, 1968). First, it appears that some fibers connect directly to neurons in the spinal cord and some lie between secondary neurons. Thus, the ratio of stimulation of one central neuron to another is a way of encoding spatial data.

Second, it is rare that a peripheral pain receptor is stimulated without other adjacent sensory receptors being stimulated as well. This information may be transmitted via the lateral spinothalamic tract or via the ascending dorsal tracts. Patients who have interruption of the ascending dorsal tracts have diffuse, dull, poorly localized pain in response to discrete peripheral stimuli, indicating that information from both tracts is integrated in the cerebral cortex to perceive sharp, discrete pain.

At the peripheral level there are many branches and multiple connections in sensory neural circuits. Some of these connections loop upon themselves to provide a positive feedback circuit (Livingston, 1943). These reverberating circuits may be responsible for the continued perception of pain even after a painful stimulus is no longer present, for example, a blow that is felt for several minutes after the injury. Other peripheral phenomena include facilitation and zonal inhibition (Guyton, 1968). A variety of sense receptors are located in the skin at varying levels and densities. As the axons ascend, they have many connections with other fibers in the tract that serve adjacent areas of the body. As these adjacent fibers are stimulated, the sensation of pain may spread over a larger area even though a discrete area is stimulated (facilitation). This effect is decreased by centrifugal nerve fibers, which pass down from the cortex to the neuronal pool. When a stimulus excites a central receptor, surrounding receptors are less strongly stimulated, giving a blurred spatial pattern. The lateral inhibitory neurons are activated by the strong central stimulus. These circuits inhibit stimulus propagation in the fringe neurons (zonal inhibition). Thus, the spatial pattern is preserved and sharpened in its central transmission.

This inhibitory process may account for the relief from itching gained by rubbing an irritated site, as pain sensory pathways are suppressed by circuits spreading from touch sensory pathways. Transcutaneous electrical nerve stimulators reduce pain perception by mild stimulation of a broad skin surface, activating large numbers of inhibitory neurons.

There are several identifiable paths for pain stimuli above the spinal cord (Guyton, 1968). A direct lateral spinothalamic tract terminates in the posterior lateral thalamus. Projections caudally connect to the somatic sensory areas I and II along the postcentral gyrus of the cerebrum. In addition, lateral spinothalamic tract fibers terminating in the hindbrain activate portions of the spinoreticular tract. Output from this area leads to neurons of the medial thalamus. Stimulation of these neurons produces a diffuse excitation that increases the appreciation of painful stimuli. Narcotic analgesics appear to particularly affect the reticular formation neurons. This explains why narcotics reduce subjective pain while maintaining the patient's ability to localize unpleasant stimuli (Marvin & Heimbach, 1984).

The central tegmental pathway lies between the spinothalamic tract and the central gray pathway in the hindbrain and acts to suppress pain sensation. The axons of these cells descend in the dorsolateral vesiculous to the dorsal horn cells where they inhibit action potential transmission from peripheral pain fibers. The destruction of the central tegmental pathway causes extreme pain sensitivity and sometimes even the perception of continuous pain.

Only recently has the presence of opiate-like substances been suspected in the brain. There are specific tracts within the brain, including the midline raphe nuclei of the brainstem, that, when stimulated, produce a prolonged analgesia difficult to distinguish from that produced by morphine. Repeated stimulation produces tolerance, and naloxone is capable of reversing the analgesia (Goldstein, 1979).

This has led to the discovery of two endogenous pentapeptides called "enkephalins," which are capable of reducing the perception of pain. Opiate receptors have been found in a number of areas in the nervous system, including the limbic system, the medial thalamus, the periaqueductal gray areas, and the substantia gelatinosa of the spinal cord (Marvin & Heimbach, 1984). The role of these agents in modulating pain perception is currently a topic of intense neuropharmacological investigation (Levine, Scipio, McBryde, & Gordon 1984). One goal is to find pharmacologic agents that either increase enkephalin production or decrease enkephalin metabolism at the receptor site to produce prolonged effects. An alternative is synthesis of enkephalins that may more easily cross the blood–brain barrier and suppress pain perception.

PSYCHOLOGICAL ASPECTS OF PAIN

The factors that alter the perception of pain are multiple and poorly understood. Certainly fear and anxiety heighten the appreciation of pain. Relief at surviving a terrifying experience may decrease the sensation (Beecher, 1958). Individuals vary markedly in their perception of pain, and cultural or societal expectations play a great role (Perry, 1984). In many cultures acknowledgment of pain is considered a sign of weakness and entails a loss of status (Streltzer & Wade, 1981). In Western societies modern medicine interprets pain as a sign of dysfunction that mandates investigation, treatment, and elimination, so even small amounts of pain are very poorly tolerated. Older cultures have frequently interpreted pain as part of a spiritual cleansing or healing process to be tolerated stoically or even welcomed.

There is no universally definable pain scale. Childbirth has been used as the yardstick for women, but it is a variable experience for each individual dictated by pelvic anatomy, size of the fetus, and duration of labor, as well as environmental, cultural, and emotional factors. Almost all women report that subsequent births are less distressing or painful than the first. No similar painful experience has been suggested for men.

Because pain is so subjective, rating scales are difficult to formulate (Torgerson, 1984). Two have achieved some popularity. The pain thermometer is a self-reporting scale in which the patient rates no pain as zero and the most intense possible pain as 100 (Katz et al., 1984). Numerical values are then collected before and after intervention therapy. In children, the Eland Color Tool has been useful (Eland, 1982). The child is given a body diagram and asked to indicate the location of each pain on the outline, using different colors for different kinds and intensities of pain. The play aspect has been especially helpful in eliciting responses from withdrawn individuals.

There are physiologic and psychological changes that accompany the experience of pain (Klein & Charlton, 1980). The patient in pain may manifest sweating, tremor, tachycardia, hypertension, and nausea or vomiting. The patient may experience agitation, anxiety, anger, or fear. At least two observer scales have been devised in an attempt to achieve more objective measurements of pain. Eleven behaviors manifested by patients experiencing pain are rated by intensity. The Procedure Behavioral Rating Scale records the occurrence or absence of a specific behavior (Katz, Kellerman, & Siegel, 1980). The Burn Treatment Distress Scale uses a time sampling method, noting the behavior and its intensity (Elliot & Olson, 1983).

PAIN STAGES

According to one current theory of coping behavior in response to pain, there are three stages after injury—immediate, acute, and rehabilitative (Bowden, Jones, & Feller, 1979). In burn patients, these stages are quite distinct and can be described in detail.

Immediate Burn Pain

When a minor burn injury occurs, direct thermal damage to the tissue causes intense immediate pain in the affected area. Thermal receptors are most susceptible to stimulation as the temperature rises, but become inactive as the temperature falls. Free pain endings, however, remain stimulated for prolonged periods with even minor burns such as sunburn. Since the adverse effects of sunburn are ameliorated by pretreatment with aspirin, it is possible that chemical messengers like histamine or bradykinin are involved. After any severe trauma the patient is often dazed and somewhat disoriented with minimal perception of pain. It appears that this is a central effect, perhaps mediated by enkephalins. The period of hyposensitivity to pain lasts up to 8 hours (Melzack, Wall, & Ty, 1982). In very severe thermal injuries the burn extends deeply enough to completely destroy all layers of the skin including the local sensory receptors so that sensation is absent. The patient with charred extremities may not be able to comprehend that he has sustained a lethal injury because he has no pain.

Acute Burn Pain

After admission to a burn center, dressing changes and debridement are performed until skin grafting can take place. This removes the overlying protective layers of dead, anesthetic tissue and exposes the viable tissue and its nerve endings. Patients in the past often experienced excruciating pain from the burn wounds. Currently multiple modalities are used to minimize the distress that the patient feels during this period. As the patient begins to comprehend what has happened, anxiety mounts. He realizes that he will probably live but has to deal with the prospect of hospitalization, baths, therapy, and surgical procedures. Feller (1970) found that 70% of burn victims in some way contributed to their injuries. Thus the patient may have to deal with guilt regarding the cause or outcome of the fire, or adjust to the loss of property or loved ones.

Rehabilitative Phase Pain

At this stage the patient has completed his initial surgical procedures and is being prepared for release from the hospital. Now, as he leaves the protected hospital environment, he must deal with an altered body image and new physical limitations, whether temporary or permanent. A new set of sensations, many of them unpleasant, are now appreciated, including marked itching, excessive sweating, hyperesthesia or hypoesthesia of the skin, and heat and cold intolerance.

IS PAIN NECESSARY AFTER BURN INJURY?

Perry (1984) has published a very provocative paper postulating that experiencing pain is necessary after burn injury. He arrived at this startling conclusion based on his experiences as a consulting psychologist on an active burn center. Despite his concerted efforts to see that patients received adequate amounts of pain medication, he repeatedly saw that the patients were undermedicated. A variety of reasons were offered, but fears of respiratory depression, hypotension, or addiction were most common. He noted symptoms that nurses experienced anxiety after eliciting pain during burn cares, a finding observed by others (Ravencraft, 1982). Yet during dressing changes nurses frequently commented, "Your pain isn't so bad."

Perry deduced that there is an underlying need on the part of health caregivers to observe pain in burn patients, but not in a sadistic way. Certainly patients in pain require hospitalization and care, but those who are pain-free perhaps no longer need such intensive services. Perry feels that pain defines caregiver/patient roles and when pain disappears these roles become blurred. It also defines the otherness of the patient ("Since I don't feel pain, I am not the patient."). In a few isolated cases, pain is perceived consciously or unconsciously as an appropriate reward for preburn (perhaps criminal) behavior or postburn (resistive or manipulative) actions.

Perry failed to recognize, however, the most important aspect for caregivers. Pain shows that the patient is alive and has a favorable prognosis. Anesthetic skin is dead and sloughs, so the nurses are looking for the boundary where viable tissue begins. Most disturbing is the fact that patients with lethal burns are totally anesthetic; even if they are awake, alert, and talking, they will not survive. And the moribund patient lapses into an unresponsive coma before death. Therefore, if the patient reacts appropriately to painful stimuli, he is expected to survive, and the anxiety of the caregiver is reduced.

Perry also interviewed patients with severe burns who had been treated with curare to facilitate mechanical ventilation. Such patients were totally paralyzed and given considerable amounts of narcotics. To prevent drying of the corneas, the eyes were taped shut. As a result the patients were sometimes conscious but sensory-deprived. Usually they reported an initial inability to tell if they were alive. Once they began to feel pain, they were greatly relieved.

Touch, pressure, temperature, and pain are the ways we normally cutaneously sense our environment. When these disappear we lose the sense of our boundary with the outside world (the "interface" is lost). In burn patients, pain is usually preserved and supports a sense of identity. Initially the presence of pain may reinforce, for the victim, the passive patient role. He does not have to deal with the unpleasant realities of his new postburn state while still experiencing pain. He is "too sick" to be responsible. As his condition improves, the presence of pain gives the patient some control in a situation where he has little or no control. By complaining, he can elicit action from the caregivers without hearing that what he is experiencing is normal or necessary for his recovery. Occasional patients use pain as a justification for otherwise unacceptable behavior such as tantrums.

And, for some patients, pain is a way of expiating some degree of perceived guilt regarding the circumstances or results of the accident. Questions such as "Why did I survive?", "Why was I so stupid?", and "How can I go on?" are common after burn injury. Pain is often associated with punishment in childhood, and many burn victims feel a need to be punished. If this need is met, they are able to return to function after discharge.

MANAGEMENT OF ACUTE BURN PAIN

Psychological Intervention

Many burn victims are relatively unaware of their surroundings during their early hospitalization. In alert patients, a variety of techniques are used to minimize apprehension regarding burn treatment (Wernick, Jaremko, & Taylor, 1981). The following is an idealized description of modalities, any or all of which may be used in a given patient.

- Most of the pain is felt during bathing and debridement of the burn wounds. Afterwards the wounds are usually covered with silver sulfa-diazine, which is very soothing and may give immediate relief of pain.
- Because pain consistently occurs in bathing, a phobic state may easily develop (Shorkey & Taylor, 1973). A careful explanation of bathing procedures is required. Ambulatory patients are allowed to explore the bath area without the pressure of an impending treatment (Wernick et al., 1981). Thus, attempts are made to prevent association of the place with an unpleasant procedure.
- Within limits, the patient is offered options regarding the bath. He is encouraged to request the type and quantity of pain medication, but in return he must remain awake enough to participate in his care during the bath and with his physical therapy afterward. He is not allowed to return to bed and sleep until afternoon.
- In the bath, he assists in removing dressings, chooses which areas are washed first, and is encouraged to wash himself, which minimizes pain. Patients given options feel more in control of their lives and pain perception is diminished (Giuliani & Perry, 1985).
- A psychologist spends time with each patient and teaches relaxation exercises as a means of pain control (Knudson-Cooper, 1981). The nurses encourage the patient to rehearse the exercises both before and during the bath (Weinstein, 1976). A few patients can undergo hypno-sis with significant pain relief in the dissociated state (Crasilneck, Stieman, Willson, McCranoe, & Fogelman, 1955; Wakeman & Kaplan, 1978).
- Distraction techniques are also very effective (Klein, 1984). The pa-tient is asked to select a favorite radio station and music is played

throughout the bath. Children are allowed to select favorite toys for the tub or are asked to look for hidden objects in the corners of the room (Ravenscroft, 1982).

- Heroic visualization is used with children who are afraid of entering the water. The child is asked to imagine that there has been an accident where everyone is injured, but he must enter the water to save his friends, even if it hurts (Elliot & Olson, 1983). Once in the bath relaxation is stressed with focusing on pleasant thoughts, like drifting at sea and floating up to an island (Weinstein, 1976). The child is asked to describe the island he would find and what he would do there.

- A consistent program is maintained of reward for appropriate coping behavior (the children enjoy VCR tapes, extra desserts, passes, etc.). Parents are encouraged to cooperate in this program. They are asked not to be excessively protective or to reward inappropriate conduct. Children are not allowed to avoid treatment by manipulative means (Kelley, Jarvic, Middlebrook, et al., 1984). Written contracts may be required to reinforce adaptive behavior (Simmons, McFadd, Frank, et al., 1978).

Pharmacologic Intervention

Most patients experiencing pain expect pharmacologic therapy. A few will inappropriately demand general anesthesia. Some medications used to dress burn wounds, especially mafenide or iodophor foam, are very painful and require increased amounts of pain medication. These are used sparingly now that silver sulfadiazine is available.

In acutely injured patients who must undergo daily tub baths and debridements, narcotic analgesics such as morphine are appropriate (Perry & Heidrich, 1982). Most patients after major burns have an ileus and are unable to tolerate oral medication, so morphine is usually given intravenously in 1 to 2 mg increments to control pain and allow patient cooperation. Intramuscular injection results in erratic absorption and delayed effects. Morphine has a rapid onset of action, low cost, mild to moderate euphoric effects, and medium duration of action. Its disadvantages include respiratory depression (equal to other narcotic agents in equipotent doses), habituation and dependence, constipation, and occasional nausea.

On most general surgical services, meperidine (Demerol) is a more commonly used narcotic than morphine. Nurses rotating through a burn unit are much more comfortable administering this drug, especially via intramuscular injection. Liberal use of narcotic agents must be encouraged in the treatment of all burn patients while daily debridements and dressing changes are being carried out.

Fentanyl is a narcotic with a much more rapid action and shorter half-life than either morphine or meperidine (Hug, Murphy, & Rigel, 1979). It is used extensively by anesthesiologists and may become the drug of choice for suppressing the pain of daily burn wound debridement (Hilberman, 1984). Self-administered narcotic analgesics have been used successfully in general surgery patients (Graves et al., 1983). The patient activates a dose-limiting pump system to deliver intravenous narcotics. Preliminary data indicate this system is safe and provides excellent pain relief. We have minimal experience with this therapy but feel it warrants further investigation.

Nitrous oxide inhalers have been used in a number of centers for analgesia and anxiety relief during debridements and dressing changes (Filkins, Cosgrov, & Marvin, 1981). This system requires a good exhaust system to minimize anesthetic exposure to other patients and ancillary personnel. Symptomatic pain relief is excellent if these disadvantages can be overcome.

Once a patient can tolerate oral medications, methadone is routinely administered in divided doses of 10 to 15 mg per day for adults. The amount is decreased if sedation is noted and increased if the patient has continuing pain between dressing changes. A gradual tapering schedule is begun after the last skin grafts to minimize withdrawal symptoms. Methadone has facilitated pain control in burn patients. It decreases the euphoric effects of other narcotics and appears to minimize the risk of addiction. It provides baseline pain relief because of its prolonged action, reducing the requirements for other narcotics.

Oxycodone combined with acetaminophen (Percocet) or with aspirin (Percodan) is another effective pain-relief agent when given orally before debridement. Only the oxycodone/acetaminophen combination is used because aspirin causes platelet dysfunction. Prolonged intraoperative bleeding results in those patients who undergo subsequent tangential excision and split-thickness grafting. Dilaudid is also effective when given orally but appears to have no advantages over oxycodone combinations. It is not used regularly because of its potential for abuse. Similarily, pentazocine (Talwin) is only used in patients with a history of adverse reactions to narcotics.

Inpatients frequently exhibit marked anxiety (Melzack & Taenzer, 1977). Parenteral diazepam (Valium) may relieve anxiety initially, but shorter-acting agents are preferred to maintain patient alertness. Alprazolam (Xanax) has a short duration of action and has proved effective in combination with oral narcotic agents in allaying anxiety associated with baths. The adult dose is 0.25 to 0.5 mg p.o. before tubs or three times per day for ongoing anxiety.

Many patients also experience sleep difficulties, especially nightmares reliving the accident (Steiner & Clark, 1977). Oral haloperidol (Haldol) 1 to 2 mg at bedtime is quite effective in suppressing nightmares and allowing more sleep in the hospital. The nightmares may temporarily recur when

Haldol is discontinued, indicating its suppressive effect. Thorazine is occasionally required for combative or psychotic patients.

Any change in mental status requires immediate investigation, since somnolence may be the result of excessive medication or early sepsis, which is the most common cause of death after burns. Medications are adjusted so that the patients maintain socialization and the physical therapy activities necessary to restore function.

The majority of patients achieve remarkable relief from pain when skin grafts are applied. Some children are unable to tolerate removal of sutures or skin staples from grafted sites. Ketamine produces a rapid anesthesia of short duration that has proved helpful in these cases (Demling, Ellerbee, & Jarrett, 1978; Ward & Diamond, 1976). Unhealed donor sites may be quite painful, especially if dry gauze or scarlet red-impregnated gauze dressings have been used. After discharge it is common for donor sites to blister and form small open sores that are temporarily painful. These invariably close, but healing can sometimes be speeded by the application of a gelatin/zinc oxide gauze dressing (Unna boot).

As the wounds heal, every attempt is made to wean the patient from pain medications before discharge. Outpatients are routinely given only Percocet in short courses and then changed to codeine and acetaminophen combinations to minimize the risk of narcotic abuse.

MANAGEMENT OF REHABILITATION PHASE PAIN

After discharge most burn patients have a few open wounds or donor sites that heal within a few days or weeks. But they must now adjust to a new set of cutaneous sensations. Virtually all patients after thermal burns have an increased sensitivity to heat and cold. Heat or cold is felt first and feels more extreme in the burned or donor tissues. Temperatures below 40°F (4°C) or above 80°F (26°C) most frequently produce these symptoms. Heat intolerance is accompanied by sweating and itching, which are additional problems for the burn victim. Excessive sweating can occur in warm environments, or even at normal temperatures. Some patients will drip sweat from affected extremities in response to even minor stress.

Virtually all burn patients experience itching of healed donor sites and grafted areas that persists for months or years. This is most intense in areas of hypertrophic scar formation where the tissue is hard, indurated, elevated, and often hyperesthetic. The application of tight compression garments to an affected area is a relatively effective long-term treatment for hypertrophic scar. Empirically, this decreases hypertrophic burn scar formation and, in most cases, will decrease the sensation of itching.

The majority of patients report a "pins and needles" sensation with increased itching immediately after removing compression garments, associated with an increased blood flow to the scar tissue. Similarly, placing an affected limb in the dependent position will increase the sensation of itching. Hot baths or ingestion of alcoholic beverages cause vasodilation and increased blood flow to cutaneous beds and should be studiously avoided. However, a lukewarm bath is reported by a majority of patients to temporarily decrease itching sensations. Moisturizing creams alleviate skin dryness, which may contribute to itching. Application of the moisturizers includes gentle rubbing of the tissue, which stimulates lateral inhibitory sensory pathways to decrease pruritis. Removal and reapplication of compression garments allows relief of any cutaneous ischemia.

Patients must be instructed specifically not to scratch affected areas even through compression garments. The fragile skin is easily abraded by such activity. Gentle vibration of the overlying tissue either manually or with a hand-held vibrating device is helpful. Rarely will compression garments alone be adequate for control of pruritis. Intradermal triamcinolone injections may speed the maturation of hypertrophic scar tissue and decrease the complaints of itching. More commonly, oral agents such as diphenhydramine (Benadryl®), cyproheptadine (Periactin®), or hydroxazine (Atarax®) will provide partial relief. All of these agents have sedative effects and are most effective when taken at bedtime. Driving and operating dangerous equipment are contraindicated when these agents are used.

Cold sensitivity produces an aching or tightness in affected extremities, usually joints. This may feel like a toothache, "arthritis," or just decreased mobility. Specific treatment involves avoidance of exposure to cold, and protecting the affected joint with warmer garments. Most patients achieve symptomatic relief with nonsteroidal anti-inflammatory agents, especially ibuprofen (Motrin®, Advil®), but peptic ulceration is a risk. Bird and Coleborne (1980) undertook biofeedback training in a patient with severe upper extremity cold intolerance after an electrical burn. The patient was able to raise his skin temperature significantly and experienced marked alleviation of his symptoms.

An early scar contracture may also cause joint stiffness. Better fitting compression garments and more vigorous physical therapy are indicated. Other causes of joint pain and stiffness include heterotopic bone formation or joint sepsis. Heterotopic bone formation can be diagnosed by the appearance of radiodense deposits at the tendinous insertions around joints on roentgenograms. At present prophylactic disodium etidronate (oidronel) is the only specific treatment for this condition. A septic joint is usually indicated by erythema, warmth, local tenderness, and fever with associated limitation of joint motion. The diagnosis is confirmed by the aspiration of purulent material from the joint or by a positive synovial fluid culture. This complication is rare even if joint tissue has been exposed after the burn injury.

Hyperesthesia is a complaint in many patients after burn injuries (Raja, Campbell, & Meyer, 1984). This may be manifested by an extreme sensitivity to even light touch of the affected part. Previously pleasant caresses now become extremely irritating or painful (Goodstein, 1985). Hypoesthesia or loss of sensation is most common over grafted areas. If the burns have destroyed a cutaneous nerve branch, the patient will have a specific distal anesthetic area. A neuroma may be found just proximal to the anesthetic area in some patients.

Phantom pain is the perception of pain in an amputated body part. The precise mechanism is unclear but may result from stimulation of the peripheral nerve at the amputated stump or along its ascending pathway. Patients describe this as a shooting pain that is rarely prolonged or persistent. Occasionally a persistent neuroma may be resected with relief of symptoms.

Outpatients respond remarkably well to group therapy as a means of verbalizing their concerns about a changed body image, decreased earning capacity, feelings of helplessness, and dealing with the depression that may accompany these problems. Prolonged psychological intervention should be available to all burn victims to facilitate their return to normal function after discharge.

SUMMARY

Persons who have sustained thermal injury are subjected to a number of painful experiences, both during their hospitalization and after discharge. A variety of psychological and pharmacological interventions are available to the health care team that can minimize the impact of these events upon both the patient and the caregivers. An empathetic approach can significantly aid the patient in tolerating necessary, if unpleasant, procedures and returning rapidly to an optimal level of function.

REFERENCES

Beecher, H. K. (1958). Relationship of significance of wound to pain experience. *Journal of the American Medical Association, 161,* 1609–1613.

Bird, E. I., & Colborne, G. R. (1980). Rehabilitation of an electrical burn patient through thermal biofeedback. *Biofeedback and Self-Regulation, 5,* 283–287.

Bowden, M. L., Jones, C. A., & Feller, I. (1979). *Psycho-social aspects of a severe burn: A review of the literature.* Ann Arbor, MI: National Institute for Burn Medicine.

Casey, K. L. (1980). The neurobiology of pain. *Medicine, 7,* 5–11.

Crasilneck, H. B., Stirman, J. A., Wilson, B. J., McCranie, E. J., & Fogelman, M. J. (1955). Use of hypnosis in the management of patients with burns. *Journal of the American Medical Association. 158.* 103–106.

Demling, R. H., Ellerbee, S., & Jarrett, F. (1978). Ketamine anesthesia for tangentia excision of burn eschar: A burn-unit procedure. *Journal of Trauma, 18,* 269 270.

Eland, J. M. (1982). Pain. In L. Hart, J. Reese, & M. Fearing (Eds.), *Concept common to acute illness.* St. Louis, MO: Mosby.

Elliot, C. H., & Olson, R. A. (1983). The management of children's distress ir response to painful medical treatment for burn injuries. *Behavior Research and Therapy, 21,* 675-683.

Feller, I. (1970). Introduction to burn patient problems in the United States. *Fire Journal, 64,* 52-53.

Filkins, S. A., Cosgrav, P., Marvin, J. A., Engrav, L., & Heimbach, D. M. (1981) Self-administered anesthesia: A method of pain control. *Journal of Burn Care and Rehabilitation, 2,* 33-34.

Giuliani, C. A., & Perry, G. A. (1985). Factors to consider in the rehabilitation aspect of burn care. *Physical Therapy, 65,* 619-623.

Goldstein, A. (1979). Endorphins and pain: A critical review. In R. F. Beers Jr., & E. G. Bussett (Eds.), *Mechanisms of pain and analgesic compounds.* New York: Raven Press.

Goodman, C. E. (1983). Pathophysiology of pain. *Archives of Internal Medicine, 143,* 527-530.

Goodstein, R. K. (1985). Burns: An overview of clinical consequences affecting patient, staff, and family. *Comprehensive Psychiatry, 26,* 43-57.

Graves, D. A., Batenhorst, R. L., Bennett, R. L., Wettstein, J. G., Griffin, W. O., Wright, B. D., & Foster, T. S. (1983). Morphine requirements using patient-controlled analgesia: Influence of diurnal variation and morbid obesity. *Clinical Pharmacy, 2,* 49-53.

Guyton, A. C. (1968). *Textbook of Medical Physiology* (3rd ed.). Philadelphia: Saunders.

Hilberman, M. (1984). Discussion of pain control. *Journal of Trauma, 24*(9), Supplement, S179-S185.

Hug, C. C., Jr., & Murphy, M. R. (1979). Fentanyl disposition in cerebrospinal fluid and plasma and its relationship to ventilatory depression in the dog. *Anesthesiology, 50,* 342-349.

Katz, E. R., Kellerman, J., & Siegel, S. E. (1980). Behavioral distress in children undergoing medical procedures: Developmental considerations. *Journal of Consulting and Clinical Psychology, 48,* 256-265.

Katz, E. R., Varni, J. W., & Jay, S. M. (1984). Behavioral assessment and management in pediatric pain. *Progress in Behavior Modification, 18,* 163-193.

Kelley, M. L., Jarvie, G. J., Middlebrook, J. L., McNeer, M. F., & Drabman, R. S. (1984). Decreasing burned children's pain behavior: Impacting the trauma of hydrotherapy. *Journal of Applied Behavior Analysis, 17,* 147-158.

Klein, R. M., & Charlton, J. E. (1980). Behavioral observation and analysis of pain behavior in critically burned patients. *Pain, 9,* 27-40.

Knudson-Cooper, M. S. (1981). Biofeedback and relaxation therapy in the treatment of severely burned children. *Journal of Burn Care and Rehabilitation, 2,* 102-110.

Levine, J., Scipio, E., McBryde, R., & Gordon, N. C. (1984). What are the functions of endorphins following thermal injury? *Journal of Trauma, 24*(9), Supplement, S168-S172.

Livingston, W. K. (1943). *Pain mechanisms.* New York: Macmillan.

Marvin, J. A., & Heimbach, D. M. (1984). Pain management. In S. V. Fisher &

P. A. Helm (Eds.), *Comprehensive rehabilitation of burns.* Baltimore, MD: Williams & Wilkins.

Melzack, R., & Taenzer, P. (1977). Concepts of pain perception and therapy. *Geriatrics, 32,* 44-48.

Melzack, R., Wall, P. D., & Ty, T. C. (1982). Acute pain in an emergency clinic: Latency of onset and descriptor patterns related to different injuries. *Pain, 14,* 33-43.

Perry, S. W. (1984). Undermedication for pain on a burn unit. *General Hospital Psychology, 6,* 308-316.

Perry, S., & Heidrich, G. (1982). Management of pain during debridement: A survey of U.S. burn units. *Pain, 13,* 267-280.

Raja, S. N., Campbell, J. N., & Meyer, R. A. (1984). Evidence for different mechanisms of primary and secondary hyperalgesia following heat injury to the glabrous skin. *Brain, 107,* 1179-1188.

Ravenscroft, K. (1982). The burn unit. *Psychiatric Clinics of North America, 5*(2), 419-432.

Shorkey, C. T., & Taylor, J. E. (1973). Management of maladaptive behavior of a severely burned child. *Child Welfare, 12,* 543-547.

Simons, R. D., McFadd, A., Frank, H. A., Green, L. C., Malin, R. M., & Morris, J. L. (1978). Behavioral contracting in a burn care facility: A strategy for patient participation. *Journal of Trauma, 18,* 257-260.

Steiner, H., & Clark, W. R. (1977). Psychiatric complications of burned adults: A classification. *Journal of Trauma, 17,* 134-143.

Streltzer, J., & Wade, T. C. (1981). The influence of cultural group on the undertreatment of postoperative pain. *Psychosomatic Medicine, 43,* 397-403.

Torgerson, W. S. (1984). What objective measures are there for evaluating pain? *Journal of Trauma, 24*(9), Supplement, S187-S197.

Wakeman, R. J., & Kaplan, J. Z. (1978). An experimental study of hypnosis in painful burns. *American Journal of Clinical Hypnosis, 21,* 3-12.

Wall, P. D. (1979). On the relationship of injury to pain. *Pain, 6,* 253-264.

Ward, C. M., & Diamond, A. N. (1976). An appraisal of ketamine in the dressing of burns. *Postgraduate Medicine, 5,* 222-223.

Weinstein, D. J. (1976). Imagery and relaxation with a burn patient. *Behavior Research and Therapy, 14,* 481.

Wernick, R. L., Jaremko, M. E., & Taylor, P. W. (1981). Pain management in severely burned adults: A test of stress inoculation. *Journal of Behavioral Medicine, 4,* 103-109.

Cancer Rehabilitation
Introduction

Roy C. Grzesiak

Cancer remains one of the leading causes of death in the United States and in the world. Media efforts to educate the public have led to greater numbers of cancer patients being diagnosed and treated earlier. Advances in treatment, including radiation therapy, chemotherapy, and surgery have increased the number of people achieving either a cure or greatly enhanced life expectancy. Both the illness and the treatment can cause residual physical effects that suggest the need for rehabilitation medicine services. Cancer rehabilitation is a relatively new subspecialty within physiatry. Typically, the physiatrist is the link between the rehabilitation team and the clinical oncology specialists.

The physiatrist, as an expert in functional assessment, is the ideal specialist to evaluate and prescribe a program designed to minimize or ameliorate the residual physical effects of cancer or the side effects of cancer treatment. The proximity of many rehabilitation centers to major medical schools invites the participation of a host of medical specialists in the rehabilitation process. The algologist, or pain specialist, can play a central role in rehabilitation oncology. Pain is a frequent occurrence for the cancer patient, and it must be appropriately controlled to ensure the patient's optimal participation in the rehabilitation process. The psychologist is an important member of the rehabilitation team. Psychological reactions to the diagnosis of cancer have received considerable attention in the literature. How individuals cope with the diagnosis, the treatment, and the rehabilitation process appears to have effects on quality of life. There is a growing need for specialized psychosocial programs that address the myriad psychological and social problems that impact on cancer patients.

This section on cancer rehabilitation consists of three contributions written by a physiatrist, an anesthesiologist, and a psychologist, respectively. The combination of the three is intended to provide a comprehensive picture of current practices in rehabilitation for patients with cancer who have an extended life expectancy.

9

Physical Rehabilitation of the Cancer Patient

Jeanne M. Pelensky

The number of Americans surviving cancer is steadily increasing (Page & Ardyce, 1985) and will continue to grow due to (1) increasing incidence of new cancer cases (Seidman, Mushinski, Gelb, & Silverberg, 1985), (2) improved cancer prevention (Public Health Service, 1979), (3) improved surveillance (American Cancer Society, 1985), and (4) improved treatment techniques. A proportion of cancer survivors and patients with active disease develop functional impairments amenable to rehabilitation. However, the rehabilitation of these patients differs from patients with other chronic disease processes in that disease prognosis, which determines treatment goals, is quite variable. Also, the patient's functional status may rapidly change from disease progression or treatment effects (Mayer, 1976). Following passage of the National Cancer Act in 1971, a unique, comprehensive approach to the rehabilitation of the cancer patient evolved in the early 1970s (Harvey, Jellinsky, & Habek, 1982). A number of model systems were initiated and supported through the NCI Cancer Control Program during that decade (McLaughlin, 1984). More recently, a survey of 36 cancer rehabilitation programs in different settings (community, cancer, or university hospitals) indicated that program structures were roughly equivalent with limited NIH grant support (Harvey et al., 1982).

It is the purpose of this chapter to review the general structure of cancer rehabilitation programs, methods of assessing treatment outcome, and problems requiring physiatric intervention. It is assumed that the reader has an understanding of basic rehabilitation principles, which are reviewed elsewhere. Finally, future areas of investigation will be suggested.

ASSESSMENT OF REHABILITATION OUTCOME

>hysical performance scales initially were developed to assess the effects of hemotherapy in cancer patients (Karnofsky & Burchenal, 1949) and have >een shown to be reliable (Heinrich & Schag, 1984). The Karnofsky Scale >f Performance Status and other indices of physical performance of cancer >atients require an objective rater (Spitzer et al., 1981). However, indices of >sychosocial function are generally self-rated (Derogatis, Rickels, & Rock, 976; Heinrich & Schag, 1984). Combined administration of scales measur->g physical and psychosocial function provide a complete, objective measurement of cancer rehabilitation outcome (Chang & Howes, 1983). In ddition, self-rated assessment forms identify cancer patients requiring reha->ilitation (Romsaas, Juliani, Brigg, Wysocki, & Moorman, 1983).

A review of the literature reveals few studies investigating outcome of ehabilitation programs for cancer patients. Lehman's original study of 800 ·ancer inpatients indicated that one half of those with rehabilitation prob-ems responded to treatment (Lehman, DeLisa, & Warren, 1978). In one etrospective study a subgroup of cancer patients discharged from a rehabil-tation institute continued to improve functionally postdischarge (Forer & Viller, 1980). Further work is required to assess and quantify effectiveness >f rehabilitation for cancer patients.

TEAM APPROACH

Comprehensive cancer rehabilitation, which treats psychosocial and physi-:al dysfunction, requires a multidisciplinary team working together (Ston-iington, 1983). The cancer rehabilitation team has been extensively de-;cribed elsewhere (DeLisa, Miller, & Melnick, 1985; Dietz, 1981; Stonnington, 1983). Briefly, the comprehensive cancer rehabilitation team s directed by a physiatrist or medical oncologist and is composed of a psychologist, social worker, oncology nurse, physical therapist, and occu-pational therapist. In addition, a chaplain, vocational rehabilitation coun-selor, speech pathologist, dietician, psychiatrist, rehabilitation nurse, maxil-lofascial prosthetist, continuity of care coordinator, and recreation therapist may extend the team (Harvey et al., 1982). The comprehensive cancer rehabilitation team interacts with the clinical oncology team (medical oncol-ogist, surgical oncologist, radiation oncologist, and other surgical special-ties) via the physiatrist in the model described by Lehman (Lehman et al., 1978). This linkage is essential to establish appropriate rehabilitation goals and coordinate patient care. Team conferences attended by rehabilitation team members are regularly provided for each patient receiving rehabilita-

tion, to discuss functional and psychosocial problems, set goals, and arrang
plans for successful discharge of the patient (Stonnington, 1983). Goal
may often need redefinition depending on patient response to tumor treat
ment, disease progression, etc.

ROLE OF PHYSIATRIST

The physiatrist, generally the leader of the comprehensive cancer rehabilita
tion team, is frequently consulted to evaluate cancer patients with (1) weak
ness, (2) bone lesions, and (3) pain syndromes. The physiatrist will deter
mine the patient's functional problems, set realistic rehabilitation goals
outline a treatment program, and, where appropriate, perform electrodiag
nostic tests to define the problem and predict recovery. In addition, the
physiatrist is involved in functional outcome assessment of rehabilitated
cancer patients, and in evaluation and management of cancer pain. Some
problem areas requiring physiatric intervention are described below.

WEAKNESS IN CANCER PATIENTS

Weakness may be the most frequent functional problem in cancer patients
prompting a physiatric consultation or referral to a cancer rehabilitation
program. Weakness may be classified as generalized or focal, and caused by
any of the following: (1) direct tumor effects, (2) remote tumor effects
(3) treatment effects, (4) systemic effects (anemia, hypoxemia), (5) inani-
tion, or (6) unrelated to the cancer. The etiology of the patient's weakness
must be identified and treated prior to or concomitant with a therapy
program in an attempt to halt progression.

Generalized Weakness

Deconditioning Syndrome

Inactivity and bed rest produces multiorgan deleterious effects, defined as
the deconditioning syndrome. Decreased cardiovascular tolerance to exercise (Saltin, Blomqvist, & Mitchell, 1968) and orthostatism rapidly develop
(Convertino, Hung, Goldwater, & DeBusk, 1982), producing generalized
weakness and decreased endurance once activity is resumed. In addition,
patients restricted to bed rest rapidly lose muscle strength (1% to 1.5% loss
of initial strength per day) (Muller, 1970); limb immobilization in a plaster
cast further accelerates the loss of muscle strength (3.0% loss per day)
(Hettinger, 1960). The effects of disuse on muscle function and structure

have been extensively reviewed (Booth & Gollnick, 1983). A few effects of muscle disuse include: rapid muscle atrophy (Eccles, 1944), atrophy of type I and type II fibers (Sargeant, Davies, Edwards, Maunder, & Young, 1977), decreased high-energy phosphates and muscle glycogen content (MacDougall, Ward, Sale, & Sutton, 1977), decreased muscle oxidative enzyme activity (Henrickson & Reitman, 1976), and increased glucocorticoid receptors in muscle cytosol (Dubois & Alman, 1980). Antigravity muscles are more severely affected by disuse (Eccles, 1944; Sargeant et al., 1977).

Cancer patients frequently develop the deconditioning syndrome because the effects of disease (pain, anemia, etc.) or disease–treatment side effects confines them to bed. Weakness secondary to deconditioning may be prevented by instituting preferably isotonic exercise of antigravity muscles (iliopsoas, quadriceps, ankle dorsiflexors) (Eccles, 1944). A single, brief daily contraction, at one-half maximal contraction force, maintains muscle strength in healthy subjects (Hettinger, 1955). Type II fiber atrophy has been reversed with DeLorme exercise training of affected muscles following cast immobilization (Kristensen, Hanser, & Satin, 1980).

In addition to specific resistive exercises, the patient should be encouraged to perform transfers, bed mobility, and ambulation as soon as possible, to maintain muscle endurance. If orthostatism is present, use of a tilt table will allow gradual cardiovascular adaptation to elevation. An exercise program should begin while the patient is at bed rest. Vigorous exercise initiated following bed rest does not hasten recovery of cardiovascular fitness (DeBusk, Convertino, Hung, & Goldwater, 1983).

Systemic Effects

Systemic effects secondary to cancer, such as anemia, hypoxemia, congestive heart failure, and, rarely, ectopic hormone production by tumor produce generalized weakness. Anemia in cancer patients is quite common and may occur from a variety of causes, including marrow invasion by tumor, blood loss, treatment effects, depressed erythropoiesis, etc., and has been reviewed by Schnider and Manalo (1979). Depleted red blood cells transport fewer oxygen molecules as fuel to working muscle in the anemic state. This results in a state of inadequate aerobic muscle metabolism and decreased endurance of the anemic patient to perform functional activities.

Hypoxemia per se may occur in cancer patients secondary to brain tumor (decreased respiratory drive), mediastinal obstruction of blood flow (superior vena cava syndrome), or pulmonary compromise (by tumor invasion, malignant effusion, or pneumonia). Congestive heart failure may occur and produce a state of relative hypoxemia and decreased muscle endurance. In all cancer patients with generalized weakness, hematocrit values, arterial blood gases, chest x-rays, and electrocardiograms must be reviewed and corrective action taken (oxygen supplementation, digitalization, etc.) prior to initiating rehabilitation.

Paraneoplastic endocrinopathies from ectopic hormone production by tumors (Schnider & Manalo, 1979) are rare causes of generalized weakness Hypercortisolemia and hypokalemia (secondary to ectopic ACTH secretion), hypoglycemia, hyponatremia, hypercalcemia, and ectopic parathyroid hormone secretion have been associated with a variety of tumors Changes in serum electrolytes, calcium, and blood glucose concentrations may depress neuromuscular function and produce generalized weakness When suspected, endocrine suppression tests and radioimmunoassays to detect ectopic hormone confirm the diagnosis. Irradiation of tumor, whenever possible, is most effective in treatment (Bunn & Minna, 1985; Schnider & Manalo, 1979).

Cervical Myelopathy

Five percent of patients with systemic cancer develop epidural spinal cord compression (Posner, 1979). Cord compression may occur from a variety of mechanisms: (1) primary or secondary vertebral tumor expansion into the spinal canal, (2) vertebral body collapse with column angulation, (3) direct spinal canal invasion by a paravertebral tumor, or, rarely, (4) hematogenous, direct cord metastasis (Constans et al., 1983; Manz, Moore, & Schold, 1981). In cervical myelopathy secondary to cancer a presentation of neck pain alone or with radicular pain is typical (Gilbert, 1978; Klein, 1984). Thereafter generalized paresis, sensory deficits, and bowel and bladder disturbance gradually evolve (Constans et al., 1983; Gilbert et al., 1978). Occasionally, the initial presentation may be painless, with progressive weakness, paresthesias, or bladder disturbance mimicking other disease processes (Klein, 1984; Posner, 1978). Diagnosis is confirmed by bone x-rays, myelogram, and/or cervical CT scan. Primary treatment of carcinomatous cervical myelopathy generally involves high-dose Decadron (dexamethasone) administration and palliative tumor radiation (Constans, 1983). Surgical decompression and spine fusion, steroids and radiation are reserved for select patient groups (Klein, 1984; Tang et al., 1983; Tomita & Sunderesan, 1983). Chemotherapy or hormonal therapy for responsive tumors is also helpful (Jameson, 1983).

Radiation myelopathy rarely occurs following radiation for head and neck cancer, esophageal cancer, or lymphoma (Lambert, 1978). High doses in the vicinity of the spinal cord (5,000 rads) produce a slowly progressive, painless irreversible myelopathy months to years following treatment. Radiation myelopathy is a diagnosis of exclusion; tumor recurrence must be firmly ruled out by myelogram and/or spinal cord computed tomography (CT) scan.

Quadriplegia and neurogenic bowel and bladder rarely have been reported in patients with acute leukemia treated with intrathecal methotrexate
nd cervical radiation (Baum, Kock, Gorby, & Plunket, 1971; Blayer,
Drake, & Chabner, 1973). The onset of symptoms rapidly follows chemotherapy injection, with an irreversible clinical picture. Necrotizing myelop-
thy, an extremely rare paraneoplastic syndrome, also may occur at the
ervical level, most often associated with lymphoma (Ojeda, 1984). Cord
ompromise by tumor must be excluded in all cases of myelopathy.

Once the cause of cervical myelopathy has been identified and appropriate treatment initiated, intensive rehabilitation may begin. Fitting the
patient with a Philadelphia collar prevents spine movement, decreases pain,
nd is well tolerated. Prevention of joint contractures with range-of-motion
exercise, splinting, and positioning; initiation of a bowel program; and
external urinary drainage all should begin immediately. Training in performance of bed mobility, transfers, ambulation, and activities of daily living
begins promptly after the spinal lesion is rendered stable. Assistive devices,
such as a sliding board, wheelchair, or orthoses may improve functional
performance. Retraining bladder function generally is not pursued since
survival may be limited and neurologic deterioration is frequent in patients
with carcinomatous myelopathy (Constans, 1983). Sexual and psychosocial counseling should be provided for both patient and family. Vocational
counseling is appropriate if the patient responds to primary treatment and
prognosis is favorable.

Polyneuropathy

Peripheral polyneuropathy, a common finding in cancer patients, may progress to generalized weakness. This frequently is due to chemotherapeutic
agents, with loss of Achilles tendon reflexes the first sign of neuropathy
(Weiss, Walker, & Wiernik, 1974). Vincristine, a widely used chemotherapeutic agent with neurotoxic effects, has been extensively studied (Caccia,
Comoti, Ubiali, & Lucchetti, 1977; Chan, 1980; Green, 1977). With
continued drug administration, weakness of toe and ankle dorsiflexors is
observed. Abdominal pain, constipation, and paresthesias of the hands and
feet are common presenting symptoms of vincristine neurotoxicity (Holland et al., 1973). The neuropathy secondary to vincristine is dose-related,
slowly progressive, and reversible after stopping drug administration (Holland et al., 1973). However, rapidly progressive quadriplegia has been
reported when the drug is given to patients with Charcot Marie Tooth
syndrome (Hogan-Dann, Fellmeth, McGuire, & Kiley, 1984). Elderly
patients (Whitelaw & Cowan, 1963), those with malignant lymphomas
(Watkins & Griffin, 1978), and those receiving prior radiation (Cassady,
Tonnesen, & Wolfe, 1980) are more susceptible to develop neuropathy. Of
the *Vinca* alkaloids, vincristine is the most neurotoxic, followed by vinde-

sine and vinblastine (Donuso, Green, Heller-Bettinger, & Samson, 1977) Administration of VP16 with the vincas intensifies the neurotoxic effects (Thant et al., 1982); physical activity may limit neurotoxicity (Sakamoto 1974). The neurotoxic effects of chemotherapeutic agents have been extensively reviewed (Kaplan & Wiermik, 1984). Hexamethylenamine (Vogl, Berenzweig, & Kaplan, 1979), procarbazine (Oliverio, Denham, & DeVita, 1964), and VP16 (Falkson et al., 1975) produce peripheral neuropathies, reversible on discontinuing the agent(s). The neurotoxicity of cis-platinum (DDP) is less frequent in occurrence than ototoxicity, appears dose-related, and is a demyelinating sensory neuropathy without motor weakness (Kedar, Cohen, & Freeman, 1978; Thompson, Davis, Kornfield, Hilgers, & Standefer, 1984). Adriamycin has produced dorsal root ganglionitis in rats (Jortner & Cho, 1980). The nitroimidazole radiosensitizers desmethylmisonidazole and SR-2508, which sensitize tumor cells to radiation effects, produce a primary axonal peripheral neuropathy that is dose limiting (Wasserman, 1984). Laetrile (amygdalin) produces a mixed form of peripheral neuropathy with axonal degeneration and demyelination of peripheral nerves which has been noted on biopsy (Kalyanaraman, Kalyanaraman, Cullenan, & McLean, 1983).

Peripheral neuropathy occurs less frequently as a remote effect of cancer. Neuropathy associated with plasma cell neoplasm (multiple myeloma, osteosclerotic myeloma) clinically occurs in less than 5% of patients (Kelly, Kyle, Miles, O'Brien, & Dyck, 1981). However, in the small osteosclerotic subgroup, neuropathy occurs in 50 to 80% of patients and neuropathic symptoms often are the patient's presenting complaint (Driedger & Pruzanski, 1980; Kelly, Kyle, Miles, & Dyck, 1983). In multiple myeloma without amyloidosis, the associated neuropathy may be a mild sensorimotor, pure sensory, or severe motor variety (Kelly et al., 1981) and has features of axonal degeneration (Ohi, Kyle, & Dyck, 1985); multiple myeloma with amyloidosis is associated with a primary sensory neuropathy (Kelly et al., 1981). Osteosclerotic myeloma has an associated neuropathy that is symmetric, predominantly motor, and severely progressive, and often associated with a light-chain monoclonal serum protein (Kelly et al. 1981, 1983). Only the neuropathy associated with sclerotic myeloma improves with primary tumor treatment, particularly when a solitary lesion is present (Driedger & Pruzanski, 1980; Kelly, 1983). Mechanisms proposed for the neuropathies associated with plasma cell neoplasms include: lightchain effects (Kelly, 1983), monoclonal antibodies to peripheral nerve myelin (Latov et al., 1980), or other immunopathologic effects of the myeloma.

Peripheral neuropathy may occur as a remote effect of neoplasms (Schnider, 1979) and is of two varieties: a pure sensory neuropathy and a mixed sensorimotor neuropathy (McLeod, 1984). *Pure sensory neuropathy* is unique to cancer and may precede the appearance of cancer, with paresthesia, severe sensory loss, hyporeflexia, and aching limb pain as part of the clinical picture. Axonal degeneration and dorsal root ganglionitis and antibodies to CNS neurons have been detected (Horwich, Cho, & Porro, 1977; Wilkinson & Zeromski, 1965). The neuropathy does not improve with cancer treatment (Horwich, 1977). *Sensorimotor neuropathy* as a remote cancer effect is more common (Croft & Wilkinson, 1965) and may have several clinical patterns (McLeod, 1984): (1) a subacute or chronic form with predominantly distal weakness, hyporeflexia, and mild sensory deficits (Croft & Wilkinson, 1969), (2) an acute form resembling Guillain-Barré syndrome, and (3) a remitting relapsing neuropathy, with improvement related to steroid treatment (Croft, 1967). A mixed picture of axonal degeneration and segmental demyelination is seen on histopathology (Croft, Urich, & Wilkinson, 1967; Graus, Ferrer, & Lamarca, 1983).

From 17 to 48% of lung cancer patients have demonstrated peripheral polyneuropathy on electrodiagnostic testing (Graus, 1983; Teravainen & Larson, 1977; Trojaborg, Frantzen, & Andersen, 1969). Neuropathy has been detected in half of lung cancer patients with weight loss of 15% or greater, suggesting a nutritional etiology (Graus, 1983; Hawley, Cohen, Saini, & Armbrustmacher, 1980). Electrophysiologic evidence of neuropathy has been observed in 10 to 30% of lymphoma patients, generally in the form of a primary axonal degeneration (Graus, 1983; Walsh, 1971). Occasionally a severe, relapsing, demyelinating polyneuropathy has been observed in lymphomas (Graus, 1983), which may respond to steroid therapy (Sumi, Farrell, & Knaus, 1983).

A syndrome of proximal muscle weakness, hyporeflexia, and distal sensory loss has been observed in patients with cancer and termed "carcinomatous neuromyopathy" (Shy & Silverstein, 1965). Myopathic changes on biopsy, myopathic potentials in proximal muscles, signs of chronic denervation, and slowed nerve conduction on electrodiagnostic testing, and significant nerve fiber loss on sural nerve biopsy is part of this syndrome, which is most often associated with lung cancer patients (Campbell & Paty, 1974; Paul, Katiyar, Musra, & Pant, 1978).

The diagnosis of peripheral neuropathy requires electrodiagnostic testing to define the type of neuropathy (Asbury, 1980; Thage, Trojaborg, & Buchtal, 1963). In addition, other causes of peripheral neuropathy should be identified (i.e., diabetes, alcoholism, renal failure, pernicious anemia) with appropriate diagnostic tests. The treatment of weakness secondary to peripheral neuropathy has been reviewed by Herbison (1983). Treatment of all cancer related neuropathies consists of (1) withdrawal of the inciting agent; (2) maintenance of joint range of motion; (3) prevention of muscle disuse atrophy, with brief isometric (Muller, 1970; Lehman, 1959) or isotonic (DeLorme, Schwab, & Watkins, 1948) contractions; (4) functional retraining through compensatory mechanisms (Herbison, Jaweed, & Ditunno, 1983); and (5) prevention of muscle overstretch with use of orthoses (Huddleston, 1952).

Myopathy

Myopathy, when it occurs in cancer patients, is generally secondary to steroid treatment. The presentation is of an insidiously progressive, painless weakness of proximal muscles, with the pelvic girdle affected earlier and more severely than the shoulder girdle muscles, although all muscles may be affected (Askari, Vignos, & Moskowitz, 1976; Mandel, 1982). The patient typically complains of difficulty arising from a bed or climbing stairs. Quadriceps muscles are invariably affected on examination and on muscle force contraction measurements (Kaheeli, Edward, & Gohill, 1983). Other findings include (1) elevated 24-hour urinary 3-methylhistidine/creatinine ratio, (2) occasional myopathic potentials (BSAPPs) in proximal limb muscles on EMG without abnormal spontaneous activity, and (3) atrophy of type II fibers and, less commonly, type I fibers, on muscle biopsy (Kaheeli et al., 1983; Mandel, 1982). A severe necrotizing myopathy has been noted on muscle biopsy in some subjects treated with steroids (Ojeda, 1982).

Treatment consists of withdrawing steroids, if possible. Patients treated with relatively low doses (15 mg prednisone/day) may reverse the muscle wasting effects with exercise despite continued steroid administration (Horber, Scheidegger, Grunig, & Frey, 1985). However, with higher doses of steroid administration no significant improvement in muscle mass or function was noted with exercise.

Dermatomyositis and polymyositis, rare paraneoplastic syndromes, may produce generalized weakness. When dermatomyositis occurs with cancer the patients tend to be older than the general dermatomyositis population and more often are women with a history of ovarian or stomach cancer (Barnes, 1976; Peters, Andersen, & Thornton, 1983). Presentation is one of a subacute symmetric proximal weakness beginning in the lower extremities and progressing to involve shoulders, anterior neck muscles, and posterior pharynx. Typically, marked elevations of muscle enzymes, specific skin changes, myopathic potentials on electromyogram (EMG) [brief, small amplitude potentials (BSAPPs), spontaneous activity at rest, and repetitive high frequency discharges], and necrosis of type I and type II muscle fibers on biopsy are noted (Pearson & Bohan, 1977). The syndrome responds partially to steroids but subacutely progresses to severe dysphagia, dyspnea, respiratory insufficiency, and death. Exercises to preserve joint range of motion and prevent disuse atrophy are indicated, particularly as the inflammatory phase subsides. Simple goals are set (e.g., independent transfers, ambulation) during rehabilitation; these must be redefined as the process progresses. The family is involved early in the rehabilitation process because of the poor prognosis and progression of the myopathy.

Carcinamatous metastases to muscle have been found in patients with a progressive myopathic syndrome (Doshi & Fowler, 1983). However, muscle biopsies of systemic cancer patients tend to be abnormal (Pearson, 1959; Scelsi & Pinelli, 1977; Warmolts, Re, & Lewis, 1975), suggesting another cause for weakness in Doshi's cases.

Paraneoplastic Syndromes

Paraneoplastic syndromes other than those previously discussed (peripheral neuropathy, dermatomyositis) may produce generalized weakness and include the following: subacute cerebellar degeneration, progressive multifocal leukoencephalopathy (PML), amyotrophic lateral sclerosis (ALS), subacute motor neuropathy, Guillain-Barré syndrome, myasthenic syndrome, and myasthenia gravis (Bunn, 1985; Posner, 1979). All paraneoplastic syndromes are quite rare and may precede signs of cancer. Subacute cerebellar degeneration presents as progressive limb ataxia, dysarthria, hypotonia, and frequent dementia evolving over days or months (Brain & Wilkinson, 1965). Progressive multifocal leukoencephalopathy is a rapidly progressive syndrome of progressive paralysis, dementia, aphasia, ataxia, dysarthria, visual field defects, and associated with the reticuloses (Currie, Henson, Morgan, & Poole, 1970). Amyotrophic lateral sclerosis is associated with cancer in less than 10% of cases, with progressive weakness, hyporeflexia, fasciculations, and muscle wasting as part of the clinical picture (Norris, 1984). The progression of motor neuron disease may be more gradual than in primary ALS. Myasthenic syndrome (Eaton-Lambert syndrome) is frequently associated with oat cell lung cancer and presents with proximal leg weakness, hyporeflexia, mouth dryness, vague muscle aches, and weakness improving with exercise (Lambert & Rooke, 1965). Marked facilitation of the evoked motor response on repetitive stimulation is diagnostic. Subacute motor neuronopathy is a syndrome of progressive lower motor neuron weakness without sensory deficit, which is associated with lymphoma (Schold, Cho, Somasundaram, & Posner, 1979). Guillain-Barré syndrome also has been associated with lymphoma, with a picture of progressive ascending weakness beginning in the legs and sensory disturbance (Currie et al., 1970; Lisak, Mitchell, Sweiman, Orreshio, & Asbury, 1977). Myasthenia gravis may occur in cancer, particularly in patients with malignant thymoma, with fluctuating weakness of ocular, bulbar, limb, and/or trunk musculature. Myasthenia gravis is diagnosed by significant decrement of the motor-evoked response on repetitive muscle stimulation (Stalberg, 1980).

Removal of the primary tumor may produce remission of some paraneo plastic neurologic syndromes (subacute cerebellar degeneration, Eaton-Lam bert syndrome). Generally, however, the syndromes run their own cours (Bunn, 1985). Rehabilitation consists of training the patient in compensa tory techniques to perform functional activities, training in energy conser vation techniques (for myasthenia gravis), and providing adaptive equip ment, environmental control systems, and/or home remodeling to improv the patient's functioning.

Encephalopathy

Encephalopathy may occur in cancer patients, often secondary to treatment Intrathecal or intraventricular methotrexate administered for CNS prophy laxis of leukemia may produce subacute or chronic leukoencephalopathies with confusion, dementia, lethargy, ataxia, tremor, generalized weakness and seizures as part of the clinical picture (Price & Jamieson, 1975). The CNS changes are augmented with systemic methotrexate administra tion and/or cranial irradiation (Bleyer & Griffin, 1981). Intrathecal cyto sine arabinoside may produce similar effects in children treated for CNS prophylaxis of leukemia (Peylan-Ramu, Poplach, Pizzo, Adornato, & DiChiro, 1978). Measurement of serum electrolytes, arterial blood gases, liver function tests, serum calcium, magnesium, and blood glucose is re quired to eliminate other treatable causes of encephalopathy.

Focal Weakness

Focal weakness in cancer patients has a variable presentation ranging from hemiparesis to isolated muscle weakness, depending on the site of neuro muscular pathology. Causes of focal weakness in cancer are briefly outlined.

Brain Tumor

Brain tumor, either primary or secondary, frequently produces focal weak ness in cancer patients. In an autopsy series of 531 patients with systemic cancer, 26% had cerebral metastases (Manz et al., 1982). Another autopsy series indicated a 1% incidence of malignant gliomas in patients aged 55 and over (Annegers, Schoenberg, Okazaki, & Kurland, 1981). The main symp tom on initial presentation is early morning headache, although a smaller number of patients present with weakness, personality change, or focal seizure (Posner, 1979). If weakness is part of the early presentation, it is usually mild and focal (monoparesis or hemiparesis), or occasionally a limb ataxia (Posner, 1979). As the tumor grows, the signs and symptoms pro gress. Diagnosis requires CT scan of the brain with contrast and brain biopsy of solitary lesions or stereoencephatotomy for small or deep-seated esions (Ostertag, Mennel, & Kiessling, 1980). Metastatic and primary brain tumor treatment results have been reviewed (Markesbery, Brooks, & Gupta, 1978; Salcman, 1980, 1985). For metastatic tumors, survival rates improved following treatment (surgery, radiation, or steroids), although no modality was clearly superior (Markesbery, 1978). Increased doses of whole brain irradiation (greater than 2,000 rads) did not improve survival time (Gelber, Larson, Borgelt, & Kramer, 1981). Excision of solitary brain metastases followed by radiation therapy improved survival in select primary tumor types (Sundaresan & Galicich, 1985). Radioactive element implants placed directly into the brain tumor (interstitial brachytherapy) have produced a 68% response rate (tumor regression or neurologic stability) in primary and secondary maligant brain tumors after a 9-month follow-up (Gutin et al., 1984). In addition, enhancement of chemotherapy penetration across the blood–brain barrier with intracarotid mannitol administration (Neuwelt, 1983), potentiation of chemotherapy effects with local CNS hyperthermia (Silberman et al., 1985), and treatment with newer chemotherapeutic agents such as aziridinylbenzoquinone (AZQ) (Eagan et al., 1983) or BCNU and T2T (Eagan et al., 1984) holds promise for treatment of primary brain malignancies.

Despite improvements in diagnosis and treatment, the median survival following treatment for brain metastases is 5 to 6 months (Markesbery, 1978), and for glioblastoma multiforme 3 to 4 months (McLendon, 1985; Salcman, 1982). Thus, rehabilitation must focus on short-term functional goals (i.e., transfers, ambulation), with family training and counseling undertaken immediately. Neurologic regression requires redefinition of achievable goals; assessment for further adaptive equipment needs, and continued family training in the performance of ADL, mobility, and skin care.

Cerebrovascular Disease

Stroke may produce focal weakness in patients with systemic cancer, frequently caused by cerebral emboli from septic sources, nonbacterial thrombotic endocarditis (Min, Gyorkey, & Sato, 1980), or microvascular thrombosis from diffuse intravascular coagulopathy (DIC) (Al-Mondhery, 1975). The etiologic determination of stroke requires head CT scan and, in the appropriate setting, blood and CSF cultures, determination of fibrinogin and fibrin split product concentration, platelet count, coagulation studies, and echocardiogram. Prognosis for neurologic recovery from stroke depends on correlation of the underlying etiology: DIC in cancer has a poor prognosis (Al-Mondhery, 1975), whereas nonbacterial thrombotic endocarditis may be treated with anticoagulation, and further septic embolization prevented by appropriate early antimicrobial treatment (Chernik, Armstrong, & Posner, 1977).

Leptomeningeal Cancer

Leptomeningeal metastasis is a less frequent form of direct CNS tumor invasion producing focal weakness. Tumor seeding of the meninges has been noted to occur spontaneously in solid tumors (Wasserstrom, Glass, & Posner, 1982), non-Hodgkin's lymphomas (Griffin, Thompson, Mitchinson, DeKiewiet, & Welland, 1971; Levitt, Dawson, Rosenthal, & Moloney 1980), leukemias, and traumatically after resection of malignant gliomas (Corbett & Newman, 1981). The metastases may produce symptoms and signs of brain, spinal cord, or peripheral nerve involvement. In a series of 90 patients the most common symptoms noted were headache, mental change, and gait dysfunction (Wasserstrom et al., 1982). Diagnosis requires a high index of suspicion, CT scan of head and spinal cord at clinically indicated levels, myelogram, and CSF analysis for tumor cells and biochemical markers (Wasserstrom et al., 1982). Delayed lower extremity F-wave latencies or absent F waves in the posterior tibial nerves suggests leptomeningeal disease (Argov & Siegal, 1985). Treatment requires focal irradiation to areas with mass tumor infiltration and repeated doses of intrathecal methotrexate (Griffin et al., 1971; Wasserstrom et al., 1982). Long-term survival is measured in weeks but is improved and prolonged with aggressive treatment (Raz, Siegal, & Pollack, 1984). Due to the eventual neurologic deterioration and systemic cancer process, rehabilitation must be brief, with limited goals and immediate family involvement.

Myelopathy

Myelopathy, when occurring at thoracic or lumbar levels, may produce focal weakness. The lumbosacral spine is the major site of vertebral metastases, and breast, lung, and prostate cancer the most frequent tumor sources (Schaberg & Gainor, 1985). Due to the limited vascular supply between spinal segments T3 to T9, thoracic level bony lesions have the tendency to rapidly produce paraplegia (Constans et al., 1983). Because there is potential for rapid neurologic deterioration from cord compression at this level, and the capability to excise vertebral tumor and provide stabilization by an anterior approach, some authors recommend surgery as part of the early management of carcinomatous spinal cord compression (Constans et al., 1983; Sundaresen, Bains, & McCormack, 1985). Radiation, high-dose steroids, and chemotherapy/hormonal manipulation are also indicated in epidural cord compression (Jameson, 1983).

Radiculopathies

Radiculopathies occur secondary to epidural root compression by vertebral metastases, local tumor masses, direct (endoneural) hematogenous spread (Johnson, 1977), or radiation fibrosis. The clinical picture is one of back pain, unilateral pain and paresthesias in a dermatomal pattern, and progresive focal muscle weakness. However, when roots and spinal cord have been radiated together (receiving greater than 5,000 rads), the signs of myelopathy will predominate (Bradley, 1984). The diagnosis requires EMG, CT scan of appropriate spine and root levels, and, occasionally, myelogram to rule out leptomeningeal tumor. Ulnar F-wave conduction velocity determinations in patients with C8 to T1 level involvement may aid diagnosis (Ongerboer de Visser, Van der Saude, & Kemp, 1982). Primary treatment of neoplastic radiculopathies includes local root irradiation and high-dose steroid administration. Rehabilitation is similar to that for peripheral neuropathies, with bracing or splinting when necessary, isometric or isotonic strengthening exercises for weakened muscles, and exercise to prevent disuse atrophy as part of the therapy program.

Plexopathy

Brachial and lumbosacral plexopathies have been extensively described in cancer patients. Plexopathies are produced by lymphatic enlargement, extrinsic tumor mass (Pancoast's syndrome), or radiation fibrosis with extradural compression. The clinical characteristics of recurrent tumor versus radiation effects producing brachial plexopathy have been studied. Severe arm pain, Horners' syndrome, and lower trunk involvement suggest tumor invasion, whereas minimal arm pain, arm lymphedema, paresthesias, and upper trunk involvement suggest radiation fibrosis (Kori, Foley, & Posner, 1981). Abnormal median sensory responses, normal median or ulnar motor responses, fasciculations, or myokymia on EMG also suggest radiation fibrosis as an etiology (Lederman & Wilbourn, 1984). Unfortunately, the clinical picture does not *definitely* indicate the etiology (Kori et al., 1981; Lederman & Wolbourn, 1984). Diagnosis requires CT scan, EMG, sensory and motor nerve conduction studies, and myelogram (in the case of panplexopathy). Additionally, somatosensory evoked potential determinations (Synek & Cowan, 1983) and H-reflex recording of the flexor carpi ulnaris muscle (Ongerboer de Visser, Schimsheimer, & Hart, 1984) have been helpful in identifying brachial plexus lesions. Occasionally surgical exploration is required to rule out tumor recurrence. Treatment requires the use of high-dose steroids, radiation, and/or chemotherapy in carcinomatous plexopathy. Narcotic analgesics or various neurosurgical procedures to disrupt pain-conducting pathways are partially effective in treating intractable pain associated with plexopathy (Kori, 1981). Good pain relief but little functional improvement has been noted following neurolysis and nerve transfer procedures to treat radiation induced plexopathy (Narakas, 1985).

Lumbosacral plexopathies have been diagnosed in 15% of cancer patients referred for evaluation of low back pain (Jaeckle, Young, & Foley, 1985). Carcinomatous plexopathies present with progressive pelvic or leg pain, followed by paresthesias and leg weakness. A positive reversed straight-leg raising test, lymphedema, rectal mass, and hydronephros suggest cancer a the etiology (Jaeckle et al., 1985; Pettigrew, Glass, Moor, & Zornoza 1984). Painless leg weakness and paresthesias with a history of abdomina radiation suggest radiation-induced plexopathy. Diagnosis requires C scan of the pelvis, including views of the lower thoracic and upper lumba spine; myelogram (particularly in bilateral plexopathies or when radiation i planned); EMG; and, occasionally, surgical exploration (Jaeckle et al. 1985). Primary treatment is similar to that of brachial plexopathies, with high-dose steroids (100 mg dexamethasone/day) effective in relieving the pain syndrome (Pettigrew et al., 1984). The rehabilitation of brachial and lumbosacral plexopathies requires treatment of lymphedema (discussed below), management of intractable pain, splinting and/or bracing, and exercise approaches (discussed under peripheral neuropathies).

Neuropathy

Focal weakness may occur from various mononeuropathies. Direct compression by local tumor mass (Kline, Garcia, & Harsh, 1984; Unsold Safran, Safran, & Hoyt, 1980), osseous metastasis (Hall, Buzdar, & Blumenschein, 1983; Massy, 1981a), lymphedema (Ganel, Engel, Sela, & Brooks, 1979), or perineural tumor spread (Morris & Joffe, 1983) have been described. Radiation (Berger & Bataini, 1977), chemotherapy (Levitt & Prager, 1975), and various surgical procedures have produced focal neuropathies. Diagnosis is made by EMG, tumor marker analysis (LaBan, Meerschaert, & Taylor, 1982), appropriate level CT scans, bone x-rays, bone marrow biopsy (Massy, 1982), and, in some cases, surgical exploration (Kline et al., 1984; Morris & Jaffe, 1983). Treatment requires local irradiation, chemotherapy (Hall et al., 1982; Morris, 1983), or, if secondary to tumor, surgical excision (Kline et al., 1984). When chemotherapy has produced neuropathy, withdrawal of the agent allows recovery.

After surgical destruction of nerves that innervate muscles controlling joint motion (i.e., destruction of spinal accessory nerve during radical neck dissection), precise rehabilitation is required. Maintenance of joint motion, avoidance of weakened muscle stretch, and strengthening of compensatory muscle groups must be performed in a stepwise fashion (DeLisa et al., 1984). In some cases nerve regrafting may be performed.

Bone and Soft Tissue Tumors

Skeletal involvement by cancer is a common problem, with metastasis to bone occurring in 32% of cancer patients (Johnston, 1970). The most frequent sites of metastatic bone disease in order of decreasing frequency are: spine, pelvis, ribs, skull, femur, and humerus (Burke & Griffiths, 1983;

Formassier & Horne, 1975). Blastic, lytic, or mixed lesions are noted on x-ray, depending on the effect of metastatic tumor on bone. Bone destruction may occur by direct tumor invasion or indirectly by tumor release of humoral substances such as prostaglandins (Bennett et al., 1977), osteoclastic activating factor (Horton, Raisz, Simmons, Oppenheim, & Mergenhagen, 1972), or other ectopic hormones (Tashjcan, 1975) that affect bone.

The earliest symptom of bone involvement is pain with movement or weight-bearing of the affected part. Diagnostically, bone scan is more sensitive than bone x-ray in detecting metastases except in myeloma (Brady & Croll, 1979). X-rays are helpful in determining the extent of cortical erosion and presence of bone fracture. CT scans have been recommended in evaluating primary or secondary bone tumors to: (1) evaluate positive bone scans with normal x-rays (Durning, 1983), (2) determine the extent of soft tissue invasion by primary bone tumor, (3) indirectly determine tumor grade by estimating fat content (Rosenthal, 1985), or (4) evaluate focal areas of bone destruction in multiple myeloma (Helms & Genant, 1982). From preliminary studies, magnetic resonance imaging (MRI) appears to improve the evaluation of bone tumors, better defining the extent of narrow invasion, cortical erosion, soft tissue invasion, and nucleus pulposus degeneration (Helms, Moon, & Genant, 1984).

The primary treatment of metastatic bone lesions is radiotherapy; this will palliate pain and allow bone healing (Allen, Johnson, & Hibbs, 1976; Ambrad, 1978). However, the optimum dose schedule for pain palliation has not been defined (Madsen, 1983). With multiple sites of bone involvement, aggressive chemotherapy has improved palliation and prolonged survival in breast cancer (Smalley, Scogna, & Melmud, 1982).

Prior to initiating rehabilitation, radiographs of the tumor site(s) must be reviewed to determine (1) the extent of cortical erosion and (2) the location of cortical erosion in reference to sites of muscle tendon insertion. Bony cortical erosion of 50% or greater has produced pathologic fracture in 61% of patients (Fider, 1981). All lytic lesions of weight-bearing bones with more than 50% cortical erosion or greater than 3 cm in diameter should be internally fixed prophylactically. Intramedullary nailing is the procedure of choice to prevent long-bone fractures or to treat painful lesions not responding to radiation (Dobozi, Dvonch, & Saltzman, 1984). Once fracture occurs, bipolar endoprosthesis placement for proximal femur involvement (Burke & Griffiths, 1983), Zickel nailing for distal long-bone fractures (Albright, Gillespie, & Butaud, 1980), or intramedullary rodding for poor operative risk patients is indicated (Moehring, 1984) to increase mobility and relieve pain. Fracture cast bracing has been an alternative approach to stabilize appropriate upper extremity and lower extremity pathologic fractures, although painful nonunion of pathologic fractures may require surgical management (Sarmiento, Kinman, & Galvin, 1977).

In providing an exercise program to prevent the effects of bedrest and improve function, it is essential to ascertain bone tumor location. In particular, patients with destruction of pelvic bones (frequent sites of metastases), proximal femur, scapula, and proximal humerus should avoid resistive exercise to muscles originating or inserting at the site of bony tumor invasion. Generally the patient complains of pain with contraction of the affected muscle, but precautions should be taken to avoid further disruption of tendinous insertion with exercise. The risk of patients with bone metastases developing pathologic fracture during rehabilitation is quite low, although females of younger age and with advanced lytic disease are at increased risk to develop fracture (Bunting, Lamont-Havers, Schweon, & Kliman, 1985).

Primary malignant tumors of bone and soft tissue are quite rare, representing less than 2% of all new adult cancer cases per year (NIH Consensus Conference, 1985). Primary bone tumors generally occur in patients less than 30 years of age (Murray, Sutow, & Martin, 1982), although soft tissue sarcomas affect an older age group (Weisenberger et al., 1981). The multidisciplinary management of these tumors has rapidly evolved, with less than limb amputation now advocated for select patient groups (NIH Consensus Conference, 1985).

In evaluation of skeletal sarcomas, a bone biopsy, oriented so that the needle tract will be excised during definitive tumor operation, is crucial (Gebhart, Lane, & McCormack, 1985). To determine the extent of osseous and extraosseous tumor and the presence of metastases prior to treatment CT has been recommended. In appropriately selected patients, limb-sparing procedures undertaken in appropriately equipped specialty centers result in excellent local tumor control with preservation of involved limb function (Gebhart, 1985; NIH Consensus Conference, 1985; Weisenberger et al., 1981). Various custom prosthetic devices (Gebhart, 1985; Johnston, Harries, & Alexander, 1983; Katzelson & Nerubay, 1980; Sim, Chao, & Pritchard, 1980), vascularized fibula bone grafts, and autogenous autoclaved bone grafts (Johnston et al., 1983) have been used to replace or supplement excised bone. Tumors located about the shoulder or pelvis are difficult to resect and still preserve limb function (Sim et al., 1980), although resections of pubic rami, ischial rami, or posterior iliac wing do not require reconstruction. Preoperative adjuvant chemotherapy is part of the initial management of osteosarcoma treated with limb-sparing surgery (Gebhart et al., 1985; NIH Consensus Conference, 1985).

Sarcomas of soft tissue are treated with high-dose radiation and wide local excision with or without limb-sparing surgery (Lindberg, Fletcher, & Martin, 1975). Shrinking field radiation techniques and preservation of a nonradiated strip of tissue are currently employed to prevent lymphedema development. The addition of adjuvant chemotherapy in combination with radiation and surgery is controversial in management of soft tissue sarcoma (Benjamin, 1985).

The functional outcome of patients treated with soft tissue sarcoma and osteosarcoma has recently been studied. Comparison of the energy cost of ambulation in osteosarcoma patients treated by amputation was significantly greater than similar patients treated with limb salvage surgery (Otis, Lane, & Kroll, 1985). Functional assessment of patients with soft tissue sarcoma treated with wide excision and radiation indicated that lower extremity tumors had poorer functional outcome (ADL, mobility); more frequent lymphedema; and altered vocational, social, or educational status (Lampert et al., 1984) compared with patients treated with upper extremity, trunk, or head and neck tumors. Evaluation of patients with pelvic osteosarcoma treated with acetabular ring resection revealed that all had significant gait deviations and leg length discrepancies, requiring walking aids (Nilsonne, Kreicbergs, Olsson, & Stark, 1982). However, their gait was generally painless and one-half the patients could walk for significant distances. Patients with Ewing's sarcoma of the lower extremity treated with radiation and chemotherapy had variable functional results (i.e., frequency of contractures, muscle function, gait quality, etc.) depending on the radiation dose, tumor location (i.e., near growing epiphysis), patient age, and sparing a soft tissue strip from radiation (Jentzsch et al., 1981). Femoral lesions tended to have a less favorable functional outcome (significant pain, edema, weakness, shortening, contractures) compared with other tumor locations, in this study.

The indications for amputation in cancer patients are decreasing, but for treatment of nonfunctional limbs (tumor invasion of major blood supply or nerve), or tumors without an adequate surgical margin following limb-sparing surgery, amputation is still appropriate (NIH Consensus Conference, 1985). Patients treated by limb amputation for cancer tend to use a prosthesis as successfully as vascular amputees, if they survive the cancer (Subbarao & McPhee, 1982). However, only two-thirds of cancer patients treated with hemipelvectomy continued to use their prosthesis 1 year posttreatment (Sneppen, Heerfordt, Dissing, & Petersen, 1978). It has been suggested that successfully rehabilitated cancer amputee visitors may definitely contribute to the rehabilitation process of the patient (May, McPhee, & Pritchard, 1979).

Breast Cancer

Breast cancer is the most common cause of cancer and cancer death in women (Silverberg, 1985). The management of primary breast cancer has been significantly modified in our generation, as exemplified by newer surgical trends. The radical mastectomy has been replaced by less deforming operations for local control of tumor (Henderson & Canellos, 1980). Tumors less than 4 cm that are confined to one breast and ipsilateral axillary lymphatics may be treated by segmental mastectomy, axillary node dissection, breast irradiation, and chemotherapy for positive nodes (Fisher et al., 1985), or excisional biopsy, axillary staging, and primary breast irradiation (Ghossein, Stacey, & Alpert, 1976; Harris, Beadle, & Hellman, 1984); and adjuvant chemotherapy for positive nodes (Danoff, Goodman, Glick, et al., 1983). The evolution to lesser surgery and refined multimodal techniques has eliminated shoulder instability postmastectomy, has improved cosmesis (Beadle, Silver, Botnick, Hellman, & Harris, 1984; Clarke, Martines, & Cox, 1983; Danoff et al., 1983), and probably decreased the frequency of lymphedema. However, functional problems still exist following primary cancer treatment.

Patients treated by modified radical mastectomy for large tumors have decreased ipsilateral shoulder range of motion and decreased upper extremity function without postoperative rehabilitation (Wingate, 1985). Ipsilateral arm lymphedema has been noted in 12% of patients treated by lumpectomy, axillary dissection, and breast and lymphatic irradiation (Beadle et al., 1984). Addition of adjuvant chemotherapy following lumpectomy and breast/node irradiation in patients with regional lymph node disease produced ipsilateral arm lymphedema in 22% of patients (Danoff et al., 1983). Finally, deep venous thrombosis involving upper or lower extremities was observed in 5% of patients treated by mastectomy and adjuvant chemotherapy (Weiss, Tormey, Holland, & Weinberg, 1981).

Whether or not to initiate exercise of the ipsilateral shoulder immediately postoperatively has been debated in the surgical and rehabilitation literature. Reports that wound drainage and wound complications increased with early postsurgical arm immobilization fueled the controversy (Flew, 1979; Lotze, Duncan, Gerber, Woltering, & Rosenberg, 1980). Other studies demonstrated improved shoulder range of motion, improved arm function, and no delay in wound healing or radiation treatment in patients receiving an early postoperative arm exercise program (Pollard, Calhum, Altman, & Bates, 1976; Wingate, 1984). Further studies should be done to resolve this issue.

The development of lymphedema of the ipsilateral arm remains a significant complication of breast cancer and its treatment. Radiation therapy premastectomy or postmastectomy (Nikkanen, Vanharanta, & Helenius-Reunanen, 1978; Swedborg & Wallgreen, 1981), and radiation plus chemotherapy postlumpectomy and axillary dissection (Danoff et al., 1983) predisposes to lymphedema development. If lymphedema persists or progresses, treatment is only partially successful with resultant poor cosmesis, limited arm use, and secondary nerve entrapments (Ganel, 1979). A variety of treatments are used, including self-range-of-motion exercises, arm elevation, isometric hand grip exercise, intermittent external pneumatic compression, gradient pressure sleeves, and prompt antibiotic treatment of skin infection (Jungi, 1981; McNair, 1976; Zeissler, Rose, & Nelson, 1972).

Newer modalities include sympathetic blockade (Swedborg, Arner, & Meyerson, 1983); heat and bandage treatment (Ti-sheng et al., 1984); new intermittent pneumatic compression devices, including Lympha-Press (Zelikovski, Manoach, Giler, & Urca, 1980) and the Wright linear pump (Alexander, Wright, Wright, & Bikowski, 1983); and microlymphatic or lymphaticovenous anastomoses (Ho & Kennedy, 1983; O'Brien, Sykes, & Threlfall, 1983). Prior to treating lymphedema, lymphatic obstruction by recurrent tumor must be determined and antineoplastic treatment begun. Early lymphedema identification and successful treatment requires patient education in proper skin care (Zeissler et al., 1972) and edema recognition.

Breast reconstruction can be performed on patients treated by radical mastectomy, modified radical mastectomy (Bostwick, 1979), or lumpectomy and radiation (Pearl & Wisnicki, 1985). However, placement of the definitive surgical scar must be carefully planned preoperatively to achieve cosmetically acceptable results with plastic surgery. Breast retraction and poor cosmesis develop if the lumpectomy incision is not made parallel to skin lines (Clarke et al., 1983). In patients treated with radiation, the final result of breast reconstruction has not been consistently acceptable (Pearl & Wisnicki, 1985). However, in the patient who is cooperative, concerned with cosmesis, and tenacious, results from breast reconstruction are generally more acceptable than use of a breast prosthesis.

Head and Neck Cancer

New developments, detection methods, and surgical management have decreased the morbidity associated with head and neck cancer treatment (Jahn, 1985). Use of CT scan and MRI have greatly improved the evaluation of tumor extent and lymph node metastases. Early glottic cancer may be successfully treated by radiation alone (Harwood et al., 1980). Newer surgical techniques and multimodal treatments have decreased the number of total laryngectomies performed (Gates, Ryan, Cantue, & Hearne, 1982a; Gates, Ryan, Cooper, et al., 1982b; Weaver, 1978). Myocutaneous flap reconstruction has been used to reconstruct the mandible (Lam, Wei, & Siu, 1984), correct oral defects, and close fistulas (Bryce, 1981). However, life expectancy has not significantly changed for head and neck malignancies over the past several decades. Early referral and early diagnosis are the requirements for cure.

Treatment of head and neck malignancies may result in disfigurement, dysarthria, dysphagia, aspiration (Weaver & Fleming, 1978), altered taste (Chencharick & Mossman, 1983), limited cervical movement, and shoulder weakness. Newer surgical procedures developed to avoid or limit such complications include partial laryngectomy for amenable tumors (Weaver et al., 1978), epiglottic reconstruction procedures following supraglottic laryngectomy (Calcatera, 1985), and modified radical neck dissection sparing destruction of the spinal accessory nerve (Lingeman, Helmus, Stephens, & Ulm, 1977). Postsurgical teflon injection of paralyzed vocal cords (Woodson & Miller, 1981) has been advocated to improve voice and prevent aspiration. Cricopharyngeal myotomy following total glossectomy for advanced tongue cancer has prevented aspiration during swallowing (Effron et al., 1981). A palatal prosthesis to fill in palatal defects and lift or reshape the palate may be made from preoperative impressions and improves voice, prevents regurgitation, and assists in swallowing (Wurster, Krepsi, Davis, & Sisson, 1985). Posttreatment rehabilitation of head and neck cancer patients has been reviewed extensively (Dudgeon, DeLisa, & Miller, 1980; Villaneuva & Ajmani, 1977). Intensive cooperation between surgeon(s), radiation therapist, prosthodontist, and therapists is required in initial patient management (Wurster et al., 1985). Pretreatment baseline measurements of shoulder and cervical spine range of motion and neuromuscular function are helpful in planning future goals. Successful rehabilitation of deglutition is inversely related to the extent of surgery and the number of malfunctioning swallowing phases (Aguilar, Olson, & Shedd, 1979). Radiologic assessment of swallowing function is most beneficial in designing compensatory swallowing techniques (Redmond, Berkliner, Ambos, & Horowitz, 1982) or surgical intervention to aid the process (Effron et al., 1981). Barium cineradiographs of patients with pharyngeal cancer treated with radiation have demonstrated epiglottic dysfunction, delayed closure of the laryngeal vestibule, paresis of pharyngeal constrictors, and esophageal webs in certain patients (Ekberg & Nylander, 1983). Additionally, cineradiographs reveal that patients treated with total glossectomy for advanced tongue cancer may protect their airway when swallowing by glottic closure and adapted pharyngeal function (Effron et al., 1981).

Dysphagia and hypermetabolism secondary to cancer or surgical management often results in nutritional problems and weight loss. Radiation therapy, although impairing taste and salivation, does not result in additional weight loss (Chencharich et al., 1983). Nutritional problems must be identified and treated concomitant with a rehabilitation program.

Speech function is frequently affected in patients with head and neck cancer. Partial laryngectomy (hemilaryngectomy, subtotal supraglottic laryngectomy, and partial laryngopharyngectomy) used to treat resectable tumors does preserve the larynx but also affects voice quality and intelligibility. In one study 82% of patients reported speaking effectively in most situations with little effect on vocational activities (Klein, Wasserstrom, & McFerson, 1977). The vocal changes most frequently noted have been breathiness, harshness, and hoarseness; partial laryngopharyngectomy has affected intelligibility most severely. Total laryngectomy now is reserved for patients with more extensive laryngeal cancer, often combined with other forms of treatment. Compensatory vocalization following total laryngectomy may be achieved by esophageal speech. In this compensatory technique the patient learns to inject and trap air in the upper esophagus and erupt it back into the pharynx for use as voice (Dudgeon et al., 1980). Less than one-half of total laryngectomees achieve successful esophageal speech, probably because of the greater extent of disease in patients so treated (Gates et al., 1982b). Positive factors influencing successful achievement of esophageal speech include (1) the presence of a spouse as facilitator (Gibbs & Achterberg-Lawlis, 1979), (2) younger patient age (Dhillon, Palmer, Pittam, & Shaw, 1982), (3) less postoperative radiotherapy, and (4) dysphagia (Gates et al., 1982a). In appropriately selected total laryngectomees the tracheoesophageal puncture of Blom-Singer, to divert pulmonary air into the pharynx via a voice prosthesis, has rapidly restored voice without requiring prolonged speech rehabilitation (Pretsfelder, Izzo, & Mohr, 1985; Singer & Blom, 1980). External electrolarynxes are also used to facilitate speech, although the quality of voice produced is harsh. Spectral analysis of the voice quality and intelligibility produced by these devices should assist in future design (Rizer, Schechter, & Coleman, 1984).

The psychosocial effects of head and neck cancer treatment have been studied. Often, due to the diagnosis of cancer and the effects of treatment, patients make poor psychological adjustment (Harris, Vogtsberger, & Mattox, 1985; Johnson, Casper, & Lesswing, 1979). Interviews with patients and families of patients treated by total laryngectomy have indicated that inadequate information regarding effects of surgery was provided preoperatively (Johnson et al., 1979). In another study, patients treated with radiation and definitive surgery were more dependent on others than a similar group not treated with radiation (Schuller et al., 1983). Additionally, patients treated with modified neck dissection tended to socialize more than those with radical neck dissection. Only one-half of laryngectomees returned to full-time employment following treatment (Johnson et al., 1979). Group psychotherapy has proven effective in treating patients and their families as an adjunct to treatment of head and neck cancer (Harris et al., 1985). However, a large proportion of patients with depression in this group have underlying organic brain disease related to age and prior ethanol abuse (Adams, Larson, & Goepfert, 1984). It is recommended that all patients demonstrating a change in mental status, particularly following treatment, undergo a thorough neuropsychological evaluation to diagnose and treat degenerative brain disease.

CONCLUSION

The evaluation and management of some current functional problems encountered by cancer patients have been reviewed. Emphasis has been placed on areas that prompt a physiatric evaluation, such as weakness or bone lesions. The physiatrist usually is the first to define the patient's functional and psychosocial problems and direct an appropriate program of management via the cancer rehabilitation team. The physiatrist may suggest further diagnostic studies when appropriate, serve as intermediary to the clinical oncology and rehabilitation teams, and provide information regarding treatment effects and functional outcome.

Cancer treatment has markedly changed in the past 10 years, with new developments in radiation therapy, surgery, and chemotherapy demanding a team approach to patient management. So, too, cancer rehabilitation has evolved and requires a multidisciplinary team approach. General rehabilitation principles are used to treat cancer patients with a clear perspective of the prognosis for recovery or deterioration. Rehabilitation goals may require rapid modification, depending on treatment effects or disease progression. Unfortunately, few studies have scientifically examined the functional outcome of patients receiving comprehensive cancer rehabilitation. Further controlled studies to determine the efficacy and cost effectiveness of rehabilitating cancer patients are required.

REFERENCES

Adams, F., Larson, D. L., & Goepfert, H. (1984). Does the diagnosis of depression in head and neck cancer make organic brain disease? *Otolaryngology—Head and Neck Surgery, 92,* 618–624.

Aguilar, N. V., Olson, M. L., & Shedd, D. P. (1979). Rehabilitation of deglutition problems in patients with head and neck cancer. *American Journal of Surgery, 138,* 501–507.

Al-Mondhery, H. (1975). Disseminated intravascular coagulation: Experience in a major cancer center. *Thrombosis et Diathesis Haemorrhaigica, 34,* 181–193.

Albright, J., Gillespie, T. E., & Butaud, T. R. (1980). Treatment of bone metastases. *Seminars in Oncology, 7,* 418–434.

Alexander, M. A., Wright, E. S., Wright, J. B., & Bikowski, J. B. (1983). Lymphedema treated with a linear pump: Pediatric case report. *Archives of Physical Medicine and Rehabilitation, 64,* 132–133.

Allen, K. L., Johnson, T. W., & Hibbs, G. G. (1976). Effective bone palliation as related to various treatment regimens. *Cancer, 37,* 984–987.

Ambrad, A. J. (1978). Single-dose and short, high-dose fractionation radiation therapy for osseous metastases (Abstract). *International Journal of Radiation, Oncology, Biology, Physics, 4,* 207–208.

American Cancer Society, Ohio Division (1985). Survey of physician's attitudes and practices in early cancer detection. *Cancer, 35,* 197–213.

Annegers, J. F., Schoenberg, B. S., Okazaki, H., & Kurland, L. T. (1981). Epidemiologic study of primary intracranial neoplasms. *Archives of Neurology, 38,* 217–219.

Argov, Z., & Siegal, T. (1985). Leptomeningeal metastases: Peripheral nerve and root involvement—clinical and electrophysiologic study. *Annals of Neurology, 17,* 593–596.

Asbury, A. K. (1980). The clinical view of neuromuscular electrophysiology. In A. J. Sumner (Ed.), *The physiology of peripheral nerve disease* (pp. 484–491). Philadelphia: Saunders.

Askari, A., Vignos, P. J., & Moskowitz, R. W. (1976). Steroid myopathy in connective tissue disease. *American Journal of Medicine, 61*, 485–491.

Barnes, B. E. (1976). Dematomyositis and malignancy. A review of the literature. *Annals of Internal Medicine, 84*, 68–76.

Baum, E. S., Koch, H. F., Gorby, D. G., & Plunket, D. C. (1971). Intrathecal methotrexate. *Lancet, 1*, 649.

Beadle, G. F., Silver, B., Botnick, L., Hellman, S., & Harris, J. R. (1984). Cosmetic results following primary radiation therapy for early breast cancer. *Cancer,* 2911–2918.

Benjamin, B. S. (1985). Limb salvage surgery for sarcoma: A good idea receives formal blessing. *Journal of American Medical Association, 245*, 1765–1766.

Bennett, A., McDonald, A. M., Stamford, I. F., Charlier, E. M., Simpson, J. S., & Zebro, T. (1977). Prostaglandins and breast cancer. *Lancet, 2*, 624–626.

Berger, P. S., & Bataini, J. P. (1977). Radiation-induced cranial nerve palsy. *Cancer, 40*, 152–155.

Bleyer, W. A., Drake, J. C., & Chabner, B. A. (1973). Neurotoxicity and elevated cerebrospinal fluid methotrexate concentration in meningeal leukemia. *New England Journal of Medicine, 289*, 770–773.

Bleyer, W. A., & Griffin, T. W. (1980). White matter necrosis, mineralizing microangiopathy and intellectual abilities in survivors of childhood leukemia: Associations in central nervous system irradiation and methotrexate therapy. In H. A. Gilbert & A. R. Kagan (Eds.), *Radiation damage to the central nervous system* (pp. 155–174). New York: Raven Press.

Booth, F. W., & Gollnick, P. D. (1983). Effects of disease on the structure and function of skeletal muscle. *Medicine and Science in Sports Exercise, 15*, 415–420.

Bostwick, J. (1979). Breast reconstruction: A comprehensive approach. *Clinical Plastic Surgery, 6*, 143–162.

Bradley, W. G. (1984). Diseases of the spinal roots. In P. J. Dyck, P. K. Thoma, E. M. Lampert, & R. Bunge (Eds.), *Peripheral neuropathy* (pp. 1368–1382). Philadelphia: Saunders.

Brady, L. W., & Croll, M. N. (1979). The role of bone scanning in the cancer patient. *Skeletal Radiology, 3*, 217–222.

Brain, L., & Wilkinson, M. (1965). Subacute cerebellar degeneration associated with neoplasms. *Brain, 88*, 465–478.

Bryce, D. P. (1981). Unique features of head and neck malignancies which relate to their management. *Journal of Otolaryngology, 10*, 3–9.

Bunn, P. A., & Minna, J. D. (1985). In V. T. DeVita, S. Hellman, & S. A. Rosenberg (Eds.), *Cancer principles and practice of oncology* (pp. 1797–1842). Philadelphia: Lippincott.

Bunting, R., Lamont-Havers, W., Schweon, D., & Kliman, A. (1985). Pathologic fracture risk in rehabilitation of patients with boney metastases. *Clinical Orthopaedics and Related Research, 192*, 222–227.

Burke, J., & Griffiths, H. (1983). Pathologic fracture of the femoral neck with multiple intramedullary metastases in the shaft of the femur. *Orthopedics, 6*, 1484–1487.

Caccia, M. R., Comoti, B., Ubiali, E., & Lucchetti, A. (1977). Vincristine polyneuropathy in man. A clinical and electrophysiological study. *Journal Neurology, 216*, 21–26.

Calcatera, T. C. (1985). Epiglottic reconstruction after supraglottic laryngectomy. *Laryngoscope*, *95*, 786–789.

Campbell, M. J., & Paty, D. W. (1974). Carcinomatous neuromyopathy: I. Electrophysiological studies. *Journal of Neurology, Neurosurgery and Psychiatry*, *37*, 131–141.

Cassady, J. R., Tonnesen, G. L., & Wolfe, L. C. (1980). Augmentation of vincristine neurotoxicity by irradiation of peripheral nerves. *Cancer Treatment Reports*, *64*, 963–965.

Chan, S. Y., Worth, R., & Ochs, S. (1980). Block of axoplasmic transport in vitro by *Vinca* alkaloids. *Journal of Neurobiology*, *11*, 251–264.

Chang, S. K., & Hawes, K. A. (1983). The adequacy of the Karnofsky Rating and Global Adjustment to Illness Scale as outcome measures in cancer rehabilitation and continuity care. In P. Engstrom, P. N. Anderson & L. E. Mortenson (Eds.), *Advances in cancer control: Research and development* (429–443). New York: Alan R. Liss.

Chencharick, J. D., & Mossman, K. L. (1983). Nutritional consequences of the radiotherapy of head and neck cancer. *Cancer*, *51*, 811–815.

Chernick, N. L., Armstrong, D., & Posner, J. B. (1977). Central nervous system infections in patients with cancer. *Cancer*, *40*, 268–274.

Clarke, D., Martines, A., & Cox, R. S. (1983). Analysis of cosmetic results and complications in patients with stage I and II breast cancer treated by biopsy and irradiation. *International Journal of Radiation, Oncology, Biology, Physics*, *9*, 1807–1813.

Constans, J. P., DeVitiis, W., Donzelli, R., Spaziante, R., Meder, J. F., & Haye, C. (1983). Spinal metastases with neurologic manifestations. Review of 600 cases. *Journal of Neurosurgery*, *59*, 111–118.

Convertino, V., Hung, J., Goldwater, D., & DeBusk, R. F. (1982). Cardiovascular responses to exercise in middle-aged men after ten days of bedrest. *Circulation*, *65*, 134–140.

Corbett, J. J., & Newman, N. M. (1981). Symptomatic leptomeningeal metastases preceding other manifestations of occult primary brain tumors. *Surgical Neurology*, *15*, 362–367.

Croft, P. B., & Wilkinson, M. (1969). The course and prognosis in some types of carcinomatous neuromyopathy. *Brain*, *92*, 1–8.

Croft, P. B., Urich, H., & Wilkinson, M. (1967). Peripheral neuropathy of sensorimotor type associated with malignant disease. *Brain*, *90*, 31–66.

Croft, P. B., & Wilkinson, M. (1965). The incidence of carcinomatous neuromyopathy in patients with various types of carcinoma. *Brain*, *88*, 427–434.

Currie, S., Henson, R. A., Morgan, H. G., & Poole, A. J. (1970). The incidence of the non-metastatic neurological syndromes of obscure origin in the reticuloses. *Brain*, *93*, 629–640.

Danoff, B. F., Goodman, R. L., Glick, J. H., et al. (1983). The effect of adjuvant chemotherapy on cosmesis and complications in patients with breast cancer treated by definitive irradiation. *International Journal of Radiation, Oncology, Biology, Physics*, *9*, 1625–1630.

Debusk, R. F., Convertino, V. A., Hung, J., & Goldwater, D. (1983). Exercise conditioning in middle-aged men after ten days of bed rest. *Circulation*, *68*, 245–250.

DeLisa, J. A., Miller, R. M., & Melnick, R. R. (1985). Rehabilitation of the cancer patient. In V. DeVita, S. Hellman, & S. A. Rosenberg (Eds.), *Cancer principles and practices of oncology* (pp. 2155–2188). Philadelphia: Lippincott.

DeLorme, T. L., Schwab, R. S., & Watkins, A. L. (1948). The response of the quadriceps femoris to progressive-resistance exercises in poliomyelitis patients. *Journal of Bone and Joint Surgery, 30,* 834–847.

Derogatis, L. R., Rickels, K., & Rock, A. F. (1976). The SCL-90 and the MMPI: A step in the validation of a new self-report scale. *British Journal of Psychiatry, 128,* 280–289.

Dhillon, R. S., Palmer, B. V., Pittam, M. R., & Shaw, H. J. (1982). Rehabilitation after major head and neck surgery—The patient's view. *Clinical Otolaryngology, 7,* 319–324.

Dietz, J. H. (1981). *Rehabilitation Oncology.* New York: Wiley.

Dobozi, W. R., Dvonch, V. M., & Saltzman, M. L. (1984). Treatment of impending pathologic fractures of the femur with flexible intramedullary nails. *Orthopedics, 7,* 1682–1688.

Donuso, A. J., Green, L. S., Heller-Bettinger, I. W., & Samson, F. E. (1977). Action of the *Vinca* alkaloids vincristine, vinblastine, and desacetyl vinblastine amide on axonal fiber organelles in vitro. *Cancer Research, 37,* 1401–1407.

Doshi, R., & Fowler, T. (1983). Proximal myopathy due to discrete carcinomatous metastases in muscle. *Journal of Neurology, Neurosurgery and Psychiatry, 46,* 358–360.

Driedger, H., & Pruzanski, W. (1980). Plasma cell neoplasia with peripheral polyneuropathy. *Medicine, 59,* 301–310.

DuBois, D. C., & Almon, R. E. (1980). Disuse atrophy of skeletal muscle is associated with an increase in number of glucocorticoid receptors. *Endocrinology, 107,* 1649–1651.

Dudgeon, B. J., DeLisa, J. A., & Miller, R. M. (1980). Head and neck cancer, a rehabilitation approach. *American Journal of Occupational Therapy, 34,* 243–251.

Eagan, R. T., Dinapoli, R. P., Hermann, R. C., Groger, R. V., & Layton, D. D. Jr. (1983). Preliminary communication-treatment of primary brain tumors recurrent after irradiation with aziridinylbenzoquinone (AZQ; NSC-182986). *American Journal of Clinical Oncology, 6,* 577–578.

Eagan, R. T., Dinapoli, R. P., & Hermann, R. C. (1984). Chemotherapy for primary brain tumors progressive after radiation and chemotherapy. *Cancer Treatment Reports, 68,* 431–433.

Eccles, J. C. (1944). Investigations on muscle atrophies arising from disease and tonotomy. *Journal of Physiology, 103,* 253–266.

Effron, M. Z., Johnson, J. T., Myers, E. N., Curtin, H., Beery, Q., & Sigler, B. (1981). Advanced carcinoma of the tongue management by total glossectomy without laryngectomy. *Archives of Otolaryngology, 107,* 694–697.

Ekberg, O., & Nylander, G. (1983). Pharyngeal dysfunction after treatment for pharyngeal cancer with surgery and radiotherapy. *Gastrointestinal Radiology, 8,* 97–104.

Falkson, G., Van Dyk, J. J., Van Eden, E. B., van der Merwe, A. M., Van Den Bergh, J. A., & Falkson, H. C. (1975). A clinical trial of the oral form of 4-'-dimethyl-epipodophyllotoxin-B-Dethylidene glucoside (NSC 141540). VP/-6-21, *Cancer, 35,* 1141–1144.

Fidler, M. (1981). Incidence of fracture through metastases in long bones. *Acta Orthopaedica Scandinavica, 52,* 623–627.

Fisher, B., Bauer, M., Margolese, R., Poisson, R., Pilch, Y., Redmond, C., Fisher, E., Wolmark, N., Deutsch, M., & Montague, E. (1985). Five-year results of a randomized clinical trial comparing total mastectomy and segmental mastectomy with or without radiation in the treatment of breast cancer. *New England Journal of Medicine, 312,* 665–672.

Flew, T. J. (1979). Wound drainage following radical mastectomy: The effect of restriction of shoulder movement. *British Journal of Surgery, 66*, 302–305.

Forer, S. K., & Miller, L. S. (1980). Rehabilitation outcome: Comparative analysis of different patient types. *Archives of Physical Medicine Rehabilitation, 61*, 359–365.

Fornasier, V. L., & Horne, J. G. (1975). Metastases to the vertebral column. *Cancer, 36*, 590–594.

Ganel, A., Engel, J., Sela, M., & Brooks, M. (1979). Nerve entrapments associated with post-mastectomy lymphedema. *Cancer, 44*, 2254–2259.

Gates, G. A., Ryan, W., Cantue, E., & Hearne, E. (1982a). Current status of laryngectomee rehabilitation: II. Causes of failure. *American Journal of Otolaryngology, 3*, 8–14.

Gates, G. A., Ryan, W., Cooper, J. C., Lawlis, G. F., Cantue, E., Hayashi, T., Lauder, E., Welch, R. W., & Hearne, E. (1982b). Current status of laryngectomee rehabilitation: I. Results of therapy. *American Journal of Otolaryngology, 3*, 1–7.

Gebhart, M. J., Lane, J. M., & McCormack, R. R. (1985). Limb salvage in bone sarcomas—Memorial Hospital experience. *Orthopedics, 8*, 626–635.

Gelber, R. D., Larson, M., Borgelt, B. B., & Kramer, S. (1981). Equivalence of radiation schedules for the palliative treatment of brain metastases in patients with favorable prognosis. *Cancer, 48*, 1749–1753.

Ghossein, N. A., Stacey, P., & Alpert, S. (1976). Local control of breast cancer with tumorectomy plus radiotherapy or radiotherapy alone. *Radiology, 121*, 455–459.

Gibbs, H. W., & Achterberg-Lawlis, J. (1979). The spouse as facilitator for esophageal speech: A research perspective. *Journal of Surgical Oncology, 11*, 89–94.

Gilbert, H., Apuzzo, M., Marshall, L., Kagan, A. R., Crue, B., Wagner, J., Fuchs, K., Rush, J., Rao, A., Nussbaum, H., & Chan, P. (1978). Neoplastic epidural spinal cord compression. A current perspective. *Journal of American Medical Association, 240*, 2771–2773.

Goldberg, R. T. (1975). Vocational and social adjustment after laryngectomy. *Scandinavian Journal of Rehabilitation Medicine, 7*, 1–8.

Graus, F., Ferrer, I., & Lamarca, J. (1983). Mixed carcinomatous neuropathy in patients with lung cancer and lymphoma. *Acta Neurology Scandinavica, 68*, 40–48.

Griffin, J. W., Thompson, R. W., Mitchinson, M. J., De Kiewiet, J. C., & Welland, F. H. (1971). Lymphomatous leptomeningitis. *American Journal of Medicine, 51*, 200–208.

Gutin, P. H., Phillips, T. L., Wara, W. M., Leibel, S. A., Hosobuchi, Y., Levin, V. A., Weaver, K. A., & Lamb, S. (1984). Brachytherapy of recurrent malignant brain tumors with removable high activity iodine—125 sources. *Journal of Neurosurgery, 60*, 61–68.

Hall, S. M., Buzdar, A. U., & Blumenschein, G. R. (1983). Cranial nerve palsies in metastatic breast cancer due to osseus metastasis without intracranial involvement. *Cancer, 52*, 180–184.

Harris, J. R., Beadle, G. F., & Hellman, S. (1984). Clinical studies on the use of radiation therapy as primary treatment of early breast cancer. *Cancer*, 705–711.

Harris, L. L., Vogtsberger, K. N., & Mattox, D. E. (1985). Group psychotherapy for head and neck cancer patients. *Laryngoscope, 95*, 585–587.

Harvey, R. F., Jellinek, H. M., & Habeck, R. V. (1982). Cancer rehabilitation. An analysis of program approaches. *Journal of American Medical Association, 247,* 2127-2131.

Harwood, A. R., Hawkins, N. V., Keane, T., Cummings, B., Beale, F. A., Rider, W. D., & Bryce, D. P. (1980). Radiotherapy of early glottic cancer. *Laryngoscope, 90,* 465-470.

Hawley, R. J., Cohen, M. H., Saini, N., & Armbrustmacher, V. W. (1980). The carcinomatous neuromyopathy of oat cell lung cancer. *Annals of Neurology, 7,* 65-72.

Heinrich, R. L., & Schag, C. C. (1984). Living with cancer: The cancer inventory of problem situations. *Journal of Clinical Psychology, 40,* 972-980.

Helms, C. A., & Genant, H. K. (1982). Computed tomography in the early detection of skeletal involvement with multiple myeloma. *Journal of American Medical Association, 248,* 2886-2887.

Helms, C. A., Moon, K. L., & Genant, H. K. (1984). Magnetic resonance imaging. Skeletal applications. *Orthopedics, 7,* 1429-1435.

Henderson, I. C., & Canellos, G. P. (1980). Cancer of the breast the past decade (Part II). *New England Journal of Medicine, 302,* 17-88.

Henricksson, J., & Reitman, J. S. (1977). Time course of changes in human skeletal muscle succinate dehydroginase and cytochrome oxidase activities and maximal oxygen uptake with physical activity and inactivity. *Acta Physiologica Scandinavica, 99,* 91-97.

Herbison, G., Jaweed, M. M., & Ditunno, J. F. (1983). Exercise therapies in peripheral neuropathies. *Archives of Physical Medicine and Rehabilitation, 64,* 201-205.

Hettinger, T. (1955). Untersuchungen zur bestimmung der muskelatrophieschwelle. *Internationale Zeitschrift fur Angewandte Physiologie Einschliesslich Arbeitsphysiologie, 16,* 52-56.

Hettinger, T. (1960). Das verhalten der kraft eines trainierten muskels wahrend und nach mehrtagiger ruhestellung. *Internationale Zeitschrift fur Angewandte Physiologie Einschliesslich Arbeitsphysiologie, 18,* 357-360.

Ho, L. C., & Kennedy, P. J. (1983). Micro-lymphatic bypass in the treatment of obstructive lymphoedema of the arm: Case report of a new technique. *British Journal of Plastic Surgery, 36,* 350-357.

Hogan-Dann, C. M., Fellmeth, W. G., McGuire, S. A., & Kiley, V. A. (1984). Polyneuropathy following vincristine therapy in two patients with Charcot-Marie-Tooth syndrome. *Journal of American Medical Association, 252,* 2862-2863.

Holland, J. F., Scharlau, C., Gailani, S., Krant, N. J., Olson, K. B., Horton, J., Shnidr, B. I., Lynch, J. J., Owens, A., Carbone, P. P., Colsky, J., Grob, D., Miller, S. P., & Hall, T. C. (1973). Vincristine treatment of advanced cancer: A cooperative study of 392 cases. *Cancer Research, 33,* 1258-1264.

Horber, F. F., Scheidegger, J. R., Grunig, B. E., & Frey, F. J. (1985). Evidence that prednisone-induced myopathy is reversed by physical training. *Journal of Clinical Endocrinology and Metabolism, 61,* 83-88.

Horton, J. E., Raisz, L. G., Simmons, H. A., Oppenheim, J. J., & Mergenhagen, S. E. (1972). Bone resorbing activity in supernatant fluid from cultured peripheral leukocytes. *Science, 177,* 793.

Horwich, M. S., Cho, L., & Porro, R. S. (1977). Subacute sensory neuropathy: A remote effect of carcinoma. *Annals of Neurology, 2,* 7-19.

Jaeckle, K. A., Young, D. F., & Foley, K. M. (1985). The natural history of lumbosacral plexopathy in cancer. *Neurology, 35,* 8-15.

Jahn, A. F. (1985). Head and neck cancer—A changing disease. *Oncology Times,* *10,* 2.

Jameson, R. M. (1983). Paraplegic and prostatic cancer. *European Urology, 9,* 267–269.

Jentzsch, K., Binder, H., Craner, H., Glaubiger, D. L., Kessler, R. M., Bull, C., Pomeroy, T. C., & Gerber, N. L. (1981). Leg function after radiotherapy for Ewing's sarcoma. *Cancer, 47,* 1267–1278.

Johnson, P. C. (1977). Hematogenous metastases of carcinoma to dorsal root ganglia. *Acta Neuropathologica, 38,* 171–172.

Johnson, J. T., Casper, J., & Lesswing, N. J. (1979). Toward the total rehabilitation of the alaryngeal patient. *Laryngoscope, 89,* 1813–1819.

Johnston, A. D. (1970). Pathology of metastatic tumors in bone. *Clinical Orthopaedics and Related Research, 73,* 8–32.

Johnston, J., Harries, T. J., & Alexander, C. E. (1983). Limb salvage procedure for neoplasms about the knee by spherocentric total knee arthroplasty and autogenous autoclaved bone grafting. *Clinical Orthopaedics and Related Research, 181,* 137–145.

Jortner, B. S., & Cho, E. S. (1980). Neurotoxicity of adriamycin in rats: A low-dose effect. *Cancer Treatment Reports, 64,* 257–261.

Jungi, W. H. (1981). The prevention and management of lymphedema after treatment for breast cancer. *International Rehabilitation Medicine, 3,* 129–134.

Kaheeli, A. A., Edwards, R. H., & Gohil, K. (1983). Corticosteroid myopathy: A clinical and pathological study. *Clinical Endocrinology, 18,* 155–166.

Kalyanaraman, U. P., Kalyanaraman, K., Cullenan, S. A., & McLean, J. M. (1983). Neuromyopathy of cyanide intoxication due to "Laetrile" (amygdalin). A clinicopathologic study. *Cancer, 51,* 2126–2133.

Kaplan, R. S., & Wiermik, P. H. (1984). Neurotoxicity of antitumor agents. In M. C. Perry & J. W. Yarbro (Eds.), *Toxicity of chemotherapy* (pp. 365–431). Florida: Grune & Stratton.

Karnofsky, D. A., & Burchenal, J. H. (1949). The clinical evaluation of chemotherapeutic agents in cancer. In C. M. Macleod (Ed.), *Evaluation of chemotherapeutic agents* (pp. 199–205). New York: Columbia University Press.

Katzelson, A., & Nerubay, J. (1980). Total femur replacement in sarcoma of the distal end of the femur. *Acta Orthopaedica Scandinavica, 51,* 845–851.

Kedar, A., Cohen, M. E., & Freeman, A. I. (1978). Peripheral neuropathy as a complication of cis-dichlorodiamineplatinum (11) treatment: A case report. *Cancer Treatment, 62,* 819–821.

Kelly, J. J., Kyle, R. A., Miles, J. M., & Dyck, P. J. (1983). Osteosclerotic myeloma and peripheral neuropathy. *Neurology, 33,* 202–210.

Kelly, J. J., Kyle, R. A., Miles, J. M., O'Brien, P. C., & Dyck, P. J. (1981). The spectrum of peripheral neuropathy in myeloma. *Neurology, 31,* 24–31.

Klein, A. D., Wasserstrom, D. G., & McFerson, R. (1977). Rehabilitation of partial laryngectomy patients. *Transactions of American Academy of Ophthalmology and Otolaryngology, 84,* 324–335.

Klein, H. J., Richter, H. R., & Schafer, M. (1984). Extradural spinal metastases—A retrospective study of 197 patients. *Advances in Neurosurgery, 17,* 35–43.

Kline, L. B., Garcia, J. H., & Harsh, G. R. (1984). Lymphomatous optic neuropathy. *Archives of Ophthalmology, 102,* 1655–1657.

Kori, S. H., Foley, K. M., & Posner, J. B. (1981). Brachial plexus lesions in patients with cancer: 100 cases. *Neurology, 31,* 45–50.

Kristensen, J. H., Hanser, T. I., & Saltin, B. (1980). Cross-sectional and fiber size changes in the quadriceps muscle of man with immobilization and physical training. *Muscle Nerve, 3,* 275–276.

LaBan, M. M., Meerschaert, J. R., & Taylor, R. S. (1982). Electromyographic evidence of inferior gluteal nerve compromise: An early representation of recurrent colorectal carcinoma. *Archives of Physical Medicine and Rehabilitation, 63,* 33–35.

Lam, K. H., Wei, W. I., & Siu, K. F. (1984). The pectoralis major costomyocutaneous flap for mandibular reconstruction. *Plastic Reconstructive Surgery, 73,* 904–910.

Lambert, E. H., & Rooke, E. D. (1965). Myasthenic state and lung cancer. In W. Brain & F. H. Norris (Eds.), *The remote effects of cancer in the nervous system* (pp. 67–80). New York: Grune & Stratton.

Lambert, P. M. (1978). Radiation myelopathy of the thoracic spinal cord in long-term survivors treated with radical radiotherapy using conventional fractionation. *Cancer, 41,* 1751–1760.

Lampert, M. H., Gerber, L. H., Glatstein, E., Rosenberg, S. A., & Danoff, J. V. (1984). Soft tissue sarcoma: Functional outcome after wide local excision and radiation therapy. *Archives of Physical Medicine and Rehabilitation, 65,* 477–480.

Latov, N., Sherman, W. H., Nemni, R., Galassi, G., Shyonos, J. S., Penn, A. S., Chess, L., Olarte, M. N., Roland, L. P., & Osserman, E. F. (1980). Plasma-cell dyscrasia and peripheral neuropathy with a monoclonal antibody to peripheral-nerve myelin. *New England Journal of Medicine, 303,* 618–621.

Lederman, R. J., & Wilbourn, A. J. (1984). Brachial plexopathy: Recurrent cancer or radiation? *Neurology, 34,* 1331–1335.

Lehman, J. F., DeLisa, J. A., & Warren, C. G. (1978). Cancer rehabilitation: Assessment of need, development, and evaluation of a model of care. *Archives of Physical Medicine and Rehabilitation, 59,* 410–419.

Lenman, J. A. (1959). Clinical and experimental study of effects of exercise on motor weakness in neurological disease. *Journal Neurology, Neurosurgery, and Psychiatry, 22,* 182–194.

Levitt, L. J., Dawson, D. M., Rosenthal, D. S., & Moloney, W. C. (1980). CNS involvement in the non-Hodgkin's lymphomas. *Cancer, 45,* 545–552.

Levitt, L. P., & Prager, D. (1975). Mononeuropathy due to vincristine. *Neurology, 25,* 894–895.

Lindberg, R. D., Fletcher, G. H., & Martin, R. G. (1975). Management of soft tissue sarcomas in adults: Surgery and post operative radiotherapy. *Journal de Radiologie, D'Electrologie et de Medecine Nucleaire, 56,* 761–767.

Lingeman, R. E., Helmus, C., Stephens, R., & Ulm, J. (1977). Neck dissection: Radical or conservative. *Annals of Otology, 86,* 737–744.

Lisak, R. P., Mitchell, M., Sweiman, B., Orrechio, E., & Asbury, A. K. (1977). Guillain-Barré Syndrome and Hodgkin's disease. Three cases with immunological studies. *Annals of Neurology, 1,* 72–78.

Lotze, M. T., Duncan, M. A., Gerber, L. H., Woltering, E. A., & Rosenberg, S. A. (1980). Early versus delayed shoulder motion following axillary dissection. A randomized prospective study. *Annals of Surgery,* 288–295.

MacDougall, J. A., Ward, G. R., Sale, D. G., & Sutton, J. R. (1977). Biochemical adaptation of human skeletal muscle to heavy resistance training and immobilization. *Journal of Applied Physiology, 43,* 700–703.

Madsen, E. L. (1983). Painful bone metastases: Efficacy of radiotherapy assigned by the patients: A randomized trial comparing 4 Gy × 6 versus 10 Gy × 2. *International Journal of Radiology, Oncology, Biology, Physics, 9,* 1775–1779.

Mandel, S. (1982). Steroid myopathy insidious cause of muscle weakness. *Postgraduate Medicine, 72*, 207–215.

Manz, E. W., Moore, J., & Schold, S. C. (1981). Mental neuropathy from systemic cancer. *Neurology, 31*, 1277–1281.

Markesbery, W. R., Brooks, W. H., & Gupta, G. D. (1978). Treatment for patients with cerebral metastases. *Archives of Neurology, 35*, 754–756.

Massy, H. J. (1982). Neuropathology of systemic malignant neoplasia. In H. L. Ioachim (Ed.), *Pathobiology Annual* (Vol. 12, pp. 233–265). New York: Raven Press.

May, C. H., McPhee, M. C., & Pritchard, D. J. (1979). An amputee visitor program as an adjunct to rehabilitation of the lower limb amputee. *Mayo Clinic Proceedings, 54*, 774–778.

Mayer, N. H. (1976). Physical rehabilitation. In A. Sutnick & P. F. Engstrom (Eds.), *Oncologic medicine—clinical topics and practical management* (pp. 59–90). Baltimore, MD: University Park Press.

McLendon, R. E., Robinson, J. S., Chambers, D. B., Grufferman, S., & Burger, P. C. (1985). The glioblastoma multiforme in Georgia. *Cancer, 56*, 894–897.

McLeod, J. C. (1984). Carcinomatous neuropathy. In P. J. Dyck, P. K. Thomas, E. H. Lampert, & R. Bunge (Eds.), *Peripheral neuropathy* (pp. 2180–2191). Philadelphia: Saunders.

McLoughlin, W. J. (1984). Cancer rehabilitation: People investing in people. *Hospital Practice, 19*, 177–183.

McNair, T. J. (1976). Intermittent compression for lymphedema of the arm. *Clinical Oncology, 2*, 339–342.

Min, K., Gyorkey, F., & Sato, C. (1980). Mucin-producing adenocarcinomous and nonbacterial thrombotic endocarditis. Pathogenetic role of tumor mucin. *Cancer, 45*, 2374–2382.

Moehring, H. D. (1984). Closed flexible intramedullary fixation for pathologic lesions in long bones. *Orthopedics, 7*, 829–834.

Morris, J. G., & Joffe, R. (1983). Perineural spread of cutaneous basal and squamous cell carcinomas. The clinical appearance of spread into the trigemenal and facial nerves. *Archives of Neurology, 40*, 424–429.

Muller, E. A. (1970). Influence of training and of inactivity on muscle strength. *Archives of Physical Medicine and Rehabilitation, 50*, 449–462.

Murray, J. A., Sutow, W. W., & Martin, R. G. (1982). Bone and cartilage tumors. In J. F. Holland & E. Frei (Eds.), *Cancer medicine* (pp. 2159–2179). Philadelphia: Lea & Febiger.

Narakas, A. O. (1985). The treatment of brachial plexus injuries. *International Orthopedics, 9*, 29–36.

Neuwelt, E. A. (1983). Successful treatment of primary central nervous system lymphomas with chemotherapy after osmotic blood-brain barrier opening. *Neurosurgery, 12*, 662–671.

NIH Consensus Conference (1985). Limb-sparing treatment of adults with soft tissue sarcomas and osteosarcomas. *Journal of the American Medical Association, 254*, 1791–1796.

Nikkanen, T. A., Vanharanta, H., & Helenius-Reunanen, H. (1978). Swelling of the upper extremity function and muscle strength of shoulder joint following mastectomy combined with radiotherapy. *Annals of Clinical Research, 10*, 273–279.

Nilsonne, U., Kreicbergs, A., Olsson, E., & Stark, A. (1982). Function after pelvic tumour resection involving the acetabular ring. *International Orthopedics, 6*, 27–33.

Norris, F. H., McMenemey, W. H., & Barnard, R. O. (1984). Anterior horn pathology in carcinomatous neuromyopathy compared with other forms of motor neuron disease. In F. H. Norris & L. T.1 Kurland (Eds.), *Motor neuron diseases: Research on amyotrophic lateral sclerosis and related disorders* (pp. 1525–1533). New York: Grune & Stratton.

O'Brien, B., Sykes, P. J., & Threlfall, G. N. (1983). Microlymphaticovenous anastomoses for obstructive lymphedema. *Journal of Microsurgery, 3*, 197–211.

Ohi, T., Kyle, R. A., & Dyck, P. J. (1985). Axonal attenuation and secondary segmental demyelination in myeloma neuropathies. *Annals of Neurology, 17*, 255–261.

Ojeda, V. J. (1982). Necrotizing myopathy associated with steroid therapy. Report of two cases. *Pathology, 14*, 435–438.

Ojeda, V. J. (1984). Necrotizing myelopathy associated with malignancy. A clinopathologic study of two cases and literature review. *Cancer, 53*, 1115–1123.

Oliverio, V. T., Denham, D. C., & DeVita, D. T. (1964). Some pharmacologic properties of a new antitumor agent, N-isopropyl-(2-methyl-hydrazino)-P-tolusmide hydrochloride (NSC-77213). *Cancer Chemotherapy Reports, 42*, 1–7.

Ongerboer deVisser, B. W., Schimsheimer, R. J., & Hart, A. M. (1984). The H-reflex of the flexor carpi radialis muscle. A study in controls and radiation-induced brachial plexus lesions. *Journal of Neurology, Neurosurgery, and Psychiatry, 47*, 1098–1101.

Ongerboer deVisser, B. W., Van der Saude, J. J., & Kemp, B. (1982). Ulnar F-wave conduction velocity in epidural metastatic root lesions. *Annals of Neurology, 11*, 142–146.

Ostertag, C. B., Mennel, H. D., & Kiessling, M. (1980). Sterotactic biopsy of brain tumors. *Surgical Neurology, 14*, 275–283.

Otis, J. C., Lane, J. M., & Kroll, M. A. (1985). Energy cost during gait in osteosarcoma patients after resection and knee replacement and after above the knee amputation. *Journal of Bone and Joint Surgery, 67-A*, 606–611.

Page, H. S., & Ardyce, A. J. (1985). *Cancer rates and risks* (NIH Publication No. 85-691). Bethesda, MD: U. S. Department of Health and Human Services.

Paul, T., Katiyar, B. C., Musra, S., & Pant, G. C. (1978). Carcinomatous neuromuscular syndromes. A clinical and quantitative electrophysiological study. *Brain, 101*, 53–63.

Pearl, R. M., & Wisnicki, J. (1985). Breast reconstruction following lumpectomy and irradiation. *Plastic and Reconstructive Surgery, 76*, 83–86.

Pearson, C. M. (1959). Incidence and type of pathological alterations observed in muscle in a routine muscle autopsy survey. *Neurology, 9*, 757–766.

Pearson, C. M., & Bohan, A. (1977). The spectrum of polymyositis and dermatomyositis. *Medical Clinics of North America, 61*, 439–457.

Peters, W. A., Andersen, W. A., & Thornton, W. N. (1983). Dermatomyositis and coexisting ovarian cancer: A review of the compounding clinical problems. *Gynecologic Oncology, 15*, 440–446.

Pettigrew, L. C., Glass, P., Moor, M., & Zornoza, J. (1984). Diagnosis and treatment of lumbosacral plexopathies in patients with cancer. *Archives of Neurology, 41*, 1282–1285.

Peylan-Ramu, N., Poplach, D. G., Pizzo, P. A., Adornato, B. D., & Di Chiro, G. (1978). Abnormal CT scans of the brain in asymptomatic children with acute lymphocytic leukemia after prophylactic treatment of the central nervous system with radiation and intrathecal chemotherapy. *New England Journal of Medicine, 298*, 815–818.

Pollard, R., Callum, K. G., Altman, D. G., & Bates, T. (1976). Shoulder movement following mastectomy. *Clinical Oncology, 2,* 343–349.

Posner, J. B. (1979). Neurological complications of systemic cancer. *Medical Clinic of North America, 63,* 783–800.

Pretsfelder, L. H., Izzo, K. L., & Mohr, R. (1985). Speech rehabilitation outcome after Blom-Singer tracheoesophageal puncture. *Archives of Physical Medicine o, Rehabilitation, 66,* 814–817.

Price, R. A., & Jamieson, P. A. (1975). The central nervous system in childhood leukemia: II. Subacute leukoencephalopathy. *Cancer, 35,* 306–318.

Public Health Service (1979). *Smoking and health: A report of the Surgeon Genera* (DHEW Publication No. PHS 79-50066). Washington, D. C.: U. S. Government Printing Office.

Raz, I., Siegal, T., & Polliack, A. (1984). A CNS involvement by non-Hodgkin's lymphoma: Response to a standard therapeutic protocol. *Archives of Neurology 41,* 1167–1171.

Redmond, P., Berkliner, L., Ambos, M., & Horowitz, L. (1982). Radiological assessment of pharyngoesophageal dysfunction with emphasis on cricopharyngeal myotomy. *American Journal of Gastroenterology, 77,* 85–92.

Rizer, F. M., Schechter, G. L., & Coleman, R. F. (1984). Voice quality and intelligibility characteristics of the reconstructed larynx and pseudolarynx. *Otolaryngology—Head and Neck Surgery, 92,* 635–638.

Romsaas, E. P., Juliani, L. M., Brigg, A. L., Wysocki, G., & Moorman, J. (1983). A method for assessing the rehabilitation needs of oncology outpatients. *Oncology Nursing Forum, 10,* 17–21.

Rosenthal, D. I. (1985). Computer tomography of orthopedic neoplasms. *Orthopedic Clinics of North America, 16,* 461–471.

Sakamoto, A. (1974). Physical activity: A possible determinant of vincristine (NSC-67574) neuropathy. *Cancer Chemotherapy Reports, 58,* 413–415.

Salcman, M. (1980). Survival in glioblastoma: Historical perspective. *Neurosurgery, 7,* 435–439.

Salcman, M. (1985). The morbidity and mortality of brain tumors: A perspective on recent advances in therapy. *Neurology Clinics, 3,* 229–257.

Saltin, B., Blomqvist, G., & Mitchell, J. H. (1968). Response to exercise after bedrest and after training. *Circulation, 38, (suppl. 17),* 1–78.

Sargeant, A. J., Davies, C. T., Edwards, R. H., Maunder, C., & Young, A. (1977). Functional and structural changes after disuse of human muscle. *Clinical Science and Molecular Medicine, 52,* 337–342.

Sarmiento, A., Kinman, P. P., & Galvin, E. G. (1977). Functional bracing of fractures of the shaft of the humerus. *Journal of Bone and Joint Disease, 59,* 596–601.

Scelsi, R., & Pinelli, P. (1977). Subclinical myopathic findings in patients affected by malignant tumors. An autopsy study. *Acta Neuropathologica, 38,* 103–108.

Schalberg, J., & Gainor, B. J. (1985). A profile of metastatic carcinoma of the spine. *Spine, 10,* 19–20.

Schnider, B. J., & Manalo, A. (1979). Paraneoplastic syndromes: Unusual manifestations of malignant disease. *DM. Disease-A-Month, 25,* 1–60.

Schold, S. C., Cho, E., Somasundaram, M., & Posner, J. B. (1979). Subacute motor neuronopathy: A remote effect of lymphoma. *Annals of Neurology, 5,* 271–287.

Schuller, D. E., Reiches, N. A., Hamaker, R. C., Lingeman, R. E., Weisberger, E. C., Suen, J. Y., Conley, J. J., Kelly, D. R., Miglets, A. W. (1983). Analysis of disability resulting from treatment including radical neck dissection or modified neck dissection. *Head and Neck Surgery, 6,* 551–558.

Seidman, H., Mushinski, M. H., Gelb, S. K., & Silverberg, E. (1985). Probability of eventually developing or dying of cancer—United States. *Cancer, 35*, 36–56.

Shy, G. M., & Silverstein, I. (1965). A study of the effects upon the motor unit by remote malignancy. *Brain, 85*, 515–528.

Silberman, A. W., Rand, R. W., Storm, K., Drury, B., Benz, M. L., Morton, D. L. (1985). Phase 1 trial of thermochemotherapy for brain malignancy. *Cancer, 56*, 48–56.

Silverberg, E. (1985). Cancer statistics. *Cancer, 35*, 19–35.

Sim, F. H., Chao, E. Y., & Pritchard, D. J. (1980). Replacement of the proximal humerus with a ceramic prosthesis: A preliminary report. *Clinical Orthopaedics and Related Research, 146*, 161–174.

Singer, M. I., & Blom, E. D. (1980). An endoscopic technique for restoration of voice after laryngectomy. *Annals of Otology, Rhinology, and Laryngology, 89*, 529–533.

Smalley, R. V., Scogna, D. M., & Malmud, L. S. (1982). Advanced breast cancer with bone-only metastases: A chemotherapeutically responsive pattern of metastases. *American Journal of Clinical Oncology, 5*, 161–166.

Sneppen, O., Johansen, T., Heerfordt, J., Dissing, I., & Petersen, O. (1978). Hemipelvectomy: Postoperative rehabilitation assessed on the basis of 41 cases. *Acta Orthopaedica Scandinavica, 49*, 175–179.

Spitzer, W. O., Dobson, A. J., Hall, J., Chesterman, E., Levi, J., Shepherd, R., Battista, R. N., & Catchlove, B. R. (1981). Measuring the quality of life of cancer patients: A concise QL-Index for use by physicians. *Journal of Chronic Disease, 34*, 585–597.

Stalberg, E. (1980). Clinical electrophysiology in myasthenia gravis. *Journal Neurology, Neurosurgery and Psychiatry, 43*, 622–633.

Stonnington, H. H. (1983). Rehabilitation. In F. H. Sim (Ed.), *Diagnosis and treatment of bone tumors* (pp. 281–292). Thorofare, NJ: Charles B. Black.

Subbarao, J. V., & McPhee, M. C. (1982). Prosthetic rehabilitation. Comparison of the outcome in patients with cancer and vascular amputation of extremities. *Orthopedic Review, 11*, 43–51.

Sumi, S. M., Farrell, D. F., & Knauss, T. A. (1983). Lymphoma and leukemia manifested by steroid-responsive polyneuropathy. *Archives of Neurology, 40*, 577–582.

Sundaresan, N., & Galicich, J. H. (1985a). Surgical treatment of brain metastases. Clinical and computerized tomography evaluation of the results of treatment. *Cancer, 55*, 1382–1388.

Sundaresan, N., Bains, M., & McCormack, P. (1985b). Surgical treatment of spinal cord compression in patients with lung cancer. *Neurosurgery, 16*, 350–356.

Swedborg, I., Arner, S., & Meyerson, B. A. (1983). New approaches to sympathetic blocks as treatment of postmastectomy lymphedema: Report of a successful case. *Lymphology, 16*, 157–163.

Swedborg, I., & Wallgren, A. (1981). The effect of pre- and postmastectomy radiotherapy on the degree of edema, shoulder-joint mobility, and gripping force. *Cancer, 47*, 877–881.

Synek, V. M., & Cowan, J. C. (1983). Somatosensory-evoked potentials in patients with metastatic involvement of the brachial plexus. *Electromyography and Clinical Neurophysiology, 23*, 545–551.

Tang, S. G., Byfield, J. E., Sharp, T. R., Utley, J. F., Quinol, L., Seagren, S. L. (1983). Prognostic factors in the management of metastatic epidural spinal cord compression. *Journal of Neuro-oncology, 1*, 21–23.

Tashjan, A. H. (1975). Prostaglandins, hypercalcemia, and cancer. *New England Journal of Medicine, 293,* 1317–1318.

Teravainen, H., & Larsen, A. (1977). Some features of the neuromuscular complications of pulmonary carcinoma. *Annals of Neurology, 2,* 495–502.

Thage, O., Trojaborg, W., & Buchtal, F. (1963). Electrophysiologic findings i polyneuropathy. *Neurology, 13,* 273–278.

Thant, M., Hawley, R. J., Smith, M. T., Cohan, M. H., Minna, J. D., Bunn, P. A. Ihde, D. C., West, W., Matthews, M. L. (1982). Possible enhancement o vincristine neuropathy by VP-16. *Cancer, 49,* 859–864.

Thompson, S. W., Davis, L. L., Kornfield, M., Hilgers, R. D., & Standefer, J. C (1984). Cisplatin neuropathy. Clinical electrophysiologic, morphologic, an toxicologic studies. *Cancer, 54,* 1269–1275.

Ti-sheng, Z., Wen-yi, M., Liang-Yu, H., & Wu-Yi, L. (1984). Heat and bandag treatment for chronic lymphedema of extremities. *Chinese Medical Journal, 97* 567–577.

Tomita, T., Galicich, H. H., & Sundaresan, N. (1983). Radiation therapy for spina epidural metastases with complete block. *Acta Radiologica Oncology, 22,* 135 143.

Trojaborg, W., Frantzen, E., & Andersen, I. (1969). Peripheral neuropathy an myopathy associated with carcinoma of the lung. *Brain, 92,* 71–82.

Unsold, R., Safran, A. B., Safran, E., & Hoyt, W. F. (1980). Metastatic infiltratio of nerves in the cavernous sinus. *Archives of Neurology, 37,* 59–61.

Villanueva, R., & Ajmani, C. (1977). The role of rehabilitation medicine in physica restoration of patients with head and neck cancer. *Cancer Bulletin, 29,* 46–54

Vogl, S. E., Berenzweig, M., & Kaplan, B. H. (1979). The CHAD and HAL regimens in advanced ovarian cancer: Combination chemotherapy including cyclophosphamide, hexamethylmelamine, adriamycin and cis-dichlordiamino platinum (11). *Cancer Treatment Reports, 63,* 311–317.

Walsh, J. C. (1971). Neuropathy associated with lymphoma. *Journal Neurology Neurosurgery and Psychiatry, 34,* 42–50.

Warmolts, J. R., Re, P. K., & Lewis, R. J. (1975). Type II muscle fiber atrophy: A early systemic effect of cancer (Abstract). *Neurology, 25,* 375.

Wasserstrom, W. R., Glass, J. P., & Posner, J. B. (1982). Diagnosis and treatment o leptomeningeal metastases from solid tumors: Experience with 90 patients *Cancer, 49,* 759–772.

Watkins, S. M., & Griffin, J. P. (1978). High incidence of vincristine-induce neuropathy in lymphomas. *British Medical Journal, 1,* 610–612.

Weaver, A. W., & Fleming, S. M. (1978). Partial laryngectomy: Analysis of associated swallowing disorders. *American Journal of Surgery, 136,* 486–489.

Weisenberger, T. H., Eilber, F. R., Grant, T. T., Morton, D. L., Mirra, J. J. Steinberg, M., & Rickles, D. (1981). Multidisciplinary "limb salvage" treatment of soft tissue and skeletal sarcomas. *International Journal of Radiation Oncology, Biology, Physics, 7,* 1495–1499.

Weiss, H. D., Walker, M. D., & Wiernik, P. H. (1974). Neurotoxicity of commonly used antineoplastic agents (II). *New England Journal of Medicine, 291,* 127–133.

Weiss, R. B., Tormey, D. C., Holland, J. C., & Weinberg, V. E. (1981). Venous thrombosis during multimodal treatment of primary breast carcinoma. *Cancer Treatment Reports, 65,* 677–679.

Whitelaw, D. M., & Cowan, D. (1963). Clinical experience with vincristine. *Cancer Chemotherapy Reports, 30,* 13–20.

Wilkinson, P. C., & Zeromski, J. (1965). Immunofluorescent detection of antibodies against neurones in sensory carcinomatous neuropathy. *Brain, 88,* 529–538.

Wingate, L. (1985). Efficacy of physical therapy for patients who have undergone mastectomies. A prospective study. *Physical Therapy, 65,* 896–900.

Woodson, G. E., & Miller, R. H. (1981). The timing of surgical intervention in vocal cord paralysis. *Otolaryngology—Head and Neck Surgery, 89,* 264–267.

Wurster, C. F., Krepsi, Y. P., Davis, J. W., & Sisson, G. A. (1985). Combined functional oral rehabilitation after radical cancer surgery. *Archives of Otolaryngology, 111,* 530–533.

Zeissler, R. H., Rose, G. B., & Nelson, P. A. (1972). Postmastectomy lymphedema: Late results of treatment in 385 patients. *Archives of Physical Medicine and Rehabilitation, 53,* 159–166.

Zelikovski, A., Manoach, M., Giler, S., & Urca, I. (1980). Lympha-press. A new pneumatic device for the treatment of lymphedema of the limbs. *Lymphology, 13,* 68–73.

10

Psychological Considerations in Rehabilitation of the Cancer Patient

Roy C. Grzesiak

In spite of the anxiety and morbid fear associated with terms such as cancer, neoplasm, and malignancy, the facts are that an ever-increasing percentage of people are surviving cancer. After radical surgery, extensive radiation, and/or chemotherapy, these survivors often suffer from prolonged or permanent functional losses. However, many of them do have a better life expectancy than prior to their cancer treatment. The issue then becomes how to optimize the quality of that life. For many, a rehabilitation program will improve function, maximize independence, and eliminate or minimize untoward psychological reactions. It is the psychological reactions that this chapter will address. After some introductory comments on defenses and emotions, life-style, self-injurious habits, and stress as they relate to cancer, the focus will be on the psychological and psychosocial issues that are an inherent part of the clinical picture for the person with cancer.

Since our primary concern is for individuals who have already been diagnosed and treated for their malignancy, no attempt has been made to differentiate between the various kinds of cancer. Suffice it to acknowledge that different kinds of cancer have different prognoses, require different types of treatment, have varying residual effects, and are accompanied by psychological reactions that occur at different times during the course of the disease.

Before that, however, a brief look at the evidence with respect to the role of psychological factors in the etiology of cancer will be presented. This excursion into contemporary psychosomatics is sparked by the recent dialogue in the *New England Journal of Medicine* on whether psychological factors play any role whatsoever in the course of cancer.

THE MIND–BODY PROBLEM AND CANCER

n recent years there has been a resurgence of interest in mind–body nteractions, based primarily on the significant advances being made in the reurosciences. We all acknowledge that life-style (self-injurious habits, oxic environments, etc.) plays an important role in health and disease. What about personality factors? Intuitively, personality style and emotional expression have been implicated by clinicians as important in the development of cancer. A thorough review of retrospective and prospective studies by Temoshok and Heller (1984) has demonstrated that certain emotional patterns are consistently implicated in individuals with certain kinds of cancer. A thorough review of this literature is beyond the scope of this chapter, and only selected research will be presented to illustrate these common components.

Loss of a Close Relationship

We are all familiar with stories about how the loss of a beloved spouse is often followed by the onset of serious illness in the survivor. In fact, we all could probably cite examples from our personal experiences. Parkes (1972), n his introduction to studies on bereavement, noted that in the 17th century grief was actually listed as a cause of death. Rosch (1984) provided an excellent review of both historical and current findings. While impressive, most reports of this nature are anecdotal. Recent research in psychoneuroimmunology lends strong credence to loss of a close relationship as a precursor of illness. Locke (1982) reviewed the two relevant studies on postbereavement immune suppression. Briefly, these studies indicate that bereavement is accompanied by a loss of immune competence that leaves the survivor at risk for serious illness. An even more provocative finding is that n neither of the studies could the immunosuppression be tied to changes in neuroendocrine function. Locke (1982) concludes that a direct brain–immune system link is quite likely.

Inability to Express Feelings

Clinicians and researchers alike have found the inability to express feelings to be an integral aspect of the personality of many cancer patients (Kissen, 1966; LeShan, 1977; Temoshok & Heller, 1984). In their review, Temoshok and Heller, while noting that the role of psychosocial factors in cancer remains complex and obscure, emphasize "one consistently appearing theme: that cancer patients have difficulty in expressing emotions, or even feeling them" (1984, p. 255). A major longitudinal study was initiated about 35 years ago by Thomas and associates (Thomas, 1977; Thomas & Duszynski, 1974). They conducted a psychosocial study of medical students, monitoring their health and illness patterns over the years. Referring to the Thomas data, Rosch (1984) stated: ". . . cancer tends to occur in individuals who are low-key, nonaggressive, and unable to adequately express their emotions" (p. 6). In another review, Greer and Watson (1985) noted that if one considers only controlled studies, the same consistent pattern continues. Namely, cancer patients have a personality attribute that is variously called emotional suppression, repression, or inhibition. Extensive experience doing psychotherapy with cancer patients led Renneker (1981) to define the "Pathological Niceness Syndrome." In this syndrome, cancer patients are described as submissive, compliant, passive, selfless, and anxious to please so as not to be disliked. However, as Greer and Watson (1985) have noted, emotional suppression has been implicated in a number of psychosomatic disorders. They caution that while emotional suppression may be implicated as a risk factor for development of cancer, precise mechanisms remain unclear but probably involve the interaction of emotional suppression with physiological activation channeled into specific biological response patterns.

Inability to Cope

In addition to loss of a significant other, additional stressful life events have been implicated as precursors of cancer. Greer and Watson (1985) have reported that no controlled studies have demonstrated a significant association between stressful life events and diagnosis of cancer. Yet there are a number of studies comparing cancer patients with other medical patients. Smith and Sebastian (1976), utilizing a structured interview approach, compared the emotional history of 44 cancer patients with 44 medical patients without cancer. As Cooper (1984) pointed out, this study was far more open-ended than traditional life-event research that relies heavily on self-report and psychometric properties. Smith and Sebastian (1976) found that cancer patients had a history of significantly more frequent and intense emotional events than did the control group. In another study, Witzel (1970) compared a group of cancer patients with a group of patients with serious but nonmalignant disease. He found significantly more past illnesses in the lives of the cancer patients. Overall, even prior to the diagnosis of cancer, the cancer group had more extensive histories of medical illness.

At this juncture it must be emphasized that the entire life-stress literature is plagued with definitional problems. For example, Locke (1982) has noted that "it is not stress itself that is immunosuppressive, but stress coupled with poor coping" (p. 56). There is a conceptual problem here. Can you have stress if you cope well? It is generally believed that to understand the

nterrelationships between so-called stressful life events and coping pro-
esses, one must distinguish between coping and adaptation (Lazarus &
'olkman, 1984a). Drawing on both their work and that of others, Lazarus
nd Folkman have pointed out that adaptation is a much broader concept
hat involves everyday, routine, automatic modes of getting along in life,
vhile the concept of coping always involves some degree of stress. A life
ituation that demands drawing on something extra is one that requires
oping. Coping always involves a mobilization of effort. In other words, for
nost of us the process in dealing with ordinary life events is nonstressful,
lot requiring coping. We simply do what we have to do. A major problem
vith some of the early stressful life event research was that it relied heavily
on check-list forms of self-report. It is now clear that the persons' percep-
ion or appraisal of the meaning of an event is what makes it either a stressor
or nonstressor. Lazarus and Folkman (1984b) define coping as "constantly
hanging cognitive and behavioral efforts to manage specific external and/
or internal demands that are appraised as taxing or exceeding the resources
of person" (p. 141). They note that this definition of coping serves three
mportant functions. First, it emphasizes coping as a process; second, it
tresses management rather than mastery; third, it emphasizes the central
mportance of appraisal in defining whether or not an event is stressful. It is
he individual's cognitive appraisal of the situation that determines whether
t is viewed as a harm, threat, or challenge (Lazarus & Folkman, 1984a).
Vhile this short discourse on the nature of coping may, at first glance,
ppear out of place here, it is of critical importance. When studies attempt-
ng to link stress, psychoneuroimmunology, and cancer are examined, a
undamental finding is that "it is not exposure to a stressor *per se*, but the
bility to cope with it effectively which is most likely to influence neopla-
ia" (Bieliauskas, 1984, p. 44).

A number of studies have attempted to link psychological features such as
lepression, helplessness–hopelessness, and disposition to the development
of cancer. Problems of definition plague the depression and cancer research
is well. Bieliauskas (1984) noted that there is minimal evidence suggesting
hat cancer patients are more depressed, from a psychiatric perspective, than
inyone else. Attempts to link onset of cancer with premorbid depressive
llness have had equivocal results. In a longitudinal investigation, Shekelle,
Raynor, Ostfeld, et al. (1981) found that a group of men who had scored
iighest on the depression scale of the Minnesota Multiphasic Personality
nventory (MMPI) were at double the risk of death from cancer. This
iignificant difference was present even when additional risk factors, for
example, smoking, alcohol use, and age, were controlled. It is important to
iote that the elevation on the depression scale was not in what was gener-
illy considered the pathological range. In an additional study, Bieliauskas
ind Shekelle (1983) found two behavioral characteristics in patients with a

high depression MMPI profile. They noted a decreased percentage of tim
in bed spent sleeping and an increased percentage of time feeling nervous o
upset. As the authors noted, these two behavioral factors are consistentl
found in patients with depression but are also found in individuals wit
other psychiatric and medical illnesses. That depression is a frequent precur
sor of cancer diagnosis is not strongly supported by research. Bieliauska
(1984) does note that a chronic mild depressive-like state is probably both
risk factor for mortality from cancer and a clinical sign in patients with
diagnosis of cancer.

The concept of helplessness, in particular, "learned helplessness," ha
been advanced as an alternative definition of depression (Seligman, 1974)
Helplessness–hopelessness implies a profound deficit in coping capacity. I
a frequently cited study, Schmale and Iker (1971) were able to predict wit
astounding accuracy the presence of cervical cancer in women who wer
asymptomatic but with suspicious PAP smears. The women with malig
nancies had a helpless-prone personality style. This "giving-up-given-up"
complex has been advanced by Engel (1968) as a general precursor t
susceptibility to all types of illness. As with most of the so-called psychoso
matic formulations of illness, some biological predisposition is assume
(Krantz & Glass, 1984).

Coping Style and Prognosis

Just as inability to cope is viewed by some as a precursor of cancer, so too i
ability to cope viewed as capable of influencing the course of neoplasti
disease. Reviewing animal studies, Levy (1985) noted that acute behaviora
helplessness is correlated with, and most likely causal in, suppression o
lymphocyte function and faster tumor growth. In the clinical literatur
much of the evidence is again anecdotal and poorly controlled, althoug
provocative. The same factors as mentioned above appear to also play a rol
in the course of illness. One of the earliest studies compared two groups o
cancer patients that were matched for age, intelligence, and state of disease
All patients knew their diagnoses. Both groups were followed from initia
treatment on. When those patients that died in less than 2 years wer
compared with those that survived for more than 6 years, a lack of adequat
emotional expression was found in those with short survival time (Blum
berg, West, & Ellis, 1954).

A surprising number of studies have similar findings (Bacon, Rennecker
& Cutler, 1952; Booth, 1964; Kissen, 1963; LeShan & Worthington
1953). Derogatis and associates (Derogatis, Abeloff, & Melisaratos, 1979
found that women with breast cancer who reported less negative emotio
and adjusted positively to their illness had shorter survival times. Studying

sample of women with diagnoses of breast cancer but no evidence of metastases, Greer, Morris, and Pettingale (1979) used interview findings to divide the women into four groups: those who denied their illness, those who were initially optimistic but demonstrated a desire to fight their illness, those who were stoic about the disease, and those who displayed helplessness and passivity. On 5-year follow-up both the deniers and the fighters had more favorable outcomes. Among their findings, Greer et al. observed that women who were "bitchy" or antagonistic appeared to have a better prognosis.

The investigation of premorbid personality factors is always difficult but, using a sample of VA patients with available pre-illness MMPI profiles, Dattore, Shontz, and Coyne (1980) were able to compare a group with cancer to a group of noncancer patients. They found significant differences on three MMPI scales, namely Repression, Depression, and Denial of Hysteria. Cancer patients showed significantly more repression but less depression. Rogentine and associates (1977) found that relapse did not occur in patients who had their malignant melanomas excised surgically if they maximized, rather than denied, the significance of their problem.

The above studies do strongly suggest some common features, both premorbid and in terms of coping with illness, regarding the possible roles of psychological and psychosocial factors in neoplastic disease. An extensive review of this literature can be found in Cooper (1984). Little attention was given to the physiological functions that correlate with emotional status although there is a growing body of evidence that truly reflects psychobiological or, if you prefer, biopsychological interactions. That certain personality patterns or emotional responses occur consistently across a multitude of studies does bear further investigation. What is troubling, however, is the fact that the same psychological signs that indicate a favorable disease course should have prevented the occurrence of the disease in the first place. Barofsky (1981) presented a cogent assessment of both the strong and weak versions of psychogenic models of cancer. He concluded that the nature of the evidence thus far mitigates against drawing any firm conclusions.

COPING WITH CANCER—THE CLINICAL PICTURE

How individuals cope with a diagnosis of cancer has received considerable attention in the clinical literature. Although certainly not the first to address the psychology of dying, Kübler-Ross (1969) pioneered in efforts to afford the terminally ill more humane health care. Of course, a discussion of cancer is not a discussion of dying, but for most of us, the two are equivalent. As Ruitenbeck (1973) noted, Kübler-Ross is credited with confronting mental health professionals with their uneasiness about death and dying. More than that, she appears to have elevated the public consciousness as well. Many authors have addressed the psychology of loss, and, significantly, they all describe a similar series of phenomenological experiences. They describe a process that begins with denial and ultimately ends with acceptance or resolution.

In this section and, indeed, in the remainder of the chapter, attention is primarily on clinical matters. What can the rehabilitation specialist expect in the way of emotional reactions from the patient with cancer? What are their primary defenses? How do they think? What kinds of obstacles do they encounter? What are their principal concerns? How should their problems be handled?

Coping and Accepting: A Stage Approach

Although familiar to most health professionals, Kübler-Ross's (1969) stage approach to coping with one's terminal illness will be briefly described. Theorists have criticized this approach as too concrete and simple, suggesting that the patient is somehow pigeon-holed into "stages." As happens too often in practice, clinical guidelines are invariably transformed into rules. For example, the patient must be depressed; if not, he or she must be denying that he or she is depressed (Trieschmann, 1980). It must be emphasized that the stages to be described below are guidelines to assist the clinician in empathic assessment of the patient's state of mind.

Denial

Most people react to unpleasant news with some variation of denial. Comments such as "oh no," "it can't be," "I don't believe it!" even "what did you say?" all serve the same purpose—to buffer reality. Almost all patients react with denial or, at least, partial denial. Denial can be a very adaptive defense; it is not pathological early on in the course of significant illness. There are times when denial can negatively influence treatment; for example, when the patient decides to shop around hoping for better news elsewhere and delays what would be appropriate care.

Denial is usually a short-lived defense because it is emotionally expensive to maintain in the face of reality. It is not an all-or-none defense either; it does take a variety of forms, tends to shade and color meanings, and waxes and wanes. Kübler-Ross (1969) used as an example the fact that one cannot stare directly at the sun. Similarly, one cannot confront one's death all the time. Often patients will refuse to talk about their illness at the time but will leave the topic open for later discussion. The clinician must be attuned to covert messages. Even bad news can be properly timed. Anxious denial is frequently a consequence of poor timing or a response to the rather clumsy attempt of the physician to get the unpleasantness over with.

Anger

As denial gives way to reality, "not me" is replaced with "why me?" The patient reacts with feelings of anger, bitterness, and resentment. It is generally believed that the anger expressed by patients with a potentially terminal illness is related only to the diagnosis. However, Kübler-Ross (1969) observed that many factors come into play to generate anger. If we place ourselves in the patient's position, it is easier to imagine what these factors might be: loss of privacy, isolation from family and friends, loss of income and financial drain, painful medical tests, uncomfortable and debilitating treatments, and loss of independence and control. In addition, there is the ever-present fear associated with potential death.

A frequent consequence of the patient's anger is further alienation from family, friends, and staff. Angry patients are usually indiscriminate in expressing their discontent. Too often alienation supercedes understanding, and those who should stand by the patient fall victim to injured feelings. Although ideally above it, health professionals sometimes take the patient's anger personally and quality of care is compromised. For the majority of patients the anger stage is just that, a stage that is usually short-lived. Unfortunately, the already alienated family and staff may not see that the patient has moved beyond anger and is more open to emotional support and reassurance.

Bargaining

Chaplains and psychotherapists are most likely to hear about the patient's more magical attempts to deal with terminal illness. Patients must bargain with their God because only one's God can negotiate for such high stakes. When anger fails to solve the problem, the patient often resorts to a trial of "good behavior" in an attempt to gain reprieve. Bargains typically involve promises to engage in good behavior, dedicate remaining years to good causes, or expiate for real or imagined past failures. Kübler-Ross (1969) observed that bargains usually involve either a postponement of death or relief from pain and suffering. To strike a bargain, one must set a time limit on the bargaining period. When there has been no dramatic improvement in circumstances at the end of the time period, the patient must acknowledge failure of the bargain. What happens next is variable; the patient may revert to denial, become angry, experience greater sadness, or, in some cases, attempt to renegotiate another bargain. Failure in bargaining is often signaled by marked changes in behavior and/or mood.

Depression

Some degree of depression is generally the rule in cancer patients. While the term "depression" is used here, a more appropriate term might be "sadness" or "grief." Convention dictates continuing to use the term "depression." Kübler-Ross (1969) has pointed out that there are really two depressive processes going on in the terminally ill. *Reactive depression* involves mourning what has been lost while *preparatory depression* involves taking into account what is going to be lost. Patients must be allowed to mourn these losses. Unless the depression is complicated by premorbid depressive trends, it is a self-limiting process that does not require formal psychiatric intervention. If the patient is so inclined, he or she can benefit from having someone to talk with. That person need not be a psychotherapist but they should be capable of maintaining a psychotherapeutic attitude, namely, to listen, accept, and understand.

There are two ways in which the staff can complicate an appropriate mourning process. First, many people, professionals as well as lay people, are often acutely uncomfortable when faced with a very sad patient. There is an unfortunate tendency to want to do something, to fix the problem. Too often they resort to banal phrases such as: "cheer up," "look on the bright side," or "it can't be that bad." The implicit message is to stop feeling sad. The patient's reaction to such communication is likely to be negative with a subsequent withdrawal from further interaction. Second, there are times when the patient has accepted the situation but the staff has not. The patient's acceptance should be respected.

Acceptance

Acceptance of one's imminent death usually only comes after one has worked through some variation of the above "stages." At this point the patient is neither angry nor sad. The dominant feeling tone is one of quiet acceptance; there is no need to talk for there is nothing left in the world for the patient to be interested in. Similarly, there is often a quiet withdrawal from personal attachments, in effect, from the living. Family, significant others, and staff should be respectful and accepting of the patient's state of mind.

For the patient in a rehabilitation setting, one would hope for a more optimistic, albeit realistic, state of affairs because, by definition, a more prolonged survival time is anticipated. Nevertheless, the rehabilitation oncology patient has had to deal with the very same personal issues during the acute treatment. Acceptance that one has cancer requires a major review of one's life and often a significant reordering of priorities. It is inappropriate for rehabilitation staff to assume the patient's emotional status will remain static through the course of their program. One final caution about Kübler-

Ross's stage approach: The patient should not be expected to come to terms with cancer "by the numbers," so to speak. The stages are simply a set of guidelines.

The Existential Plight

While it has certainly been acknowledged that cancer patients have to face issues of life and death, Weisman and Worden (1977) attempted to differentiate between those who coped well and those who coped poorly with a diagnosis of cancer. Their concept of *existential plight* refers to a distinct phase that is characterized by an exacerbation of thoughts about life and death; it indicates a "luckless predicament in which one's very existence seems endangered" (p. 3). Generally it refers to any and all emotional distress in the newly diagnosed cancer patient. For some the period of emotional distress is brief, while for others it spreads to encompass a variety of psychosocial and emotional problems that would have otherwise remained hidden.

The Weisman and Worden (1977) study is reported here for a number of reasons: it provides a clear picture of the relative incidence of emotional distress; ties it to diagnostic groupings; demonstrates factors involved in emotional vulnerability; and, important to this presentation, provides the clinician with insight into common cognitive coping strategies regardless of their effectiveness. They studied 120 newly diagnosed cancer patients (Breast = 37; Hodgkin's = 18; lung = 23; colon = 23; and malignant melanoma = 19) for the first 100 days of their illness with particular attention to coping, vulnerability, and emotional distress.

General coping strategies were examined and their effectiveness noted. Because these strategies indicate how the patient thinks and attempts to problem solve, they will be presented in detail:

General Coping Strategies (from Weisman & Worden, 1977, p. 6)
- Rational-intellectual—Seek more information about the situation.
- Shared concern—Talk with others to relieve distress.
- Reversal of affect—Laugh it off; make light of situation.
- Suppression—Try to forget; put it out of mind.
- Displacement—Do other things to distract self.
- Confrontation—Take firm action based on present understanding.
- Redefinition—Accept, but find something favorable.
- Fatalism—Submit to and accept the inevitable.
- Acting out—Do something, anything, however reckless.
- If X, then Y—Negotiate feasible alternatives.
- Tension reduction—Reduce tension by drinking, overeating, drugs.
- Stimulus reduction—Withdraw socially into isolation.

• Disowning responsibility—Blame someone or something.
• Compliance—Seek direction from an authority and comply.
• Self-pity—Blame yourself, sacrifice, or atone.

Findings indicated that "good copers" were accepting of diagnosis and treatment, talked with others both to relieve distress and gain information, and displayed an optimistic mood. In terms of specific strategies, good copers relied most on confrontation, redefinition, and compliance with authority. By contrast, the poor copers were pessimistic, not only regarding their illness but in general, reported more marital distress, lack of familial support, and more recent life changes. Poor copers relied on strategies of suppression, stoic submission (fatalism), and tension-reducing measures. It is important to note that, in many cases, even the so-called good coping strategies do not work simply because the problem defies resolution. For some, seeking information and sharing concern does minimize emotional distress, but for others it is not enough. Weisman and Worden noted that one must differentiate between whether the strategy is being used to cope or used as a defense; the latter always involving avoidance of the problem.

Even though all participants in this study were told their diagnosis and provided with a treatment plan, it is interesting that 10% still claimed no knowledge of their diagnosis. As an observation, the older patients were more open about the possibility of death while the younger patients were more preoccupied with disrupted life plans, that is, career, marriage, etc. Patterns were noted between time of high emotional distress and type of cancer. Over the first 100 days level of emotional distress steadily rose for the lung cancer group. Those with Hodgkin's disease started with high existential plight that continued to escalate up to the point of 2-month follow-up, after which it diminished somewhat. Patients with colon cancer and malignant melanoma showed peak emotional upset at the time of initial assessment, usually just after the first treatment (surgical excision), followed by a decline in symptoms of plight. Women with breast cancer did not show peak vulnerability until 2-month follow-up, followed by a decline in emotionality. Not only do patients bring a variety of coping repertoires to the clinical situation but the nature of the specific cancer makes variable demands as well. Generally, peak emotional vulnerability appears partly a function of whether or not, and how, the cancer is being treated and response to that treatment.

As they anticipated, Weisman and Worden (1977) found that life and death concerns were the overriding issues for the new cancer patient. Degree of vulnerability to high emotional distress does appear related to premorbid personal resources; "poor copers" have had more life difficulties and possess fewer emotional resources to handle problems. Although begging the issue of whether optimism, good coping skills, and minimal emotional distress actually enhance outcome, Weisman and Worden (1977) believe that the improved capacity to identify who will cope poorly should enable more timely and appropriate psychological interventions and, thereby, minimize suffering.

Elements of Adaptation

That effective coping in the face of cancer may actually involve the use of illusion was suggested by Taylor (1983) in her cognitive theory of adaptation. She maintains that adaptation or readjustment involves dealing with 3 specific issues: a search for meaning; an attempt to regain mastery over the health problem and life in general; and an effort to enhance self-esteem.

Taylor's (1983) observations are based on intensive study of 78 women with breast cancer and their family members. In describing her sample, she noted that some of the women had a good prognosis while others did not. Some made a satisfactory adaptation and achieved a good quality of life; some did not. Regardless of outcome, Taylor (1983) observed that virtually all of the women made some attempt at resolving issues involving meaning, mastery, and self-enhancement.

Search for Meaning

When stressful events such as cancer strike, we need to make sense of them. We grapple for understanding with the hope that prediction and control are possible. Although there are known causes of cancer, the ability to attribute causation in individual cases is not possible. Nevertheless, 95% of the patients studied made some attempt to understand why they had developed cancer. Spouses were asked if they held any particular notions as to why their partners developed cancer. Spouses were less likely to make causal attributions (63%). Forty-one percent of the women attributed their cancer to either general stress or a particular kind of stress. Specific stressors noted were ongoing marital problems or recent divorce. Thirty-two percent attributed their condition to either ingested carcinogens or environmental cancer-causing substances. Heredity was blamed in 26% of the sample. Seventeen percent attributed cancer to dietary factors. Another 10% blamed specific trauma. Many women held multiple attributions, accounting for the greater than 100% total. Taylor made the point that with the exception of heredity, events labeled as causal are either historical or refer to processes over which the patients believe they have some degree of control; for example, stress or diet. The search for meaning often interacts with the striving for mastery.

None of the attributions mentioned above correlated with better adjustment. It appears that the process of searching for a causal meaning is a goal in itself; even if erroneous, the ability to attribute causation appears important. Part of the search for understanding involves a reappraisal of one's life. Slightly over one-half of the sample reported that they had reviewed their lives and many of them spoke of reordering their priorities, giving more attention to relationships, personal projects, and simple enjoyment. For those who can construe a positive meaning to the cancer experience, psychological adjustment is enhanced.

Mastery

An illness of the magnitude of cancer often is accompanied by a sense of loss of personal control. A second major issue in adaptation is gaining a sense of control over the illness and believing that they can prevent a recurrence of disease. In Taylor's (1983) sample, two thirds believed they had a modicum of control over either disease course or recurrence. The remaining third did not believe that they personally had control over the illness but did believe that their doctors and continued treatment would control the cancer. Whether true or not, these beliefs do enhance adjustment and attitude. Many patients practiced self-regulatory techniques such as relaxation, meditation, and positive thinking. Those patients who attributed the cause of their cancer to past events were usually steadfast in their belief that their lives were different now, thereby eliminating the risk factor. A sense of mastery is more important to the patient than to the spouse. Spouses were not so quick to accept the patients' or the doctors' role in control of cancer.

In addition to attempting to control the disease itself, further mastery was afforded many by understanding the nature of the treatment. Patients who received either chemotherapy or radiation therapy often used self-control techniques to control side effects. Being able to take active steps toward either the treatment proper or management of side effects affords the illusion of control and optimizes adjustment.

Self-enhancement

The final component to successful adaptation involves enhancing one's self-esteem. The occurrence of serious illness is often followed by a precipitous drop in self-regard. Some patients have the personal wherewithal to initiate self-enhancing cognitive statements on their own. Many make social comparisons to bolster their view of the situation. People can make either upward or downward social comparisons. If they observe patients who are apparently doing better, that is an upward comparison. It can serve to either improve motivation or demoralize. In the downward comparison the patient observes others who do not appear to be doing as well, which leads to enhanced self-evaluation. In Taylor's (1983) sample virtually all of the women viewed themselves as well as or better off than their peers. Citing a recent review by Wills (1981), Taylor (1983) noted the following: ". . . when faced with threat, individuals will usually make self-enhancing comparisons in an effort to bolster self-esteem" (p. 1165). She goes on to note: "The point, of course, is that everyone is better off than someone as long as one picks the right dimension" (p. 1166).

The Role of Illusion in Adaptation

As the reader has probably noted, the basis for much of the evidence on which the patients build meaning, mastery, and self-esteem is illusory. There is in fact little evidence to substantiate the idea that one can personally control cancer. Taylor (1983) argues that these illusions serve psychological adaptation. That this position runs counter to generally accepted theories of mental health is certainly true; the psychotherapist would never advocate distortion of reality or self-deception to patients. Yet there is a formidable literature, particularly in the cognitive theory of depression, that would support Taylor's position. The crucial point is that what one believes is actually more important than what actually is. For example, if one believes that one can control pain, they often can, regardless of the biological processes that contribute to nociception (Grzesiak, 1984).

A major drawback of Taylor's (1983) theory of cognitive adaptation is that the person is left quite open to having their belief systems disconfirmed. If things do not go well, the belief system is shattered. But people do tend to be resilient and adaptive when faced with setbacks. To quote again from Taylor: "One does not, for example, react calmly to a recurrence of cancer. What I mean is that people who believed they understood the cause of their cancer, believed they could control it, or believed that they were handling it well, and who then discover their beliefs are untrue, are not worse off for having thought so. In fact, they may be better off" (p. 1170).

What can the rehabilitation psychologist do with such provocative theorizing when faced with cancer patients in actual clinical work? Two formulations come to mind. First, while there is a paucity of hard "scientific" evidence to support psychological factors as being able to alter the course of cancer, there is a substantial clinical literature that lends support (Achterberg, Lowlis, Simonton, & Matthews-Simonton, 1976; Cousins, 1976; Simonton & Simonton, 1975). The answers are not in, and it would be foolhardy to stop asking the questions. In clinical practice a position that optimizes adjustment, even if illusory, will minimize suffering at the very least. Second, in our clinical work a balance must be maintained between reality and illusion so that the patient is never damaged, either emotionally or physically. Customary and appropriate treatment must never be dismissed in favor of illusory control.

PROBLEMS IN REHABILITATION ONCOLOGY

What problems does the cancer patient have that could best be handled in a rehabilitation medicine setting? In an effort to define rehabilitation problems in a cancer population, Lehmann, DeLisa, Warren, et al. (1978) studied a randomly selected sample of 805 patients who were referred to four participating hospitals. It should be noted that this sample closely approximates the national distribution. Interviews were conducted with patients and families, physical examinations were performed, and a detailed evaluation protocol was followed by the rehabilitation team. On the basis of the team's findings, a program of rehabilitation interventions was recommended for each patient. This "ideal" program was then compared with the actual rehabilitation services patients had received. The purpose was to identify gaps in service delivery.

The number of patients with one or more rehabilitation problems was determined and the types of problems were then ranked on the basis of frequency. Psychological problems led the list; approximately 40% of the sample displayed significant psychological difficulty. Examination of the type of psychological problem revealed that moderate to severe depression was the major difficulty. In approximate order of frequency, additional psychological problems included the following: isolation and body image concerns, intellectual deficits, organic brain syndrome—behavior change, increased marital stress, excess dependency, excess inactivity, sexual dysfunction, and postillness divorce or separation. Surprisingly, excessive pain behavior was at the bottom of the list. Because of the relatively high level of psychological disturbance, the sample was reexamined in terms of those who did and those who did not have physical rehabilitation problems. Parenthetically, Lehmann et al. (1978) did not include generalized weakness as a specific physical rehabilitation problem. Of the 438 patients with rehabilitation (physical) problems, 52% had psychologic difficulty compared with only 29% of the remaining patients with no physical rehabilitation problem. The authors concluded that psychological disturbance is greater when the patient is left with residual physical difficulties. When patients with psychological problems were examined with respect to site of cancer, it was found that the above-mentioned psychological problems were common to virtually all cancer sites, although somewhat more pronounced in those with malignancy involving the central nervous system. The latter finding explains the surprisingly high incidence of intellectual deficit and organic brain syndrome.

Although this particular presentation is concerned with the psychological aspects of cancer rehabilitation, it is informative to describe the other rehabilitation problems as well. Functional limitations did tend to cluster around site and type of cancer. Problems with activities of daily living (ADL) were prominent in patients with breast cancer, cancer of the respiratory system, and cancer of the nervous system. In these patients the limitations were due to contractures, shortness of breath, paresis, and paralysis. Ambulation problems were found in those with respiratory and nervous system cancers. Communication problems were found in head/neck and nervous system malignancies. Vocational problems were found in the majority of patients with physical problems. Generalized weakness and pain were common to all cancer sites.

On the basis of these findings a model rehabilitation program was developed that linked the Clinical Oncology Team and the Rehabilitation Team. The physiatrist served as the connecting link. A formal in-service educational program was instituted with both teams sharing knowledge from their areas of expertise. When gaps in service delivery were again measured and compared with the findings prior to the model program, a statistically significant difference was noted.

Diller and associates (Diller, Gordon, Freidenbergs, et al., 1979; Gordon, Freidenbergs, Diller, et al., 1980) conducted a comprehensive survey of cancer patients from a problem-oriented perspective. On the basis of their problems survey of 136 cancer patients, they were able to identify eight general problem areas.

1. Discomfort due to medical treatments, including the side effects of surgery, chemotherapy, and radiation treatment.
2. Dissatisfaction with medical services.
3. Difficulty with activities of daily living.
4. Vocational concerns, including the need to change jobs, find jobs, lost time, and reactions of boss and co-workers.
5. Financial problems.
6. Consequential changes in family relationships, including problems communicating with family members and family anxieties about illness.
7. Intrapsychic problems; for example, anxiety, depression, irritability, sleep disturbance, etc.
8. Changes in social relationships.

With these problem areas identified, a modified team approach to psychosocial intervention was developed based on the use of "oncology counselors." Oncology counselors were either psychologists or social workers especially trained for providing services in this program. The oncology counselor met with each patient on a daily basis and served, in effect, as a case manager. The type of intervention provided depended on the patient's needs at the time. The degree and type of psychosocial intervention varied but three general types of psychosocial intervention were offered: education, counseling, and environmental modification.

The Educational Component
- Clarifying or providing information about the medical system, explaining hospital procedures, teaching patient's rights, and clarifying available outpatient services.
- Clarifying the patient's medical conditions, including type of cancer, meaning of tests, etc.
- Educating the patient about cancer and anticipated side effects from both illness and treatment.
- Teaching self-regulatory skills such as relaxation training, self-hypnosis, etc.
- Reinforcing what other medical personnel have said, encouraging compliance, explaining need for treatment, and reinforcing what the physician had explained to the patient.
- Educating about the emotional reactions to cancer, what the patient can expect in terms of feelings and reactions from others.

The Counseling Component
- Encouraging the patient to ventilate feelings.
- Offering verbal support and reassurance.
- Helping patients to clarify personal feelings, including psychodynamic interpretation of thoughts, feelings, and behavior.
- Encouraging the patient to act on personal environment; for example, encouraging discussion with medical personnel and family.
- Exploring past and current situations.
- Providing indirect support, for example, by discussions about events unrelated to cancer and illness.

The Environmental Component
- Speaking with health care personnel about the patient.
- Making a formal health service referral.

A total of 308 cancer patients were seen with 157 receiving the full psychosocial intervention program and 151 receiving evaluation only and serving as controls. Patients had diagnoses of breast, lung, or melanoma malignancy. All were essentially the same on both demographics and stage of illness.

The patients who completed the psychosocial intervention program and follow-up showed many significant differences when compared with the control group. They were more positive in their feelings and perceptions;

participated more in active as opposed to passive activities; were more realistic but adjusted; experienced a more rapid decline in feelings of anxiety, hostility, and depression; and a slightly greater number were able to return to work. Another finding, similar to that of Weisman and Worden (1977), was that site of cancer did affect both adjustment and service demands. Lung cancer patients required the most assistance and were most concerned with physical discomfort and overall medical status. Breast and melanoma patients voiced more concern over physical appearance. Breast cancer patients were concerned with family reaction and support. Melanoma patients required the least intervention.

It appears that for selected cancer patients participation in a rehabilitation program or in a specialized psychosocial program does afford the patient better adjustment, more stable and satisfying interpersonal interactions, an enhanced sense of having control of their lives, and a greater degree of activity and normalcy. What is also clear is that cancer cannot be considered as a unitary disease. Each site and type of cancer carries with it somewhat different emotional concerns, varying times of peak emotional disturbance, and requires differing degrees of psychological intervention.

SUMMARY

The diagnosis of cancer is usually accompanied by a variety of emotional or defensive reactions that precipitate the need for coping strategies. Common "defenses" such as denial are discussed, as is the pervasive presence of depressive-like reactions. Coping strategies are reviewed with particular emphasis on how the patient's distortion of reality, through illusion, can actually enhance adaptation and adjustment. There is a contradictory literature on the psychology of cancer. Some have implicated psychological, psychosomatic, and psychoneuroimmunological factors as important in the etiology, course, response to treatment, and ultimate survival of cancer patients. Given our knowledge at this time, there are few questions that can be answered definitively. However, the literature does display strong trends. Does cancer have a strong psychosomatic component? The scientific support is weak. Does life-style play a role with regard to risk of cancer? There is fairly strong correlational support. Does psychological status correlate with disease course, response to treatment, and survival? There is weak correlational support. Do psychological services improve the quality of survival time? It appears so. Do psychological services significantly affect survival time? There is no convincing evidence to support this at this time. However, with only a few exceptions, psychologists and behavioral scientists have only recently become involved in the various areas of oncology. We appear to be at a time in the history of both medicine and psychology where the accumulating evidence from both the clinic and the laboratory virtually mandates increased cooperation and collaboration. Studies from relatively new areas of collaboration such as psychoneuroimmunology are pointing to mind–body interactions, in both health and illness, that would have been considered pure science fiction a mere decade ago.

REFERENCES

Achterberg, J., Lawlis, G. F., Simonton, O. C., & Matthews-Simonton, S. (1977). Psychological factors and blood chemistries as disease outcome predictors for cancer patients. *Multivariate Experimental Clinical Research, 3*, 107–122.

Bacon, C. L., Rennecker, R., & Cutler, M. (1952). Psychosomatic survey of cancer of the breast. *Psychosomatic Medicine, 4*, 453–460.

Barofsky, I. (1981). Issues and approaches to the psychosocial assessment of the cancer patient. In C. K. Prokop, & L. A. Bradley (Eds.), *Medical psychology: Contributions to behavioral medicine.* New York: Academic Press.

Bieliauskas, L. A. (1984). Depression, stress and cancer. In C. L. Cooper (Ed.), *Psychosocial stress and cancer.* New York: Wiley.

Bieliauskas, L. A., & Shekelle, R. B. (1983). Stable behavior associated with high-point D MMPI profiles in a non-psychiatric population. *Journal of Clinical Psychology, 39*, 422–426.

Blumberg, E. M., West, P. M., & Ellis, F. W. (1954). A possible relationship between psychological factors and human cancer. *Psychosomatic Medicine, 16*, 277–286.

Booth, G. (1964). *Cancer and culture: Psychological disposition and environment* (A Rorschach Study). Unpublished.

Cooper, I. L. (1984). *Psychosocial stress and cancer.* New York: Wiley.

Cousins, N. (1976). Anatomy of an illness (as perceived by the patient). *New England Journal of Medicine, 295*, 1458–1463.

Dattore, P., Shontz, F., & Coyne, L. (1980). Premorbid personality differentiation of cancer and non-cancer groups. *Journal of Consulting and Clinical Psychology, 48*(3), 388–394.

Derogatis, L. R., Abeloff, M. D., & Melisaratos, N. (1979). Psychological coping mechanisms and survival time in metastatic breast disease. *Journal of the American Medical Association, 242*, 1504–1508.

Diller, L., Gordon, W. A., Freidenbergs, I., et al (1979). *Demonstration of benefit of early identification of psychosocial problems and early interventions toward rehabilitation of cancer patients.* Final Report, New York University Medical Center Rehabilitation R & T Center, No. 1.

Engel, G. L. (1968). A life setting conducive to illness: The giving up-given up complex. *Bulletin of the Menninger Clinic, 32*, 355–365.

Gordon, W. A., Freidenbergs, I., Diller, L., et al (1980). Efficacy of psychosocial intervention with cancer patients. *Journal of Consulting and Clinical Psychology, 48*, 743–759.

Greer, S., Morris, T., & Pettingale, K. W. (1979). Psychological response to breast cancer: Effect on outcome. *Lancet, 2*, 785–787.

Greer, S., & Watson, M. (1985). Towards a psychobiological model of cancer: Psychological considerations. *Social Science & Medicine, 20*, 273–277.

Grzesiak, R. C. (1984). Biofeedback in the treatment of chronic pain. *Current Concepts in Pain, 2,* 3–8.

Kissen, D. (1963). Personality characteristics in males conducive to lung cancer. *British Journal of Medical Psychology, 36,* 27–36.

Kissen, D. M. (1966). The significance of personality in lung cancer in men. *Annals of the New York Academy of Science, 125,* 820–826.

Krantz, D. S., & Glass, D. C. (1984). Personality, behavior patterns, and physical illness: Conceptual and methodological issues. In W. D. Gentry (Ed.), *Handbook of behavioral medicine.* New York: Guilford.

Kübler-Ross, E. (1969). *On death and dying.* New York: Macmillan.

Lazarus, R. S., & Folkman, S. (1984a). *Stress, appraisal and coping.* New York: Springer.

Lazarus, R. S., & Folkman, S. (1984b). Coping and adaptation. In W. D. Gentry (Ed.), *Handbook of behavioral medicine.* New York: Guilford.

Lehmann, J. F., DeLisa, J. A., Warren, G., et al (1978). Cancer rehabilitation: Assessment of need, development and evaluation of a model of care. *Archives of Physical Medicine and Rehabilitation, 59,* 410–419.

LeShan, L. L. (1977). *You can fight for your life.* New York: M. Evans.

LeShan, L., & Worthington, R. E. (1955). Some psychological correlates of neoplastic disease: A preliminary report. *Journal of Clinical and Experimental Psychopathology, 16,* 281.

Levy, S. M. (1985). Behavior as a biological response modifier: The psychoimmunoendocrine network and tumor immunology. *Behavioral Medicine Abstracts, 6,* 1–4.

Locke, S. E. (1982). Stress, adaptation, and immunity: Studies in humans. *General Hospital Psychiatry, 4,* 49–58.

Parkes, C. M. (1972). *Bereavement: Studies of grief in adult life.* New York: International Universities Press.

Renneker, R. (1981). Cancer and psychotherapy. In J. G. Goldberg (Ed.), *Psychotherapeutic treatment of cancer patients.* New York: Free Press.

Rogentine, G. N., Docherty, J. P., van Kammen, D. P., Fox, B. H., & Bunney, W. E. (1977). Psychosocial and biological factors in the prognosis in clinical stage II melanoma. Paper presented at the Annual Meeting, American Psychosomatic Society, Atlanta.

Rosch, P. J. (1984). Stress and cancer. In C. L. Cooper (Ed.), *Psychosocial stress and cancer.* New York: Wiley.

Ruitenbeck, H. M. (Ed.). (1973). *The interpretation of death.* New York: Aronson.

Schmale, A. H., Jr., & Iker, H. P. (1971). Hopelessness as a predictor of cervical cancer. *Social Science & Medicine, 5,* 95–100.

Seligman, M. E. P. (1974). Depression and learned helplessness. In R. J. Friedman, & M. M. Katz (Eds.), *The psychology of depression: Contemporary theory and research.* New York: Wiley.

Shekelle, R. B., Raynor, W. J., Ostfeld, A. M., et al (1981). Psychological depression and 17-year risk of death from cancer. *Psychosomatic Medicine, 43,* 117–125.

Simonton, O. C., & Simonton, S. (1975). Belief systems and management of the emotional aspects of malignancy. *Journal of Transpersonal Psychology, 7,* 29–48.

Smith, W. R., & Sebastian, H. (1976). Emotional history and pathogenesis of cancer. *Journal of Clinical Psychology, 32*(4), 63–66.

Taylor, S. E. (1983). Adjustment to threatening events: A theory of cognitive adaptation. *American Psychologist, 38,* 1161–1173.

Temoshok, L., & Heller, B. W. (1984). On comparing apples, oranges, and frui
salad: A methodological overview of medical outcome studies in psychosocia
oncology. In C. L. Cooper (Ed.), *Psychosocial stress and cancer.* New York
Wiley.

Thomas, C. B. (1977). *Habits of nervous tension: Clues to the human condition.* Th
Precursors Study, 725 N. Wolfe St., Baltimore, MD.

Thomas, C. B., & Duszynski, K. R. (1954). Closeness to parents and the famil
constellation in a prospective study of five disease states: Suicide, mental illness
malignant tumor, hypertension, and coronary heart disease. *Johns Hopkin
Medical Journal, 134,* 251–270.

Trieschmann, R. B. (1980). *Spinal cord injuries: Psychological, social and vocationa
aspects.* Elmsford, NY: Pergamon.

Weisman, A. D., & Worden, J. W. (1977). The existential plight in cancer: Signifi
cance of the first 100 days. *International Journal of Psychiatry in Medicine, 7,* 1
15.

Wills, T. A. (1981). Downward comparison principles in social psychology. *Psycho
logical Bulletin, 90,* 245–271.

Witzel, L. (1970). Anamnese und zweiterkrankungen bei patienten mit bosartige
neubildungen (Anamnesis and second diseases in patients with malignan
tumors). *Med. Klin, 63,* 876–879.

11

Pain Management in Cancer Rehabilitation

Wen-hsien Wu

The magnitude of the cancer pain problem is enormous. The newly diagnosed cases per year are approximately 15 million in the world, 700,000 in the United States, and 200,000 in Canada (American Cancer Society, 1981; Bonica, 1979). Cancer is responsible for 10% of the 50 million deaths annually worldwide and for approximately 400,000 deaths in the United States. Twenty percent of the total deaths occur in North America and Europe (American Cancer Society, 1981). The estimated incidence of pain varies from 60% to 80%, dependent on the patient populations studied (Bonica, 1982). The prevalence of pain in advanced cancer varies with the different types of cancer. Bonica summarized various series and showed that pain occurred in 85% of patients with bone lesions, 85% with cervical cancer, 70% to 75% with gastric cancer, 50% to 70% with lung cancer, 70% to 75% with male genitourinary cancer, 70% with pancreatic cancer, 55% to 68% with breast cancer, 58% with intestinal cancer, 70% with female genitourinary cancer, 55% with renal cancer, 50% to 70% with colon/rectal cancer, and 5% with leukemias.

Cleeland (1984) studied 667 patients and found that severe pain (pain intensity greater than 5 on a 0 to 10 scale) afflicted 34% of patients with breast and prostate cancer, 31% with ovarian cancer, 21% with colon/rectal cancer, and 20% with uterine cancer.

Of greater importance than the frequency is the severity of pain in the advanced cancer. One-third of adults and children with metastatic cancer have pain requiring analgesics to maintain some activity levels (Kanner & Foley, 1981). Sixty to ninety percent of patients reported severe pain in advanced cancer (Cleeland, 1984; Foley, 1985; Twycross & Lack, 1984). Pain of this severity interferes with basic daily activity and enjoyment of life. An estimated 25% of all cancer patients die with inadequate pain control. The reasons for this inadequate care are several (Bonica, 1978; Twycross & Lack, 1984):

1. Inadequate knowledge of analgesics leading to inappropriate applications of the current knowledge in medication or combination of medications. Examples are an "as required" dosing schedule, use of inadequate doses of narcotics, failure in search of optimal dose to avoid adverse effects, and failure to use adjuvant analgesics.

2. Inappropriate attitudes and behaviors by the health care team, patient, and patient's family. Examples are fear of addiction, fear of drug tolerance and respiratory depression, mistrust of the patient's description of pain, and the belief that pain must accompany cancer.

3. Inadequate access to, and availability of, appropriate services. Examples are inadequate education for care providers; geographic, cultural, language, and financial barriers; and a limited number of pain clinics and palliative care centers.

The present discussion will address various rehabilitative aspects of cancer pain management.

TYPES OF CANCER PAIN

Patients with cancer may suffer from either acute or chronic pain. It is important to recognize the difference between acute and chronic pain. Pain associated with an acute disease process or tissue injury is termed *acute pain*. It serves the host as an alarm system. The pain subsides when the injured tissue heals. When the acute pain, with or without changing its characteristics, persists beyond the duration required for tissue healing, it is termed *chronic pain*. Chronic pain serves no biological function and gradually develops psychological stress, functional limitation, attitudinal change, inactivity, overweight, depression, and isolation. These occur not only in the patient but also influence the relationship with family members and co-workers. Foley (1985) presented various types of patients with pain from cancer (Table 11.1).

Onset of acute pain may be the initial symptom leading to the diagnosis of cancer. Patients frequently associate the success or failure of therapy with the absence or presence of pain. The pain associated with cancer therapy is usually predictable and self-limiting. If the outcome is successful this self-limited pain is usually tolerated very well. However, if the outcome is unsuccessful these patients will develop significant psychological problems requiring counseling.

Patients with chronic cancer-related pain may develop increasing intensity of pain when the lesion progresses. The cause of pain produced by cancer includes bone infiltrations (with or without muscle spasm), nerve compression or infiltration, stretch of the organ capsule, visceral distension from obstruction, soft tissue infiltration, ulceration (with or without infec-

TABLE 11.1. Types of Patients with Pain From Cancer

Patients with Acute Cancer-related Pain
  a. Associated with the diagnosis of cancer
  b. Associated with cancer therapy (surgery, chemotherapy, or radiation)
Patients with Chronic Cancer-related Pain
  a. Associated with cancer progression
  b. Associated with cancer therapy (surgery, chemotherapy, or radiation)
Patients with Preexisting Chronic Pain and Cancer-related Pain
Patients with a History of Drug Addiction and Cancer-related Pain
  a. Activity involved in illicit drug use
  b. In methadone maintenance programs
  c. With a history of drug abuse
Dying Patients with Cancer-related Pain

Adapted from Foley (1985).

tion), or increased intracranial pressure. Successful treatment must consist of a combination of chemotherapy, analgesics, neurolysis, and psychological therapy. The degree of success varies from individual to individual. Acute pain caused by cancer is most often related to metastatic bone lesions, nerve compression or infiltration and hollow viscus involvement, muscle spasms, constipation, bed sores, lymphedema, candidiasis, herpatic neuralgia, and deep-vein thrombosis and pulmonary emboli. This can account for 62% of problems in an outpatient clinic and 78% in a cancer center (Daut & Cleeland, 1982; Foley, 1979). Chronic pain associated with cancer accounts for 25% of the problems in an outpatient and 19% of the problems in an inpatient population (Daut & Cleeland, 1982; Foley, 1979). When the therapy is on a palliative basis patients usually develop significant psychological problems. These include anger, anxiety, depression, isolation, sleep disturbance, anorexia, impaired concentration, and irritability and other psychological factors that can in fact lower a patient's pain threshold. (Sternbach, 1974). The pain associated with cancer therapy usually requires symptomatic treatment. It is associated with postoperative neuralgia; phantom limb pain; postradiation inflammation, fibrosis, or myelopathy; and postchemotherapy neuropathy and necrosis of the bone.

Preexisting benign chronic pain occurs in 10% of an outpatient population and 3% of an inpatient population (Daut & Cleeland, 1982; Foley, 1979). It must be differentiated from cancer-related pain, explained clearly to the patient, and treated separately. Frequently considerable effort and understanding are needed to communicate with the patient because of the patient's preoccupation with cancer. For example, musculoskeletal pain, headache (migraine, tension), arthritis, or cardiovascular pain are unrelated to cancer-related pain.

Patients with cancer-related pain and a history of drug addiction are dealt with in a special way (Foley, 1985). The emphasis is on controlling the pain adequately. Individualized medical care must be provided, along with an assessment of psychological needs (Fultz & Senay, 1975).

Dying patients with cancer-related pain should be treated with the goal of providing adequate pain control and comfort to assure the patient, the family, and medical personnel. Successful management can instill confidence and peace in all concerned.

A diagnosis of cancer does not necessarily mean that a malignant process is the direct cause of pain. Most cancer patients have more than one type of pain. Twycross & Fairfield (1982) reported that 80% of the advanced cancer patients in their study had more than one type of pain, and 34% had four or more types of pain. Each type of pain may have a different cause, requiring a different set of treatments. Various types of cancer pain will be discussed.

Bone Pain

Most of the bone metastases are not painful. However, tumor infiltration of the bone is the most common pain in cancer (Foley, 1979). Direct irritation and stimulation of the pain receptors in the periosteum and endosteum is aggravated by prostaglandins produced by the tumor. The characteristics of bone pain vary from a dull ache to a deep intense pain. It is often associated with bone tenderness. Vertebral bodies and long bones are the usual sites of involvement. Movement or weight-bearing of the involved part aggravates the pain.

Nerve Compression Pain

When a peripheral nerve or nerve root is compressed or infiltrated by tumor growth the pain is persistent in a dermatomal distribution. It is important to recognize that compression of the root can cause referred pain, numbness, motor weakness, and abnormal tendon reflexes. Usually pain precedes sensory or motor deficit by weeks or months. The pain can be a constant ache or an intermittent sharp, stabbing, or shooting pain that may radiate to a limb. Severe nerve damage is usually associated with superficial burning pain with or without hyperalgesia. When burning occurs the involvement of the sympathetic nervous system should be considered (Hubert, 1978). Compression can occur in the brachial or lumbar plexus, spinal cord, or cauda equina. Most spinal cord compressions are secondary to tumor deposits in or near the spine. Pain from unilateral root compression is common in the cervical and lumbar spine. Bilateral root pain occurs in approximately one half of the patients having thoracic involvement. The potential for neurosurgical emergency for decompression laminectomy must be kept in mind.

Dysesthesia

Dysesthesia is a constant superficial burning pain, with or without hyperalgesia. It occurs when there is acute damage of the peripheral nerve, nerve plexus, nerve root, or spinal cord. Postherpetic neuralgia occurs more frequently in immunologically suppressed patients. Postoperative neuralgia, which can occur following thoracotomy, radical neck dissection, and mastectomy, is frequently associated with dysesthesia pain. Dysesthesia does not respond to treatment with narcotic analgesics in general. The involvement of the sympathetic nervous system should be confirmed by diagnostic sympathetic blockade.

Visceral Pain

Visceral pain is usually related to local irritation, stretching of the organ capsule due to tumor growth, or partial or complete obstruction of a hollow organ or duct. The pain can be an acute intermittent colic or a constant ache. Surgical consultation should be obtained.

MANAGEMENT OF CANCER PAIN

Successful management is based on a complete assessment of the history of the pain and evaluation of the psychological status of the patient. A careful physical and neurological examination and appropriate diagnostic procedures must be used to determine the nature of the pain. One should develop an integrated total plan of management to address the cancer, the pain, and the psychological aspects of the patient. Following the initiation of therapy a continual reassessment of the patient's response and new needs and modification of the therapeutic plan, if indicated, are essential. The management plan must focus on the patient but include the entire family. Cancer pain disrupts the entire family. In order to assist the family in coping with the crisis, one must learn the family dynamics in detail. This includes the communication patterns, role shift caused by the pain, past memory and fear of the cancer pain, financial stress, and the amount of support from outside the nuclear family. One must deal with the meaning of pain (related or unrelated to cancer or to the success of therapy) and acceptability of addressing pain in a particular family. Informing the patient and family on current therapeutic methods will reduce the chance of a blind search for a miracle cure. Ethnic and religious backgrounds are also important factors. Discussion of the method to communicate with children about cancer pain and emotional support, and the time spent in sympathetic listening to family members, permitting them to express anger, guilt, and depression, will provide them with strength. Whenever possible, one should utilize a team approach. The team involves the patient, the patient's family, family physician, internist, oncologist, radiation therapist, general surgeon, anesthesiologist, neurosurgeon, neurologist, physiatrist, psychologist and psychiatrist, nurse (hospital and home care), physical therapist, occupational therapist, social worker, pharmacist, dietician, chaplain, and volunteers. This team must be under the direction of a central person who is able and willing to spend time to integrate and organize the care.

Multiple therapeutic methods must be utilized to deal with various problems of pain associated with cancer. They include those modifying the disease process (surgery, radiation therapy, hormonal therapy, or chemotherapy), those modifying the pain perception (drugs, education, psychological support, relaxation), those interrupting pain transmissions (TENS), those interrupting neural transmissions (nerve blocks, neurolysis, and neurosurgical procedures), and those modifying life-style (physiotherapy and homemaking services). Treating the underlying disease whenever possible is a fundamental rule. Optional use of analgesics and adjuvant analgesic drugs, symptomatic treatments, and supportive therapy frequently are the most effective approaches to the prevention or relief of pain. They are as important as the specific treatment directed to the cancer. The symptoms requiring treatment include nausea, vomiting, hiccups, anorexia, diarrhea, cough, constipation, weakness, insomnia, dyspnea, bedsores, and incontinence. Creative use of environment in therapy may have a dramatic impact on cancer patients. Its purpose is to create a supportive and therapeutic atmosphere for the treatment of pain. At certain stages of the pain therapy admission to the hospital may be required. One must pay attention to details, including adequacy in staffing, the use of volunteers, natural light and plants, access to nature (outside or roof garden), interest in architecture, ward traffic and quiet environment, options in music and television, colors, textures, shape, family photographs, balance between privacy and community, flexible routines (visiting hours and bath timing), meal temperature and timing, recreational activity, efficient service in radiology, and air temperature and odors. It must be emphasized that most patients with cancer pain can be treated successfully using the therapeutic methods outlined below. However, if pain persists the family physician should not hesitate to seek consultations from medical oncology, radiotherapy, pain management, or palliative care services.

The methods of pain therapy will be discussed in the following four sections, namely drug therapy, nondrug therapy, physiotherapy, and supportive therapy.

DRUG THERAPY

Analgesics are the central theme of pain control in cancer. For an effective medication program a brief review of pharmacology is necessary.

Analgesics are classified as peripherally acting and centrally acting. The latter are further subclassified as opioid agonists and antagonists (Houde, 1979) (Table 11.2).

Peripherally Acting Analgesics

This group of analgesics includes the non-steroidal anti-inflammatory drugs (NSAIDs) (see Table 11.2), which are valuable in cancer pain management, effective in treating mild pain, and useful as an adjunct to narcotics for bone pain. The NSAIDs inhibit the synthesis of prostaglandins, which sensitize the afferent nerves, enhance osteoclast activity in bone metastasis, and potentiate bradykinin-induced pain in animals. The inflammation-inducing substances released from tumors or injured tissues include prostaglandins, histamine, bradykinin, and others that increase the firing of pain receptors (Brereton, Haluska, Alexander, Keiser, & Devita, 1974; Glasko, 1976; Brodie, 1974).

Aspirin is the standard NSAID. However, its adverse effects (gastrointestinal disturbance and bleeding) limit some of its use in cancer patients. Acetaminophen is safer than aspirin but with weaker anti-inflammatory effects. Indomethacin should be used in the lowest effective dose. Increased dosage tends to increase adverse effects, particularly in doses over 150 to 200 mg/day without corresponding increase in therapeutic effects. Suppositories are available. Naproxen is as effective as aspirin but with fewer adverse effects.

Centrally Acting Analgesics

The two subgroups of centrally acting analgesics discussed here are opioid agonists and antagonists/agonists.

Narcotic Agonists

Multiple opioid receptors are present in the brain and spinal cord because opioid analgesics were unable to substitute for each other in preventing

TABLE 11.2. Classifications of Analgesics

Drug class	Drugs	Equianalgesic dose (mg)		Duration (hr)
		PO	IM**	
Peripherally acting:				
NSAID	Aspirin	650*		4–6
	Acetaminophen (Tylenol)	650*		4–6
	Indomethacin (Indocin)	400*		4–6
	Ibuprofen (Advil, Motrin)	400*		4–5
	Naproxen (Naprosyn)			2–4
	Piroxicam (Feldene)			
	Sulindac (Clinoril)			
	Zomepirac (Zomax)			
Centrally acting:				
Narcotic agonist	Codeine	30–200**	120	4–6
	Propoxyphene (Darvon)	65–240**		6
	Meperidine (Demerol)	300	75	2–6
	Oxycodone (Percodan, Percocet)	30**	15	4
	Morphine	50*–60**	10	4–6, 12⁺
	Methadone (Dolophine)	20	10	4–8
	Hydromorphone (Dilaudid)	7.5	4	4–5
	Oxymorphone (Numorphan)	6**, 5–10 (supp)**	1.0	4–6
Narcotic agonist–antagonist	Pentazocine (Talwin)	30*–180*	60	3–4
	Nalbuphine (Nubain)		10	3–6
	Butorphanol (Stadol)		2	3–4
	Buprenorphine (Buprenex)		0.3	4–6

*As compared with that of aspirin (650 mg).

**As compared with that of morphine 10 mg IM.

⁺Controlled-release morphine tablet can produce analgesia up to 12 hours.

Adapted from Houde (1979).

296

withdrawal symptoms in the dog. Martin concluded that there were three types of opioid receptors; namely, μ for morphine, κ for ketocyclazocine and σ for SKF 10,047 (N-allylnormetazocine) (Jaffe & Martin, 1980). The drug–receptor relationship is shown in Table 11.3 (Jaffe & Martin, 1980; Terenius, 1985). Each receptor is related to certain pharmacologic effects (Table 11.4). The action profile of enkephalin and β-endorphin necessitates the introduction of δ & ϵ receptors (Iwamoto & Martin, 1981; Terenius, 1985).

Codeine

Codeine is biotransformed to morphine. Its equianalgesic dose is 120 mg as compared with 10 mg of morphine. It is used in combination with peripherally acting analgesics.

Propoxyphene (Darvon)

Propoxyphene is a mild centrally acting analgesic structurally related to methadone. Its potency is half that of codeine. The dosage should be reduced in patients with hepatic and renal impairment.

TABLE 11.3. Drug Effects on Opioid Receptor

OPIOID	μ (SD, GPI)	κ (SD, GPI)	σ (SD, MVD)	δ (MVD)	ϵ (RVD)
Morphine	+	+	0		
Naloxone	−	−	−		
Leu (Met)-enkephalin (DADLE)	0	+	0		
Pentazocine	−	+	+		
Nalorphine	−	p+	+		
Buprenorphine	p+		0		
Propiram	p+		−		
N-allyl-normetazocine	−		+		
EKC (ethylketocyclizine)		+			
Dynorphin		+			
Beta-endorphin					+
Enkephalin				+	

+: Agonist
−: Antagonist
p: Partial
GPI = Guinea pig ileum
SD = Spinal cord, dog
MVD = Mouse vas deferens
RVD = Rat vas deferens
Adapted from Jaffe & Martin (1980).

TABLE 11.4. Pharmacologic Effects of Opioid Agonists in the Chronic Spinal Dog

	Opioid Receptor		
Effect	μ	κ	σ
Pupil	−	−	+
Respiratory rate	+ then −	0	+
Heart rate	−	0	+
Body temperature	−	0	0
Affect	Indifference	Sedation	Delirium
Nociceptive reflexes:			
Flexor	−	−	−
Skin-twitch	−	0	0

+: Increase; −: Decrease; 0: No change
Adapted from Jaffe & Martin (1980).

Meperidine

Meperidine is not a highly desirable drug in cancer pain management. The reasons are short duration of action (2 to 3 hours), poor oral efficacy requiring more frequent oral administration, relatively low analgesic potency, a tendency to produce tachycardia, and the possibility for excitation or convulsion, especially in the elderly because of accumulation of toxic metabolite (particularly with normeperidine). The undesirable central nervous effects increase considerably at doses over 200 mg every three hours (Kaiko, Foley, Grabinski, Heidrich, Rogers, et al., 1983; McGivney & Crooks, 1984; Twycross, 1984; Walters, 1984; World Health Organization, 1982).

Oxycodone (Percodan, Percocet)

Oxycodone resembles codeine structurally. When used in combination with a fixed dose of aspirin or acetaminophen it cannot be given in increasing doses without the risk of toxicity from the NSAID component.

Morphine

Morphine produces supraspinal analgesia, respiratory depression, and physical dependence. An oral dose of 30 mg can be initiated and can be used 3 to 8 times daily. Recently, controlled-release morphine tablets (30 mg) became available (Drug Therapy Bulletin, 1981). They are designed to be used at regularly scheduled intervals in amounts to meet individual needs without breakthrough pain. The drug can reduce the frequency of oral administration to twice daily (Arkinstall, 1984; Hanks & Trueman, 1984;

Henriksen & Knudsen, 1984; Walsh, 1984). The dose limit should be judged by central nervous depression and clinical condition of the patient.

Methadone

Methadone is well absorbed from the gastrointestinal tract, well tolerated by patients, has a long duration of action (4 to 8 hours), and is highly water-soluble, which permits use in concentrated preparations, in small volume, and by either oral or intramuscular administration. One must note that the average serum half-life of methadone is 25 hours; thus, it requires four days to three weeks to establish a steady state (McGivney & Crooks, 1984; Twycross & Lack, 1984; Twycross, 1984; Walters, 1984). Caution should be taken in giving this drug to patients with hepatic and renal dysfunction, particularly the elderly (Kaiko et al., 1982; Walters, 1984).

Hydromorphone (Dilaudid)

Hydromorphone is a highly water-soluble derivative of morphine. Its property and adverse effects are similar to those of morphine at an equianalgesic dosage level. It can be given parenterally, orally, sublingually, and rectally (suppository). Its use is more limited than morphine because of its short duration of action (McGivney & Crooks, 1984; Walters, 1984).

Oxymorphone (Numorphan)

The action and adverse effects of oxymorphone are similar to those of morphine at an equianalgesic dose. Its potency is similar to that of hydromorphone.

Narcotic Agonist–Antagonist

Pentazocine

The analgesic effect from a 30 mg oral dose of pentazocine is equal to but not greater than either aspirin or acetaminophen. Its absorption after oral administration is variable. It has a high incidence of adverse effects (nausea, vomiting, sedation, drowsiness, confusion, blurred vision, hallucinations) in cancer patients. Pentazocine should not be mixed with any agonist narcotics.

Nalbuphine (Nubain)

Nalbuphine is structurally related to naloxone and oxymorphone. Its analgesic potency is equivalent to that of morphine. It is biotransformed in the liver and excreted by the kidney. No oral preparation is available.

Butorphanol (Stadol)

Butorphanol is similar to morphine in its analgesic potency. Its narcoti
antagonist activity is 30 times that of pentazocine and 1/40 that of nalox
one in rats.

Buprenorphine (Buprenex)

Buprenorphine is an injectable narcotic agonist–antagonist analgesic. It has
high affinity to bind receptors and dissociates from receptors slowly. Its
antagonistic activity is equivalent to that of naloxone. Its analgesic potency
is approximately 30 times that of morphine.

In general, the analgesic potency of the drug chosen should be matched
with the severity of pain. Mild pain can be treated with NSAID. Mild to
moderate pain is treated with NSAID and weak narcotics, for example,
aspirin–codeine, acetominophen–codeine, or propoxyphene. Moderate to
severe pain is treated with moderate-strength narcotics, for example, codeine, propoxyphene, oxycodone, and morphine. Severe pain is treated
with a strong narcotic, including morphine, methadone, hydromorphone,
and oxymorphone.

It is practical to keep the choice of analgesics as simple as possible. It is
useful to be familiar with NSAIDs, codeine, and morphine as the basic
drugs. Then, develop additional options at each level of pain.

When the selected analgesic does not eliminate pain completely, one
should ask the following questions: Has the regular dosing schedule been
strictly adhered to? Is the interval between doses not too long? Has the
highest dosage with manageable adverse effects been reached? If the answers
to these questions are all affirmative, one should switch to an analgesic of the
next higher potency. The equianalgesic dose of various drugs (Table 11.2)
can only serve as a rough guide for switching medication, because individual
response may differ and most of the data were generated from single-dose
administrations.

Once the pain becomes severe enough to use narcotics, many practical
problems will arise. First, single agonists should be used. Second, since
increased intensity of pain requires increasing narcotic dosage, eventually a
higher initial dose will be needed to establish a pain-free state. Then the
dosage can be reduced gradually to achieve a steady state. The medication
schedule must be regular, "around the clock," to minimize the breakthrough
pain leading to a patient's anxiety and fear. Mixing two agonists is not
advised because it makes the evaluation of individual drug effects difficult,
leading to confusion in selecting other drugs subsequently. If breakthrough
pain does occur, additional doses of the same drug may be given. It is also
important to note that patients sleeping through the night may not indicate
an adequate pain control. It is possible to try to administer twice the

daytime dosage producing adequate analgesia at bedtime to ensure a painless sleep. If a patient requires 60 mg or higher doses of morphine orally, he or she needs to be awakened in order to maintain a regular medication schedule to avoid breakthrough pain. Early in the course a daily morphine dosage of 30 to 180 mg in six divided doses is usually adequate for most patients. Occasionally 900 to 1,200 mg per day in six divided doses may be necessary. If a continuous-release form of morphine is used, the dosage can be reduced to twice a day from three times a day. Should conditions aggravating the pain, such as wound dressing, weight-bearing, voluntary motion, or muscle spasm around a fracture site, be present, additional narcotic doses should be provided.

If oral morphine is not producing complete analgesia, one should examine the problem of compliance, swallowing function, dosage, intervals between doses, the nature of the pain, the need for an adjuvant analgesic, and the psychosocial, environmental, and familial elements. The adverse effects associated with morphine administration should be managed. Constipation and fecal impaction are not uncommon. Nausea and vomiting may occur in some patients after the initiation of potent narcotics, and can be caused by the stimulation of medullary chemoreceptor trigger zones, narcotic-induced delay in gastric emptying time, and an enhanced vestibular sensitivity. Prochlorperazine (5 to 10 mg tid) or haloperidol (0.5 to 1 mg bid) inhibits the chemoreceptor trigger zone. Metoclopramide (10 mg qid) improves gastric stasis and shortens emptying time. Dimenhydrinate (100 mg qid) or another antihistamine inhibits vestibular sensitivity. Nausea and vomiting tend to decrease in a week or two following oral morphine medication. At this time the medications for symptomatic relief can be gradually withdrawn. Drowsiness is frequently associated with the initiation of oral morphine. This is likely due to the compensation for physical and psychological exhaustion during the painful period. After analgesic effect is established the patient tends to sleep and rest for a prolonged period of time. Drowsiness usually clears after several days of medication. If the symptom prolongs, one should select another drug or drug combination to reduce the adverse central effect. Postural hypotension, unsteadiness, and dizziness may occur in elderly patients. In the course of narcotic administration a continuous assessment for the proper dosage is essential because the responsivity of each patient to the narcotic and the pathology may vary from time to time. If a patient develops a change of mental status in the steady state of morphine medication the possibility of cerebral metastasis should be considered. Morphine increases the tone of the detrusor muscle and the depressive central response to vesical efferent input, thus causing urinary retention. It occurs infrequently in patients receiving epidural morphine and is reversible by naloxone administration without altering the analgesia (Rawall & Wattwil, 1984).

Drug dosage should be titrated individually for optimal effects with the least adverse effects. The oral route is always the first choice of administration. In patients with difficulty swallowing, suppositories or subcutaneous or intramuscular injection can be used. In selected cases an implanted infusion pump to deliver analgesic intrathecally or epidurally (see below) may be useful in providing profound analgesia without mental clouding.

The question of ceiling dose, drug tolerance, or addiction should not be a hindrance to titrate doses toward a complete analgesia in cancer management, because the therapeutic aim is producing comfort. An arbitrary narcotic dose set as the ceiling by the physician to avoid respiratory depression and delaying initiating narcotic medication to avoid and postpone tolerance and addiction is a mistake. Actually pain and anxiety counteract narcotic-induced respiratory depression, as observed in the management of postoperative acute pain. Carefully titrated narcotic for pain control is safe, even in patients with respiratory diseases. Drug dependence involves physical and psychological elements. Cancer patients receiving an individually titrated effective narcotic dose on a regular medication schedule for a long time tend to develop drug dependence slower than drug-naive patients. Many demonstrated no physical withdrawal symptoms after sudden discontinuation of medication due to radiation or chemotherapy. While some may exhibit some degrees of physical dependence, psychological dependence does not seem to occur. When a patient with a previously established drug dose needs an increase of dose it is an indication of increase in pain rather than drug tolerance. When drug tolerance occurs another narcotic analgesic can be used because cross-tolerance is usually incomplete (Houde & Wallenstein, 1966; Interrisi & Foley, 1984). Data available do not support that a significant number of even patients with nonmalignant chronic pain develop addiction (Taub, 1982). Taub studied 2,580 patients with benign chronic intractable pain and found only 0.77% of all patients and 4.2% of patients treated with opioids thought to present a significant problem in management. These patients with benign chronic pain are thought to have greater tendencies to develop drug craving.

ROUTES OF ADMINISTRATION

The most convenient and effective route of administration is oral, which should be used whenever possible. However, other routes are considered for specific conditions.

Rectal Route

Suppositories are useful when a patient, especially a nonhospitalized patient, develops a swallowing disturbance, sore mouth, severe nausea, or vomiting from chemotherapy or has an objection to the taste of oral drugs. Suppositories are available for several analgesics (Table 11.5).

Intramuscular Route

Intramuscular (I.M.) injection is mainly used for treating acute postoperative pain. It can be used for a short time in order to establish relief from oral, rectal or other routes. Indications for use include severe and sudden breakthrough pain or acute pain from pathological fracture, severe vomiting, swallowing disturbance, and severe mental clouding and weakness in the terminal stage.

The advantages of the I.M. route are rapid onset and predictable plasma level. The disadvantages are short duration and difficulty in administration, especially for nonhospitalized patients.

Subcutaneous Route

The subcutaneous route is used in continuous infusion form with a portable pump. The reservoir can be filled by a trained family member or a visiting nurse. It is indicated when either oral or rectal administration is unsuitable, such as in esophageal or rectal cancer.

Intravenous Route

Constant intravenous infusion using a butterfly needle, an intravenous catheter, or an implantable reservoir system is indicated when the patient is unable to tolerate oral analgesics or repeated intramuscular or subcutaneous injection.

Epidural or Intrathecal Route

Since Wang first reported analgesia from spinal administration of narcotics, the field has expanded dramatically (Wang, Nauss, & Thomas, 1979). The specific binding of narcotics to the spinal opioid receptors provides excellent

TABLE 11.5. Rectal Suppositories of Narcotics

Drug	Dosage (mg)	Duration of Action (Hr)
Oxymorphone (Numorphan)	5	4
Hydromorphone (Dilaudid)	3	4
Morphine	10–20	4

analgesia without sensory, motor, or sympathetic blockade (Cousins & Mather, 1984; Yaksh, 1981). The clinical experience in spinal narcotics is still in its early stage. Table 11.6 summarizes the present experience (Cousins & Mather, 1984).

The doses used for perioperative analgesia can serve as a reference. In patients receiving lumbar intrathecal administration of preservative-free morphine the doses ranged from 0.25, 0.54, and 20 mg for general surgery (Ventafridda, Fighiuzzi, & Tamburini, 1979; Wang, 1977; Wang, 1979), and from 1.5 to 4 mg prior to open-heart surgery (Mathews & Abrams, 1980). The epidural doses range from 1 to 10 mg. We found that in patients with benign chronic pain the slope of the CO_2 response curve did not reduce at a dose below 7.5 mg and reduced at only slightly and clinically unnoticeable levels (Wu).

When high doses of narcotic are needed but cause excessive drowsiness and mental clouding, the quality of the analgesia is unsatisfactory. If family support is adequate and life expectancy is reasonable, an epidural narcotic analgesia should be considered. When necessary, 5 to 10% and 0.5 to 1% of the daily equivalent morphine dose can be used initially for epidural and intrathecal administration, respectively.

An implanted system is indicated for a patient with a life expectancy of longer than 6 months and having normal activities. A percutaneous epidural catheter or an implanted system is indicated for a patient with a life expectancy of 1 to 6 months with ambulatory status with or without pain-limited activity. A percutaneous system is indicated for a patient with an expected survival of 1 to 2 months in a bedridden state (Coombs, 1985).

Percutaneous epidural narcotic analgesia is effective in controlling cancer pain (Coombs, 1985; Cousins & Mather, 1984; Crawford, Andersen, & Augustenborg, 1983; Zenz, 1984). The reported mean doses ranged from 5 to 12.6 mg, with total daily dose of from 2 to 80 mg. A large number of patients used this route for 100 to 150 days, some for up to 300 days without major difficulties. The disadvantage is the need of catheter reinsertion because of dislodgement or infection.

The implanted system can be an epidural or intrathecal catheter connected to a subcutaneous port or pump through a subcutaneous tunnel. When an implanted reservoir is used, a special needle connected to an external syringe or infusion pump is percutaneously inserted into the subcutaneous reservoir for drug administration. With proper skin care and dressing the needle can stay in place for long periods of time. The chance of infection in this case is less than that of a transcutaneously inserted epidural catheter even through a subcutaneous tunnel. With the use of a continuous infusion approach the problem of skin breakdown from multiple percutaneous bolus injections is avoided. When an implanted pump is used the drug reservoir must be filled periodically. Thus, the patient's motivation, com-

TABLE 11.6. Epidural Opioids: Latency and Duration of Postoperative Analgesia

Drug	Dose (mg)	Onset (min) (mean ± SD or range)	Complete pain relief (min) (mean ± SD or range)	Duration (hr) (mean ± SD or range)
Meperidine	30–100	5–10	12–30	6 (median) 4–20
Morphine	5–10 5	23.5 ± 6	60 37 ± 6	6.6 ± 3.3 20 18.1 ± 6.8 12.3 ± 7.7
Methadone	5	12.5 ± 2	17 ± 3	7.2 ± 4.6 8.7 ± 5.9
Hydromorphone	1 0.1	13 ± 4	23 ± 8	11.4 ± 5.5 5.7 ± 3.7
Fentanyl	0.1	4–10	20 9	2.6 ± 4
Diamorphine	5 6	5	15	12.4 ± 6.5 2–21

Data from Zenz (1984) and Foley (1985).

mitment, and family support are essential. Psychological evaluation and counseling prior to the implantation and periodically throughout the care period are a part of the total integrated care.

Adverse effects are divided into technical and pharmacological aspects. Technical complications include dural puncture with the epidural approach; CSF leakage with the intrathecal approach; and catheter migration, knotting of the catheter, and bleeding. These effects can be minimized or eliminated by performing catheter insertion under the guidance of an image-intensifier and confirmation by contrast enhancement. A normal coagulation profile minimizes the chances of bleeding. Pharmacological adverse effects include pruritus, urinary retention, nausea, and vomiting. These adverse effects can be reversed by naloxone without altering analgesia.

The advantages of the continuous infusion approach are many: (1) The steady spinal analgesia level achieved reduces the risk of respiratory depression and adverse effects from bolus injections; (2) it provides the patient with convenience, mobility, and functional flexibility, plus less frequent need for oral medication or injections; (3) it is unlikely to produce mental clouding in average clinical doses; (4) the chance of infection is reduced, especially in immunologically suppressed patients; (5) it is not associated with motor or sensory deficit or sympathetic blockade (Cousins & Mather, 1984), so that neurolysis or ablative surgery is delayed or avoided.

CHEMOTHERAPY/HORMONAL THERAPY

When a sensitive cancer is treated with chemotherapy or hormonal therapy methods, the results are encouraging to the patient. Adverse effects are well tolerated and accepted as part of the curative therapy. However, the toxic effects of these drugs must be carefully weighed against their benefits in palliative therapy.

ADJUVANT DRUGS

Adjuvant drugs are drugs of various classes useful in treating certain cancer pain. For example, NSAIDs are useful in bone pain; tricyclic antidepressants (low dose) are good for postherpetic neuralgia (Daut, 1982) and depression (higher dose); simethicone and metoclopamine for pain of gastric distention, chlorpromazine for rectal or bladder tenesmic pain; benzodiazepines or baclofen for muscle spasms and pain; steroids and diuretics for lymphedema; NSAIDs for skin ulcer (decubitus or cancer); metronidazole or appropriate antibiotics for infected ulcers; topical anesthetic sprays for wound dressing; lidocaine viscous or jelly for a sore mouth; and nystatin for oral candiasis (Twycross & Lack, 1983). Corticosteroids are useful in treating pain associated with hepatomegaly, head and neck tumors, pelvic and retroperitoneal cancer, and metastatic arthralgia. Concomitant use of steroids and diuretics is beneficial in cases of elevated intracranial pressure, head and neck tumor, and lymphedema. After the establishment of an initial effective therapeutic dose of a benzodiazopine, continuous evaluation for possible signs of overdose must be made because accumulation may occur as a result of long half-life (e.g., diazepam half-life $= 20$ to 50 hours), especially in the elderly.

Symptomatic relief may lead to pain relief indirectly. NSAIDs can be added in treating bone pain. When the pain is not relieved by regular oral doses of codeine and oxycodone, or when one plans to switch from the parenteral route to the oral route, morphine by mouth should be considered.

Concomitant symptomatic treatment for nausea, vomiting, pruritis, anorexia, anxiety, fear, insomnia, cough, constipation, and urinary retention associated with cancer can relieve pain to some degree indirectly. One must remember that drug therapy is only a part of the total integrated treatment plan.

NON-DRUG THERAPY

Treating Underlying Pathology

Radiotherapy

Radiation can produce a cure or reduction of tumor size to reduce pain. The response should be clearly explained to the patient and family to avoid the tendency of associating the pain with prognosis, especially when pain is the initial symptom leading to the diagnosis. Pain secondary to tumor invasion of the cervical or lumbar plexus; local and ulcerating masses; and compression of the vena cava, bronchus, and ureteral and biliary tract can frequently be improved by radiation.

Bone metastasis occurs frequently in breast, lung, kidney, and thyroid tumors, and in malignant melanoma. The most frequently involved sites are the vertebrae, the proximal femur, the pelvis, the ribs, the proximal humerus, and the skull. Radiotherapy can provide partial or complete analgesia in 90% of patients with bone metastasis with and without pathological fracture.

Surgery

Palliative surgery can be very helpful. Surgery for relieving obstruction or pressure includes drainage of abscesses; debulking masses; and releasing bowel, urinary tract, or ductal obstruction. The pain from impending pathological fracture can be prevented by internal fixation. The pain from fracture can be managed by internal fixation or replacement of involved sections of bone or joint.

Stimulation Therapy

Acupuncture and electroacupuncture elicit release of β-endorphins and serotonin (Han, 1984; Han, Xie, Zhou, Folkesson, & Terenius, 1984; Kang, Zhou, Han, 1984; Xu, Zhou, & Han, 1985) to inhibit pain transmission. However, it may not be sufficient for control of severe pain and requires special skill.

Transcutaneous electrical nerve stimulation (TENS) can produce analgesia with variable degree and duration. Attention should be given to the placement of electrodes in order to optimize the effect. It is useful in treating muscle spasm.

Dorsal Column Stimulation

This modality has not been used extensively in cancer pain. The simplicity of the percutaneous placement of electrodes may offer benefits in cancer pain therapy.

Central Nervous System Stimulation

Stereotactic placement of electrodes into the internal capsule, thalamus, and hypothalamus for stimulation is still experimental (Sano, 1977).

Neural Blockade

Temporary neural blockade is achieved by using local anesthetics. Sometimes the analgesia lasts longer than the duration expected of the drug used. It is used most commonly in the case of myofacial pain syndrome (trigger points), rib metastasis, or painful bony prominence.

Neurolysis

When pain becomes too severe and persistent to be adequately controlled by surgery, chemotherapy, radiation, or potent analgesics, one should consider interruption of the pain pathways (neurolytic procedures) before extremely high dosages of narcotics are used. For patients already experiencing muscular weakness, impaired bowel and bladder activity, and sensory deficits, major neurolytic procedures can be used with less fear of the possible complications.

Neurolysis is achieved by chemicals, thermocoagulation, and freezing. These procedures can be performed at the first, second, or third sensory neuronal level and on the autonomic nervous system.

Chemical Neurolysis

Chemical neurolysis is a relatively safe procedure for the treatment of cancer pain involving somatic and visceral structures. The spinal nerves may be blocked through the intrathecal, subdural or epidural space. The most commonly used agents for subarachnoid neurolysis are phenol, absolute alcohol, and chlorocresol. The hypobaric solution includes aqueous phenol or alcohol. Hyperbaric solutions are phenol (5 to 7%) and chlorocresol (2 to 2.5%) in glycerin. After the intrathecal injection the phenol or chlorocresol is gradually released from glycerin, thus limiting the spread and achieving a better localization in the neural tissue.

Intrathecal Neurolysis

After a detailed history and physical and neurological examination, including recording the pain areas and any dysesthesia, sensory deficit, muscle weakness, or bladder and bowel dysfunction, an intrathecal neurolysis can be planned.

The neurolytic agent is introduced into the posterior nerve roots on the most dependent side by positioning the patient. Placing the spinal needle close to the vertebral outlet of the main pain-conducting nerve root improves results. Beginning with a small injectate volume to cover no more than three dermatomes and preliminary injection of water-soluble contrast medium (Amipaque) to confirm the direction of flow reduces complications. A special needle with dual tubings minimizes accidental needle movement during injection. One tubing is for injecting contrast medium and the other is for injecting the neurolytic agent.

Pain in the neck and upper limbs can be caused by cancer of the upper lobe of the lung. Intrathecal neurolysis in the neck requires special skill because of the narrow spinal canal. Subdural neurolysis is safer.

The upper chest pain can be approached at the level of the involved nerve root. Neurolysis in the midthoracic region can be difficult because of the overlapping spinous process. In the event of failure to enter the theca at this level, injection is made with a technically easier approach either from T2 or T10 with appropriate tilt of the table to allow the hyperbaric agent to flow toward the target site.

Neurolysis for the lower thoracic or lumbar region is safe. Preliminary viewing with contrast medium is essential to avoid damaging the sacral nerves (S2-4) necessary for bladder and bowel control.

Cancer of the rectum causes sacral and perineal pain frequently. Better results are obtained when a chemical neurolysis is performed before sheltering of nerves occurs. When the neurolysis of the S4-5 and coccygeal nerves is performed, the patient is kept at a 60° backward tilt to preserve the more ventrally located intervening roots (S2-4) in the sacral plexus.

Complications of intrathecal neurolysis include pain at the site of injection, motor weakness, sensory deficit or paresthesia, altered bladder and bowel control, vomiting, headaches, meningeal reaction, arachnoiditis, and thrombosis of the spinal artery.

Subdural Neurolysis

The subdural space is a potential space between the dura and the arachnoid membrane. It does not communicate directly with the subarachnoid space but extends laterally over nerve roots and dorsal root ganglia. This space is the widest in the cervical region and the only site for subdural neurolysis.

Subdural neurolysis is useful for treating pain in the neck and shoulder. It must be performed with an image intensifier with confirmation using contrast medium. Injection of 2 to 3 mL of 7% phenol can give bilateral analgesia over several dermatomes.

Epidural Neurolysis

Theoretically, epidural neurolysis is safer than the intrathecal route. Meningeal irritation, spinal cord injury, and the risk of intracranial spread are absent. It is particularly useful for patients with pain in the upper chest, upper limbs, and neck (Maher & Mehta, 1977; Papo & Visco, 1974). Limiting the injectate to 2 to 3 mL minimizes the chance of hypotension. The disadvantage of the method is that the onset of analgesia is slower than that from the intrathecal approach. A repeated injection may be necessary. A new armored epidural catheter makes the procedure easier. More than one injection through the catheter can be used to titrate for the optimal effects.

Caudal epidural neurolysis for sacral and perineal pain carries a high risk of bladder and bowel complications. Some advocate the use of a dilute solution (3 to 5% aqueous phenol) of smaller volumes.

Neurological sequelae are rare, and occasionally paraesthesia and numbness at remote sites from intended areas may occur after epidural neurolysis. Backache is fairly common.

Sympathetic Neurolysis

This method is considered when the sympathetic nervous system is involved in the pathology. Edema, cyanosis, burning, and severe pain are some of the features mimicking reflex sympathetic dystrophy (Hubert, 1978).

Stellate ganglion block lysis can be useful. A primary or secondary cancer of the upper thorax can involve a painful scar (e.g., radical mastectomy) or damage to sympathetic nerve fibers with the presentation of a reflex sympathetic dystrophy syndrome. A stellate ganglion lysis with 3 mL of 6% aqueous phenol preceded by a diagnostic block with lidocaine is valuable. Confirmation of drug spread by prior injection of a contrast medium is mandatory.

Celiac plexus neurolysis is useful for pain originating from cancer of the stomach, pancreas, liver, biliary tract, and gallbladder. It also destroys visceral efferent fibers. However, we have not observed any change in intestinal motility or glandular activity with this procedure. Systemic hypotension does occur from profound splanchnic vasodilation and is used as an indication of a successful block.

When fibrosis or neoplastic infiltration prevent even spread of the neurolytic agent one may use a higher volume of concentration or a completely separate procedure. A more accurate localization of needle tip can be guided by computed tomography (CT) (Filshie, Golding, Robbie, & Husband, 1983). When the plexus is obliterated by cancer the preganglionic fiber of splanchnic nerve can be destroyed above the diaphragm with the guidance of an image intensifier or CT (Boas, 1983).

Recently, experimental use of electrical stimulation of the plexus producing prolonged analgesia showed new hope in analgesia with preservation of the structure (Srikantha, Choi, & Wu, in press).

Cryoanalgesia

Cryoanalgesia accomplishes neurolysis by freezing a nerve, thus interrupting neural impulse transmission but not anatomy. Preservation of the framework of perineurium and epineurium allows nerve regeneration (Bernard, 1980). Duration of cryoanalgesia varies from a few weeks to 3 months and is related to the axonal regrowth rate and the distance of the lesion from the end organ (Lloyd, Bernard, & Glynn, 1976). Motor and sensory deficit are rare.

Cryoanalgesia of intercostal nerves is effective for chest well pain from lung cancer, and cryoanalgesia of sacral nerves is effective for perineal pain from rectal and pelvic cancer (Evans, Lloyd, & Jack, 1981). Cryoanalgesia, unlike alcohol, does not cause neuritis and can be safely repeated without any ill effects.

Percutaneous cordotomy is destruction of the ventrolateral spinothalamic tract. Mullan and Harper (1963), Mullan (1965), and Rosomoff, Carrol, and Brown (1965) simplified the procedure by using an insulated needle to produce a thermal lesion. It should be limited to one side to avoid respiratory failure. The procedure can be performed in terminal patients because it does not require anesthesia and can be repeated.

Transcutaneous Cervical Cordotomy

Cervical cordotomy does not relieve pain above the level of C5. It is most successful for relieving unilateral pain below the waist. Pain relief occurs in 90% of patients initially, 80% at 3 months, and 60% at 1 year.

Common complications are pain and ataxia (20%), bladder and bowel problems (10%), post-spinal-tap headache, and ipsilateral paresis of the arm or leg (5%). Contralateral pain develops in 7% to 10% of the patients. A similar number complain of previously unrecognized pain (Edem, 1963 Nathan, 1972; Ventafridda, DeConno, & Fochi, 1982). Dysesthesia (tingling or burning) is infrequent.

Thermocoagulation

Thermocoagulation of a neural tissue is achieved by insertion of a probe connected to a radiofrequency generator. It can be used to treat pain from a peripheral nerve or nerve root (rhizotomy, dorsal root ganglion lysis, and sacral spinal ganglion lysis). Unilateral neurolysis can be achieved through a caudal approach under the guidance of an image intensifier with contrast medium to visualize the neural structure and assist with accurate placement of the probe.

Pituitary Neuroadenolysis

Pituitary neuroadenolysis can be achieved chemically or by cryotherapy. Morica (1977, 1982) introduced the method of using chemicals. This technique is now used for patients with diffuse bilateral pain in any part of the body including the head.

Diabetes insipidus, when it occurs, is usually self-limiting to 2–3 weeks. Mild headache and occasional rhinorrhea occur. Ocular signs are rare.

Hypophyseal cryoablation (−50° to −70°C) produces incomplete clinical hypophysectomy (Lloyd et al., 1976). This can be repeated in a week. It is claimed that cryoablation is a more successful and safer method than alcohol injection.

PHYSIOTHERAPY

A wide variety of physical therapies are important adjuncts in the management of cancer pain. Muscle spasms are treated by massage, cold and heat, collars, traction, passive exercises, and chair/bed positioning. Pain can also be treated by applying counterirritation (mentholated ointments), heat or cold, pressure, vibration, and rubbing.

Mobilization can sometimes reduce pain. It involves stretching to prevent contractures and spasm, applying a compression cuff for lymphedema, and providing aids for transfer (board, bar) or walking (walkers, crutches, canes).

Immobilization is important to reduce the pain in certain conditions. Patients should be taught the techniques to avoid strain and fatigue and be provided with collars, corsets, splints, slings, or traction.

SUPPORTIVE THERAPY

From the time of diagnosis of cancer, the patient goes through various mental stages; namely, denial, depression and anger, and justification and acceptance (Bond, 1977). Each patient travels through these stages at different speeds and sequence. Most patients with cancer pain develop anxiety, depression, fearful thoughts, feelings of hopelessness, isolation, role shift caused by disability, and fear of impending death or treatment failure. Patients are sensitive and vulnerable. Thus, the physician must be patient and willing to spend time in communication using understandable language. It is important to have a care team to share feelings with. General relaxation techniques are helpful. These include breathing exercises, distraction/imagery, music therapy, prayer, hypnosis, and biofeedback (Eatopoulos, Graham, & Cook, 1979; Finer, 1979).

Group therapy can provide a forum for emotional support to the patient in dealing with the changes associated with cancer, for example, pain, disability, and loss of control. Family therapy provides understanding of the dynamic interaction for coping with stress, improvement of communication in expressing the feeling of fear, and realistic acceptance of the situation.

SUMMARY

The magnitude of the cancer pain problem is enormous. The prevalence of severe pain in advanced cancer is high. A significant number of cancer patients die with inadequate pain control. Reasons for this unfortunate situation have been analyzed, and various types of cancer pain with the associated pathophysiology and problems have been outlined.

Management of cancer pain is initiated by a complete assessment of the patient's status in pain, medication, emotion, family dynamics, and communication skills. Successful treatment requires an integrated team approach transcending the effort of the patient, the family, family physician, various medical specialists, paraprofessionals, and chaplain. This orchestrated treatment plan under the direction of one central person would include drug therapy, nondrug therapy, physiotherapy, and supportive therapy. Pharma-

cology of different classes of drugs and various routes of administratio
including oral, rectal, intramuscular, subcutaneous, intravenous, epidural, o
intrathecal have been discussed, and adjuvant drug therapy for pain an
symptomatic relief has been included. Drug dependence and potential ad
dictive aspects of chronic medication should be de-emphasized in order t
achieve a reasonable level of pain control. Nondrug therapy includes radio
therapy, surgery, acupuncture, transcutaneous electrical nerve stimulation
dorsal column stimulation, central nervous system stimulation, neural block
ade, neurolysis (sensory and sympathetic), cryoanalgesia, transcutaneous
cervical cordotomy, thermocoagulation, and pituitary ablation. A brie
description of physiotherapy and supportive therapy is included in th
discussion.

REFERENCES

American Cancer Society (1981). *Cancer figures and facts.* New York: America
    Cancer Society.
Arkinstall, W. W. (1984, September). Double-blind, crossover comparison betwee
    sustained release morphine tablets and oral morphine solution in patients wit
    severe pain. Paper presented at the 1984 International Symposium on Pai
    Control, Toronto, Canada.
Bernard, D. (1980). The effects of extreme cold on sensory nerves. *Annals of th
    Royal College of Surgeons, 62*, 180–187.
Boas, R. A. (1983). The sympathetic nervous system and pain relief. In *Relief o
    intractable pain (Monograph in Anesthesiology,* Vol. 13). (pp. 215–237). Amster
    dam, The Netherlands: Elsevier.
Bond, M. R. (1979). Psychologic and psychiatric techniques for the relief of pain o
    advanced cancer. In J. J. Bonica & V. Ventafridda (Eds.), *Advances in pai
    research and therapy, Vol. 2* (pp. 215–222). New York: Raven Press.
Bonica, J. J. (1979). Importance of the problems. In J. J. Bonica & V. Ventafridda
    (Eds.), *Advances in pain research and therapy, Vol. 2* (pp. 1–12). New York
    Raven Press.
Bonica, J. J. (1982). Management of cancer pain. *Acta Anaesthesia Scandinavia
    (Supplement), 74*, 75–82.
Brereton, H. D., Halushka, P. V., Alexander, R. W., Mason, D. M., Keiser, H. R.,
    & DeVita, V. T. Jr. (1974). Indomethacin-responsive hypercalcemia in a pa-
    tient with renal cell adenocarcinoma. *New England Journal of Medicine, 291*,
    83–85.
Brodie, G. N. (1974). Indomethacin and bone pain. *Lancet, 2*, 1160.
Cleeland, C. S. (1984). The impact of pain on patients with cancer. *Cancer, 54*,
    2635–2641.
Coombs, D. W. (1985). Newer approaches to chronic pain therapy. *Seminars in
    Anesthesia.* New York: Grune & Stratton.
Cousins, M. J., & Mather, L. E. (1984). Intrathecal and epidural administration of
    opiates (review). *Anesthesiology, 61*, 276–310.
Crawford, M. E., Anderson, H. B., Augustenborg, G., Bay, J., Beck, O., Ben-

veniste, D., Larsen, L., Carl, P., Djernes, M., Eriksen, J., Grell, A. M., Henriksen, H., Johansen, S. H., Jorgensen, H. O. K., Moller, I. W., Pedersen, J. E. P., & Ravlo, O. (1983). Pain treatment on out-patient basis utilizing extradural opiates: A Danish multi-center study comprising 105 patients. *Pain*, *16*, 41-46.

Daut, R. L., & Cleeland, C. S. (1982). The prevalence and severity of pain in cancer. *Cancer*, *50*, 1913-1918.

Evans, P. J. D., Lloyd, M. A., & Jack, T. M. (1981). Cryoanalgesia for intractable perineal pain. *Journal of the Royal Society of Medicine*, *4*, 803-809.

Filshie, J., Golding, S., Robbie, D. S., & Husband, J. (1983). Unilateral computerized tomography guided celiac plexus block: A technique for pain relief. *Anesthesia*, *38*, 498-503.

Finer, B. (1979). Hypnotherapy in pain of advanced cancer. In J. J. Bonica, & V. Ventafridda (Eds.), *Advances in pain research and therapy, Vol. 2* (pp. 223-229). New York: Raven Press.

Foley, K. M. (1979). Pain syndromes in patients with cancer. In J. J. Bonica, V. Ventafridda, R. B. Fink, L. E. Jones, & J. D. Loeser (Eds.), *Advances in pain research and therapy, Vol. 2* (pp. 59-75). New York: Raven Press.

Foley, K. M. (1985). The treatment of cancer pain. *New England Journal of Medicine*, *313*, 84-95.

Fotopoulos, S. S., Graham, C., & Cook, M. K. (1979). Psychophysiologic control of cancer pain. In J. J. Bonica, & V. Ventafridda (Eds.), *Advances in pain research and therapy, Vol. 2* (pp. 231-243). New York: Raven Press.

Fultz, J. M., & Senay, E. C. (1975). Guidelines for management of hospitalized narcotic addicts. *Annals of Internal Medicine*, *82*, 815-818.

Galasko, C. S. B. (1976). Mechanisms of bone destruction in the development of skeletal metastases. *Nature*, *263*, 507-510.

Han, J. S. (1984). Antibody microinjection technique as a tool to clarify the role of opioid peptides in acupuncture analgesia. *Pain*, *2*, (Supplement), 66.

Han, J. S., Xie, G. X., Zhou, Z. F., Folkesson, R., & Terenius, L. (1984). Acupuncture mechanisms in rabbits studied with microinjection of antibodies against β-endorphine, enkephalin and substance P. *Neuropharmacology*, *23*, 1-5.

Hanks, G. W., & Trueman, T. (1984). Controlled-release morphine tablets are effective in twice-daily dosage. *Advances in morphine therapy; the 1983 International Symposium on Pain Control*, *64*, 103-105. Royal Society of Medicine International Congress and Symposium Series.

Henriksen, H., & Knudsen, J. (1984, September). *Controlled evaluation and ongoing clinical experience with sustained release morphine in patients with advanced cancer.* Paper presented at the 1984 International Symposium on Pain Control, Toronto, Canada.

Houde, R. (1979). Systemic analgesics and related drugs: Narcotic analgesics. In J. J. Bonica, & V. Ventafridda (Eds.), *Advances in pain research and therapy, Vol. 2* (pp. 263-273). New York: Raven Press.

Houde, R. W., Wallenstein, S. L., & Beaver, W. T. (1966). Evaluation of analgesics in patients with cancer pain. In L. Lasagna (Ed.), *International encyclopedia of pharmacology and therapeutics, Section 6. Clinical pharmacology, Vol. 1.* (pp. 59-97). New York: Pergamon Press.

Hubert, C. (1978). *Recognition and treatment of causalgic pain occurring in cancer patients* (abstract). The Second World Congress on Pain (p. 47). International Association for the Study of Pain, Montreal, Canada.

Inturrisi, C. E., & Foley, K. M. (1984). Narcotic analgesics in the management of pain. In M. Kuhar, & G. Pasternak (Eds.), *Analgesics: Neurochemical, behavioral and clinical perspectives* (pp. 257–287). New York: Raven Press.

Iwamoto, E. T., & Martin, W. R. (1981). Multiple opioid receptors. *Medical Research Review, 1*, 411.

Jaffe, J. H., & Martin, W. R. (1980). Opioid analgesics and antagonists. In L. S. Goodman, & A. Gilman (Eds.), *The pharmacological basis of therapeutics*, (6th ed., pp. 494–534). New York: Macmillan.

Kaiko, R. F., Foley, K. M., Grabinski, P. Y., Heidrich, G., Rogers, A. G., Inturrisi, C. E., & Reidenberg, M. M. (1983). Central nervous system excitatory effects of meperidine in cancer patients. *Annals of Neurology, 13*, 180–185.

Kang, B. E., Zhou, Z. F., & Han, J. S. (1984). The involvement of serotoninergic transmission in periaquiductal grey for electroacupuncture analgesia and morphine analgesia in rabbits. *Kexue Tongbao* (Chinese), *29*, 116–122.

Kanner, R. M., & Foley, K. M. (1981). Patterns of narcotic drug use in a cancer pain clinic. *Annals of the New York Academy of Science, 362*, 161–172.

Lloyd, J. W., Bernard, J. D. S., & Glynn, G. J. (1976). Cryoanalgesia—A new approach to pain relief. *Lancet, 2*, 932–934.

Maher, R. M., & Mehta, M. (1977). Spinal (intrathecal) and extradural analgesia. In S. Lipton (Ed.), *Persistent pain, Modern methods of treatment, Vol. 1.* (pp. 61–99). New York: Grune & Stratton.

Mathews, E. T., & Abrams, L. D. (1980). Intrathecal morphine in open-heart surgery. *Lancet, 1*, 543.

McGivney, W. T., & Crooks, G. M. (1984). The care of patients with severe chronic pain in terminal illness. *Journal of the American Medical Association, 251*, 1182–1188.

Morica, G. (1977). Pituitary neuroadenolysis in the treatment of intractable pain from cancer. In S. Lipton (Ed.), *Persistent pain, Modern methods of treatment, Vol. 1.* (pp. 149–173). London: Academic Press.

Morica, G. (1982). Chemical hypophysectomy for cancer pain. In J. J. Bonica (Ed.), *Advances in neurology, Vol. 4* (pp. 707–714). New York: Raven Press.

Morphine in slo-release tablets (1981). *Drug Therapy Bulletin, 19*, 44.

Mullan, S. (1965). New techniques in neurosurgery. *Postgraduate Medicine, 37*, 636–641.

Mullan, S., & Harper, P. V. (1963). Percutaneous interruption of spinal pain tracts by means of a strontium needle. *Journal of Neurology, 20*, 932–939.

Nathan, P. W. (1972). Pain in cancer: Comparison of results of cordotomy and chemical rhizotomy. In I. Fusch & T. Kunc (Eds.), *Present limits of neurosurgery* (pp. 513–516). Amsterdam, The Netherlands: Excerpta Medica.

Papo, I., & Visco, A. (1974). Phenol rhizotomy in the treatment of cancer pain. *Anesthesia and Analgesia, 53*, 993–997.

Rawal, N., & Wattwil, M. (1984). Respiratory depression following epidural morphine: An experimental and clinical study. *Anesthesia and Analgesia, 63*, 8–14.

Rosomoff, H. L., Carroll, F., & Brown, J. (1965). Percutaneous radiofrequency cervical cordotomy technique. *Journal of Neurology, 23*, 639–644.

Sano, K. (1977). Intralaminar thalamotomy (thalamo-laminotomy) and posterior medial hypothalamotomy in the treatment of intractable pain. In H. Krayenbuhl, P. E. Maspes, & W. H. Sweep (Eds.), *Pain: Its neurosurgical management, part II: Central procedures* (pp. 50–103). Basel, Switzerland: Karger.

Srikantha, K., Choi, J. J., & Wu, W. (in press). Electrical stimulation of the celiac plexus for pain relief in chronic pancreatitis: A clinical note. *Acupuncture and Electrotherapeutics.*

Sternbach, R. A. (1974). *Pain patients: Traits and treatment.* New York: Academic Press.

Taub, A. (1982). Opioid analgesics in the treatment of chronic intractable pain of non-neoplastic origin. In L. M. Kitahata, & J. G. Collins (Eds.), *Narcotic analgesics in anesthesiology* (pp. 199–208). Baltimore, MD: Williams & Wilkins.

Terenius, L. (1985). Families of opioid peptides and class of opioid receptors. In H. L. Field, R. Duner, & R. Cervero (Eds.), *Advances in pain research and therapy, Vol. 9* (pp. 463–477). New York: Raven Press.

Twycross, R. G. (1984). Controlling pain in cancer patients. *Modern Medicine Postgraduate Series: Pain, 2–13.*

Twycross, R. G., & Fairfield, S. (1982). Pain in far-advanced cancer. *Pain, 14,* 303–310.

Twycross, R. G., & Lack, S. A. (1983). *Symptom control in far-advanced cancer, Vol. 1. Pain relief.* New York: Pitman.

Twycross, R. G., & Lack, S. A. (1984). *Therapeutics in terminal cancer.* London: Pitman.

Ventafridda, V., Fighiuzzi, M., Tamburini, M., Gori, E., Parolaro, D., & Sala, M. (1979). Clinical observation on analgesia elicited by intrathecal morphine in cancer patients. In J. J. Bonica, & V. Ventafridda (Eds.), *Advances in pain research and therapy, Vol. 3.* (pp. 559–565). New York: Raven Press.

Ventafridda, V., DeConno, F., & Fochi, C. (1982). Clinical percutaneous cordotomy. In J. J. Bonica, V. Ventafridda, C. A. Pagni, & L. E. Jones (Eds.), *Advances in pain research and therapy, Vol. 4* (pp. 185–198). New York: Raven Press.

Walsh, T. D. (1984). A controlled study of MST CONTINUS tablets for chronic pain in advanced cancer. *Advances in morphine therapy; the 1983 International Symposium on Pain Control.* Royal Society of Medicine International Congress and Symposium Series, *64,* 99–102.

Walters, J. K. (1984). Hospice care and the pharmacist. *NARD Journal,* 61–65.

Wang, J. K. (1977). Analgesic effect of intrathecally administered morphine. *Anesthesiology, 4,* 2–3.

Wang, J. K., Nauss, L. A., & Thomas, J. E. (1979). Pain can be controlled by intrathecally applied morphine in man. *Anesthesiology, 50,* 149–151.

World Health Organization (1982). *WHO Draft Interim Guidelines Handbook on Relief of Cancer Pain.* Geneva, Switzerland: World Health Organization, 30.

Wu, W. Unpublished data.

Xu, D. Y., Zhon, Z. F., & Han, J. S. (1985). Amygdaloid serotonin and endogenous opioid substances are important for mediating electroacupuncture analgesia and morphine analgesia. *Acta Physiologica Sinica, 37,* 163–171.

Yaksh, T. L. (1981). Spinal opiate analgesia: Characteristics and principles of action. *Pain, 11,* 293–346.

Zenz, M. (1984). Epidural opiates for the treatment of cancer pain. In M. Zimmerman, P. Drugs, & G. Wagner (Eds.), *Recent results in cancer research* (Vol. 89, pp. 107–115). Heidelberg, Germany: Springer-Verlag.

SECTION IV
Advances in
Rehabilitation Research

Frederica Bowden
Section Editor

Introduction

Frederica Bowden

Unfortunately, there has been a noticeable lack of data-based research conducted in the field of rehabilitation. This observation has been made repeatedly in virtually every review of rehabilitation theory and practice. The lack of such studies also has been noted by nearly every Past President of the American Congress of Rehabilitation Medicine, one of the nation's largest organizations representing rehabilitation professionals.

The purpose of this section is not to tell the reader how to conduct research. Rather, it is designed to alert the practitioner to certain pitfalls, obstacles, and problems he or she may encounter in the search for funding. In addition, it is designed to direct the practitioner–researcher to currently available data bases that should be accessed in the preparation of the proposal. Finally, the section presents information about agencies that fund rehabilitation research and that should be contacted as potential funding agents.

Information presented in Section IV, "Advances in Rehabilitation Research," is designed to be eminently practical and useful. Through use of material contained in this section, it is hoped that the potential researcher will be better able to develop methodologically and conceptually rigorous research projects and identify funding sources suitable to support their implementation.

12

Rehabilitation Research: Problems and Resources

Frederica Bowden

Rehabilitation is a complex and dynamic field characterized by constant change. Once limited to health care professionals, rehabilitation practitioners now include electronics engineers and material scientists, special educators and linguists, computer scientists and information systems specialists. As such, information about rehabilitation processes and practices now can be found in a number of very different publications. For example, federal agency publications describe research they have funded while other relevant articles are found in electronics journals, special education publications, consumer publications, and in the publications of federally funded projects.

The scope of issues embraced by persons involved in the rehabilitation process has grown considerably, and the types and numbers of publications describing results of rehabilitation research have multiplied as a result of several factors that literally have reshaped and refocused the entire field. First, where the rehabilitation field once addressed a small number of disabilities, it now deals with a much larger number of physically compromising conditions. In part, this is due to improved medical technology, which has extended the life span of the disabled person. Persons who once did not survive the initial injury now have life spans that approach that of the able-bodied population. In addition, as participation in sporting and recreational activities has increased, so has the incidence of accidents that result in disabling injuries. The needs of these persons now occupy the attention of many practitioners and researchers. Disabilities associated with old age also have increased, in part from the steadily growing numbers of the elderly in the United States and because of increased expectations about their ability to remain active and independent. Additionally, where the number of surviving multiply physically handicapped infants previously was small, persons who once did not survive to adulthood now are expected to be employed and independent.

Second, the field of rehabilitation has been affected by rapidly changing technology, which, in turn, has fostered the development of different and often better solutions to old rehabilitation problems. One example of this phenomenon is found in the improved technique used to fit lower limb prostheses. In the past this was a time-consuming and not always accurate procedure. Now electronic sensors provide a faster and more accurate measure of fit.

Third, the rehabilitation field has been affected by changing societal expectations about getting workers back into the work force and off of disability compensation. For example, the General Services Administration provides information and assistance to all federal agencies to make their work sites wholly accessible. In the private sector, the federally funded Job Accommodation Network Project provides information to employers in order to enable them to accommodate the functional limitations of employees and applicants with disabilities. The importance of vocational issues to the practice of rehabilitation is the cumulative result of recent advances made in technology that have extended and enlarged the capacity of disabled persons to lead productive and satisfying lives.

Finally, the rehabilitation field has been influenced by more knowledgeable and demanding consumers of products and services. Information networks are being developed where none previously existed. For example, consumers with spinal cord injuries inform each other of services through publications like *The Bumble Bee* (c/o Sue Owen, 412 Woodward Blvd., Pasadena, CA 91107), *Shake-A-Leg* (P.O. Box 1002, Newport, RI 02840-0009), and *The Disability Rag* (Box 145, Louisville, KY 40201). These are advocacy publications that are designed to inform disabled consumers of their rights as well as of available services and products.

PROBLEMS FACING THE REHABILITATION RESEARCHER

Each discipline involved in rehabilitation faces two kinds of problems in developing research projects: those that characterize the specific discipline and those affecting the field in general. While it is not possible to consider impediments to developing research initiatives specific to the wide range of professional disciplines engaged in the rehabilitation effort, it is possible to present a brief description of several problem areas that cross disciplinary boundaries.

Problem 1: Keeping Current with Advances in Rehabilitation

Rehabilitation is a rapidly changing field. Its scope is broadening as disciplines traditionally external or peripherally related to it now influence its practice. However, few rehabilitation professionals manage to do more than keep current in their own narrow area of expertise. In addition, only a few publications, conferences, and professional meetings cross disciplinary boundaries. As a result, the same problems may be researched simultaneously by professionals in two or more different disciplines, each approaching the problem from a different perspective. Working in isolation from each other, these professionals often lack the benefit of communicating or collaborating with others. Such communication is essential to the research process and could well accelerate the search for solutions to a research problem.

Problem 2: Design Flaws

Research that is being conducted is more often than not seriously flawed. For example, in a recent article (Thomas, 1985) it was pointed out that only 32% of applications submitted to the Medical Sciences Office of the National Institute of Handicapped Research were recommended for approval by one of six medical review panels. However, following scientific methodological evaluation only 13% were ultimately recommended for award. While many of the topics proposed for investigation were determined to be interesting, most were not supported appropriately by rigorous methodologies and research designs. Major deficiencies in these proposals included "inadequate control of important variables in experimental and control samples, sampling deficiencies, errors in methodologic conceptualization, and use of investigative methods which did not follow the hypotheses to be tested."

Problem 3: Identifying a Funding Source

Identifying an appropriate funding source presents a significant problem to the rehabilitation researcher because funding criteria may change as a response to political, economic, and societal pressures. Currently, no centralized up-to-date federal funding information data base exists, leaving many researchers unaware of funding alternatives. Rather, most researchers repeatedly attempt to secure funding from the same source even though the priorities of that funding agency may have changed dramatically.

Problem 4: Losing Funding Support

Loss of funding often occurs when the research priorities of a funding agency change or following a negative peer site evaluation. Also, some agencies only fund the research phase of a project and lose interest in continuing support as it nears the development phase. Researchers generally do not learn why their funding was discontinued, nor are they provided information about alternative funding sources.

The loss of a project's funding often results in termination of the project. If the results of the study are not disseminated, future investigations replicating the research question may have to be conducted, wasting time, energy, and funds. Research errors and problems may also be repeated by the second researcher. Expensive equipment bought or adapted for the initial project may remain unused, while a newly funded researcher must purchase identical new equipment. Currently there exists no central list of federally funded projects that would help maximize the use of such equipment or data.

Problem 5: No Funding Sources

Sometimes no funding source appears to exist to support a particular research initiative. Unfortunately it appears that as funding becomes more scarce and competition for remaining funds intensifies, agencies may be more likely to fund traditional research conducted by established researchers who work in institutions that have a record of supporting funded research. They appear increasingly less inclined to support researchers who propose investigating unusual research problems or applications originating from institutions with no established reputation as research centers.

Problem 6: Multiple Funding Sources

Sometimes a number of funding sources are utilized to investigate the same or similar problems. Multiple funding for similar research limits research money available to other researchers. Multiple funding also tends to result in duplication of effort. Duplication can be viewed as an asset during the research phase when little is known about the problem by rapidly building a broad knowledge base. However, once a broad knowledge base has been established, such duplication is wasteful.

Problem 7: Dissemination of Research Results

Inadequate dissemination of research results is a major problem in the field of rehabilitation. Few publications exist and only a limited number of conferences occur that approach rehabilitation from a holistic, multidisciplinary perspective. This reduces opportunities for cross-pollination between researchers in different disciplines. In addition, researchers are not generally compelled by a funding agency to disseminate their research results. Even some university-based researchers consistently fail to publish or present their findings. Researchers in private sector institutions are even less likely to publish or present at conferences. Finally, most of what is written appears in publications designed for small, highly specialized audiences. Further adding to the general inaccessibility of research results is the fact that results often are reported using technical terminology specific to the discipline of the researcher. This limits its accessibility to researchers in other disciplines, even though findings may be highly relevant to their work.

Problem 8: Validity of the Research Project to the Consumer

All research in the area of rehabilitation ultimately should be of some value to the disabled consumer. While a 1986 National Science Foundation report (*Women and Minorities in Science and Engineering*) indicates that 92,000 scientists and engineers report having a physical handicap, few of these potential consumers of rehabilitation research are involved in establishing research priorities, reviewing proposals for funding awards, or monitoring projects while they are being conducted. The inadequate use of this resource may result in a distorted interpretation of the project's ultimate usefulness to its consumer.

Problem 9: Technology Transfer

Lack of technology transfer can occur when results of research are not adequately developed or disseminated. In addition, because few cost-benefit analyses have been conducted for rehabilitation equipment, third party payers often remain unconvinced that such equipment would be beneficial to their clients. Manufacturers also are reluctant to produce items that have a small market, further adding to the technology transfer problem.

Problem 10: Proving the Cost Effectiveness of Rehabilitation

One of the most significant issues facing the field of rehabilitation is the need to prove its cost-effectiveness and the efficacy of treatments rendered. In the current fiscal environment of reduced budgets and constricted financial growth, health care administrators and funding agents are critically examining requests for financial support of programs whose worth has never been empirically determined.

Problem 11: Lack of Long- and Short-Term Research Priorities

At the present time no long- or short-term research agenda has been established in many federal agencies and in the field of rehabilitation as a whole. As a result, it is sometimes difficult to use short-term research results to build upon each other in a manner that meaningfully contributes to problem resolution.

FUNDING

At the time of writing there are about 30 federal agencies that fund research that in some way is related to rehabilitation. Each of these agencies has different priorities and funding criteria for rehabilitation research. In addition, these priorities and criteria regularly change. For that reason, accurate information about funding agencies is difficult to obtain. Rather, each agency likely to fund specific research must be individually contacted for current information. A listing of federal agencies that fund rehabilitation research appears below.

Department of Agriculture
14th Street and Independence
  Avenue SW
Washington, DC 20250
(202) 447-2791
Office of Grants and Program Systems
(202) 475-5720

Department of Defense
The Pentagon
Washington, DC 20301-1155
(202) 545-6700

Department of Education
400 Maryland Avenue SW
Washington, DC 20202
(202) 245-3192

Special Education Programs
400 Maryland Avenue SW
Washington, DC 20202
(202) 732-1265

Vocational Education
400 Maryland Avenue SW
Washington, DC 20202
(202) 732-2251

National Institute of Education
1200 19th Street NW
Washington, DC 20208
(202) 254-5080

National Institute of Disability
  and Rehabilitation Research
400 Maryland Avenue SW
Washington, DC 20202
(202) 732-1192

Department of Health and
  Human Services
200 Independence Avenue SW
Washington, DC 20201
(202) 245-6296

National Institutes of Health
9000 Rockville Pike
Bethesda, MD 20205
(301) 496-4000

Division of Research Grants
(301) 496-7881

National Institute on Aging
9000 Rockville Pike
Bethesda, MD 20205
(301) 496-5345

National Institute on Allergy and
  Infectious Diseases
9000 Rockville Pike
Bethesda, MD 20205
(301) 496-1521

National Institute of Arthritis,
  Diabetes, and Digestive and
  Kidney Diseases
9000 Rockville Pike
Bethesda, MD 20205
(301) 496-5741

National Institute of Child Health and
  Human Development
9000 Rockville Pike
Bethesda, MD 20205
(301) 496-3454

National Institute of Dental Research
9000 Rockville Pike
Bethesda, MD 20205
(301) 496-6621

National Institute of Neurological
  and Communicative Disorders and
  Stroke
9000 Rockville Pike
Bethesda, MD 20205
(301) 496-4677

National Cancer Institute
9000 Rockville Pike
Bethesda, MD 20205
(301) 496-5737

National Eye Institute
9000 Rockville Pike
Bethesda, MD 20205
(301) 496-7425

National Heart, Lung and
  Blood Institute
9000 Rockville Pike
Bethesda, MD 20205
(301) 496-2411

National Institute of Environmental
  Health Sciences
Research Triangle Park, NC 27709
(919) 541-3212

National Institute of General Medical
  Sciences
9000 Rockville Pike
Bethesda, MD 20205
(301) 496-7714

National Institute on Drug Abuse
9000 Rockville Pike
Bethesda, MD 20205
(301) 443-6487

National Institute of Mental Health
9000 Rockville Pike
Bethesda, MD 20205
(301) 443-3877

Health Care Financing
  Administration
200 Independence Avenue SW
Washington, DC 20201
(202) 245-6726

Social Security Administration
6401 Security Boulevard
Baltimore, MD 21235
(301) 594-1234

Health Resources and Services
  Administration
5600 Fishers Lane
Rockville, MD 20857
(301) 443-2086

National Institute for Occupational
  Safety and Health
200 Independence Avenue SW
Washington, DC 20201

Administration on Developmental
  Disabilities
348 F, Hubert H. Humphrey
  Building
200 Independence Avenue SW
Washington, DC 20201
(202) 245-2890
Grants Office
(202) 472-6712

Administration on Aging
330 Independence Avenue SW
Washington, DC 20201
(202) 245-0724

Department of Labor
200 Constitution Avenue NW
Washington, DC 20210
(202) 523-8165

National Institute for Occupational
  Safety and Health
200 Constitution Avenue NW
Washington, DC 20210
(202) 523-8017

Department of Housing and
Urban Development
451 Seventh Street SW
Washington, DC 20410
(202) 755-5600

Department of Transportation
400 Seventh Street SW
Washington, DC 20590
(202) 426-4000

National Aeronautics and Space
Administration
600 Independence Avenue SW
Washington, DC 20546
(202) 453-1000

National Science Foundation
1800 G Street NW
Washington, DC 20550
(202) 655-4000

Veterans Administration
810 Vermont Avenue NW
Washington, DC 20420

Architectural and Transportation
Barriers Compliance Board
330 C Street SW
Rm. 1010
Washington, DC 20202

Additional Funding Sources

Associations

Some associations fund rehabilitation research. The size of awards varies considerably. Each association has its own criteria for funding. Examples of a few of the associations that fund research in the area of spinal cord injury follow.

National Spinal Cord Injury
Association
149 California Street
Newton, MA 02185; (617) 964-0521
(This association funds research in the form of grants and fellowships for spinal cord injury regeneration.)

Paralyzed Veterans of America
801 18th Street NW
Washington, DC 20006;
(202) 872-1300
(This organization funds research on spinal cord restoration and regeneration. It also considers research questions that address psychosocial aspects of the spinal cord injury rehabilitation process.)

For additional information about associations that are possible sources of funding, contact the national headquarters of the individual association. A listing and detailed description of the majority of these associations can be found in the *Directory of National Information Sources on Handicapping Conditions and Related Services* (Department of Education, Washington, D.C.).

Foundations

A large number of the more than 24,000 foundations in the United States fund research in rehabilitation. They often have specific funding requirements that restrict applications to specific geographic locations, types of institutions, and disabilities. Several publications are available that consider the process of foundation funding, but few are as comprehensive as *The Funding Workbook* (available through The Funding Center, 1712 I Street, Suite 1005, Washington, DC). It includes descriptions of public and private sector foundations as well as support materials and resources.

Information identifying foundations that fund rehabilitation research also can be found in *The Handicapped Funding Directory* (Research Grant Guides, P.O. Box 357, Oceanside, NY 11572). The Directory is updated every 2 years. This and other information about foundations can be obtained from The Foundation Center, a national service organization founded and supported by foundations to provide a single authoritative source of information on foundation giving. The Center helps grant seekers as they begin to identify foundation funding sources that may be most interested in their project.

The Center has two national libraries, in New York and Washington, DC, two field libraries, in Cleveland and San Francisco, and a network of over 160 cooperating library collections across the U.S. Each library affords free public access to all the Center's publications and a wide range of other books, services, periodicals, and research documents relating to foundations and philanthropy. The Center also offers computer data bases on foundations and grants on-line through Dialog Information Services. Additional information about the Foundation Center's programs is available by calling toll free (800) 424-9836 or by writing The Foundation Center, 79 Fifth Avenue, New York, NY 10003.

Corporations

An underutilized source of funding in rehabilitation is corporations. Most corporations contribute funds to rehabilitation research because it benefits their public image. As such, they tend to support projects that provide them maximum public visibility. This is a major factor that should be considered by the researcher investigating this funding avenue.

Because of tax law revisions in 1981, corporations are allowed to contribute up to 10% of their profits, tax free, to nonprofit organizations. During 1980 approximately 30% of corporations made contributions. However, the average size of their contributions totaled only 1% of their profits. Although large corporations are inundated with requests for funding, many smaller ones are not. As such, they may be more viable as a potential funding agent.

Corporations must report their total fiscal activity annually in a 10 K Report. However, they are not required to provide detailed information concerning the recipient of contributions. Copies of these reports can be found only in the Public Reference Rooms of the Securities & Exchange

Commission (SEC) in Chicago, Los Angeles, New York City, and Washington, DC. In order to learn about the philanthropic interests of a corporation, contact must be initiated with the person within the corporation who typically makes those decisions, usually the manager of corporate contributions or the vice president of community affairs.

FUNDING APPLICATION

When deciding which federal agencies might be appropriate sources of funding for a specific project, certain basic information first must be obtained in order to determine which is most suitable. Some agencies focus on funding primary research, while others concentrate on development aspects of a project. The questions that follow are presented to serve as a guide to identifying the best funding agent.

1. How are projects awarded funds? Is funding awarded only through published requests for proposals? How often and in what form do these requests for proposals (RFPs) become public? Is funding made available only through field-initiated research proposals?
2. What is the agency's funding schedule, that is, how often are funds awarded? Is it once a year? Is it every 6 months? Is it anytime during the year?
3. How long does it usually take an application for funds to be processed and the researcher notified of the agency decision?
4. What is the duration for funding awards? Is there a minimum period of time funds are awarded? Is there a maximum period of time funds are awarded?
5. What is the process by which projects are selected by the agency for funding? Is it through a peer review panel? Is it through agency personnel? Are persons with disabilities involved in the selection process?
6. Are there eligibility requirements? Must the applicant hold United States citizenship? Must project personnel all hold United States citizenship?
7. What are the constraints on the use of project funds? Can new equipment be purchased? Can travel to other research centers and professional meetings be paid for by the grant?
8. Are there special funds available to make laboratories accessible to disabled researchers?
9. How are projects reviewed? Is it by peer visits? Is it by the funding agency project officer? Is it by a written report from the researcher? How often are projects reviewed? Are detailed review results available to the researcher?

10. Can projects be jointly funded in cooperation with another federal funding agency? What agencies can this be done with?

11. Does the federal agency produce a report describing other projects they have funded?

12. What kinds of projects are funded by the agency? Are they primarily research or development?

CLEARINGHOUSES AND INFORMATION DATA BASES

There are several national clearinghouses and data bases that provide information on rehabilitation and rehabilitation-related subjects. The most comprehensive informational data bases are listed below.

Products

ABLEDATA
National Rehabilitation Information Center (NARIC)
4407 Eighth Street NE
The Catholic University of America
Washington, DC 20017
(202) 635-5826 or (202) 635-5884 TDD
ABLEDATA is an electronic clearinghouse with information about over 13,000 commercially available assistive devices. Information often includes a description and price of the device. On-line computer access is available anywhere in the United States and internationally using the Bibliographic Retrieval System (BRS). For persons without direct computer access, ABLEDATA can be searched by information specialists at NARIC.

Assistive Device Center
6000 J Street
Sacramento, CA 95819-2694
The Assistive Device Center is associated with the School of Engineering of the California State University in Sacramento and provides product information in several ways. It has an Assistive Device Database System (ADDS), which has information about products including a description, where it may be obtained, skills necessary to operate it, and approximate price. The data base provides lists of useful resource people and resource services. The Center also has a Resource Center with an extensive library of print information.

Cheever Publishing, Inc.
P.O. Box 700
Bloomington, IL 61702-0700
Cheever Publishing provides product information three ways: through its quarterly *Accent on Living* magazine; through *Accent on Information*, a computerized listing of commercially available products; and through other special publications on products.

Research and Researchers

Interagency Rehabilitation Research Information System (IRRIS)
National Institute of Disability and Rehabilitation Research
400 Maryland Avenue, SW
Washington, DC 20202
(202) 732-1192
IRRIS is an electronic data base maintained by NIDRR. It contains information from more than 30 federal agencies about rehabilitation projects they have funded and presently fund. This information includes the researcher's name, affiliation, and highest degree held; an abstract of the research; the amount and source of funding; and the dates of funding.

Handicapped Scientists

Project on Science, Technology, and Disability
American Association for the Advancement of Science
1333 H Street NW
Washington, DC 20005
(202) 326-6667
The Project on Science, Technology, and Disability publishes a directory of scientists with disabilities and maintains this information in an electronic data base with more than 1,500 entries. The directory includes the name, address, and telephone number of the scientist; the scientific discipline and degrees attained; the most recent employment position; the nature of the disability and the age when it occurred; and the expertise and consulting interests of the individual. The directory includes listings of scientists, mathematicians, engineers, and social scientists.

Technology Transfer

Electronic Industries Foundation/Rehabilitation Engineering Center (EIF/REC)

1901 Pennsylvania Avenue NW, Suite 700
Washington, DC 20006
(202) 955-5827
The EIF/REC was established to stimulate industry in the manufacture and distribution of assistive technology designed for persons with disabilities. It serves as a liaison between the developer and the manufacturer, providing assistance in the areas of patent and licensing agreements, market identification, and technical evaluation.

Small Electronic Bulletin Boards

There are thousands of smaller electronic bulletin boards, some of which have relevant information to rehabilitation professionals. Though often elusive, they generally can be identified by contacting:

1. A professional society, especially if it has a special interest group (SIG) in microcomputers or disability.
2. A microcomputer users group, especially if it has a SIG in disability.
3. A microcomputer store, which may have a listing of local electronic bulletin boards.
4. A directory of electronic bulletin boards; for example, that available through the National Computer Bulletin Board Directory, c/o Thomas Wnorowski, 3352 Chelsea Circle, Ann Arbor, MI 48104.

Toll Free Telephone Numbers

Several organizations serving persons with disabilities have toll free telephone numbers to provide information about specific disabilities and services, products, and programs related to them. A listing of some of these and their toll free number follows:

Blind
American Council for the Blind
800-424-8666

Cancer
Cancer Information Center
800-525-3777

Cancer Information Service
800-4-CANCER

Deaf
National Crisis Center for the Deaf
800-446-9876

National Hearing Aid Society
800-521-5247

Hearing Helpline
800-424-8576

Diabetes
Juvenile Diabetes Foundation
  International
800-223-1138

American Diabetes Association
800-232-3472

Down's Syndrome
National Down's Syndrome Society
800-221-4602

Education
Center for Special Education
Technology
800-345-TECH

ERIC Clearinghouse for Adult, Career
and Vocational Education
800-848-4815

Epilepsy
Epilepsy Information Line
800-426-0660

Physical Disabilities
International Shriners Headquarters
800-237-5055

National Easter Seal Society
800-221-6827

Spina Bifida
Spina Bifida Hotline
800-621-3141

Spinal Cord Injury
Spinal Cord Injury Hotline
800-638-1733

Stuttering
National Center for Stuttering
800-221-2483

While the foregoing discussion on funding options and data bases available to the rehabilitation researcher is not complete, it does represent a source of information that can be critically important in acquiring funds and information needed to develop and conduct methodologically sound and fundable investigations. As such, accessing sources cited in this chapter may well enhance the project's competitiveness and, ultimately, determine its fundability.

REFERENCES

Thomas, J. P. (1985). Spinal cord injury research. *American Rehabilitation, 11*(4), 26–27.

Index

Ability
analysis of, 48, 51, 52, 60
vs. capability, 51
vs. performance, 60
Acetaminophen, 224, 295, 296, 298, 300
ACS Speech Pac/Epson, 93–94
Activities of daily living
in burn patients, 186, 209–210
in cancer patients, 243, 249, 283
and chronic low back pain, 20, 22, 29–30
measuring, 3, 4
and musculoskeletal pain, 139
neuropsychological assessment of, 48, 52, 55, 57
Acupuncture, 308, 314
Ad Hoc Committee on the Communicative Processes for Non-Speaking Persons, 81
Adaptation, in cancer rehabilitation, 279–281
illusion in, 281
Adaptive Behavior Scale, 59
Adriel and Evelyn Harris Toy Library for the Disabled, 81
Aerobic exercise, 118, 119, 123
Alcohol use, 27, 253
Alprazolam, 224
Ambulation, see Walking
American Academy of Physical Medicine and Rehabilitation, 11
American Congress of Rehabilitation Medicine, 10, 321
American Head Injury Foundation, 12
American Hospital Association, 9, 10
American Sign Language, 83
American Speech–Language–Hearing Association, 81
American Standard Code for Information Exchange, 100
Ameri-Ind, 83
Amputation, 249
Amyotrophic lateral sclerosis (ALS), 241
Analgesics
abuse of, 21, 224

in burn injuries, 217, 218–220, 223–225
in cancer, 290, 294, 295–312, 313–314
centrally acting, 295–299
dosages, 300–302
narcotic, 217, 218, 223–224, 245, 295–306
nonsteroidal anti-inflammatory, 295, 296, 298, 300, 306–307
peripherally acting, 295, 296
routes of administration, 302–306, 314
side effects of, 301–302, 304, 306
weaning from, 225
Anemia, 235
Anger, 275, 291
Antidepressants, 306
Antigravity positioning, in burn injuries, 182–183, 192–193
Anxiety
in cancer patients, 268, 283, 291, 313
in caregivers, 221
in chronic low back pain, 22, 27, 33, 34
medication for, 224
and muscle tension, 34, 156
and pain perception, 218, 220
Apple II computer, 94, 95, 97, 99
Areas of Change Questionnaire, 39–40
Arm pain, 245
Aspirin, 295, 296, 298, 300
Assessment
of cancer outcome, 233, 252, 271, 273
in chronic low back pain, 4, 20, 23–42
of communication skills, 102–103
diagnostic, 49–50, 55
neuropsychological, 4, 47–69
of pain, 219
of technology, 101–102
tools, xix, 6–17, 35–40, 51, 59, 61–63, 65–66, 103, 219, 233, 271, 273
Attention, disorders of, 58, 61
Augmentation communication systems, 81–95, 105
software for, 94–95
types of, 83–86
Avoidance learning, 28, 30

ORDER FORM

Save 10% on Volume 2 with this coupon.

____Check here to order ADVANCES IN CLINICAL REHABILITATION, Volume 2, at a 10% discount. You will receive an invoice requesting pre-payment.

Save 10% on all future volumes with a continuation order.

____Check here to place your continuation order for ADVANCES IN CLINICAL REHABILITATION. You will receive a pre-payment invoice with a 10% discount upon publication of each new volume, beginning with Volume 2. You may pay for prompt shipment or cancel with no obligation.

Name _____

Institution _____

Address _____

City/State/Zip _____

Examination copies for possible course adoption are available to instructors "on approval" only. Write on institutional letterhead, noting course, level, present text, and expected enrollment (include $2.50 for shipping). Prices slightly higher outside U.S.A. Prices subject to change.

Mail this coupon to:
SPRINGER PUBLISHING COMPANY
536 Broadway, New York, N.Y. 10012-3955